The evidence surrounding the skills and approaches to support good birth has grown exponentially over the last two decades, but so too have the obstacles facing women and midwives who strive to achieve good birth.

This new book critically explores the complex issues surrounding contemporary childbirth practices in a climate which is ever more medicalised amidst greater insecurity at broad social and political levels. The authors offer a rigorous, and thought-provoking, analysis of current clinical, managerial and policy-making environments, and how they have prevented sustaining the kind of progress we need. *The Politics of Maternity* explores the most hopeful developments such as the abundant evidence for one-to-one care for women, and sets these accounts against the background of changes in health service organisation and provision that block these approaches from becoming an everyday occurrence for women giving birth. The book sets out the case for renewed attention to the politics of childbirth and what this politics must entail if we are to give birth back to women.

Designed to help professionals cope with the transition from education to the reality of the system within which they learn and practise, this inspiring book will help to assist them to function and care effectively in a changing health care environment.

Rosemary Mander is Emeritus Professor of Midwifery at University of Edinburgh, UK.

Jo Murphy-Lawless teaches Sociology in the School of Nursing and Midwifery at Trinity College Dublin, Ireland.

The Politics of Maternity

Rosemary Mander and
Jo Murphy-Lawless

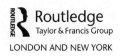
Routledge
Taylor & Francis Group

LONDON AND NEW YORK

First published 2013
by Routledge
2 Park Square, Milton Park, Abingdon, Oxon, OX14 4RN

Simultaneously published in the USA and Canada
by Routledge
711 Third Avenue, New York, NY 10017

Routledge is an imprint of the Taylor & Francis Group, an informa business

British Library Cataloguing in Publication Data
A catalogue record for this book is available from the British Library

Library of Congress Cataloging in Publication Data
Mander, Rosemary.
The politics of maternity / Rosemary Mander and Jo Murphy-Lawless.
p. ; cm.
ISBN 978-0-415-69740-8 (hbk.) - - ISBN 978-0-415-69741-5 (pbk.) - -
ISBN 978-0-203-63061-7 (ebk.)
I. Murphy-Lawless, Jo. II. Title.
[DNLM: 1. Midwifery. 2. Maternal Health Services. 3. Politics. 4. Pregnant
Women. WQ 160]
618.2--dc23
2012038678

ISBN13: 978-0-415-69740-8 (hbk)
ISBN13: 978-0-415-69741-5 (pbk)
ISBN13: 978-0-203-63061-7 (ebk)

Typeset in Bembo
by Taylor & Francis Books

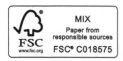

MIX
Paper from
responsible sources
FSC
www.fsc.org   FSC® C018575

Printed and bound in Great Britain by MPG Printgroup

Contents

Acknowledgements

We would like to acknowledge the many wonderful people who have supported and helped our efforts during the preparation of this book. We are particularly keen to recognise the help of Ellise Adams, Anne Brims, Members of the Birth Project Group, Margaret Carroll, Sarah Davies, Robbie Davis-Floyd, Nadine Edwards, Allison Ewing, Julika Hudson, Patricia Jeffery, Dominick Jenkins, Robin Jordan, Margaret Jowitt, IM-UK, Paul Lewis, Abigail Locke, John Low, Alwyn Lyes, Nessa McHugh, Meredith McIntyre, Liz Mogford, Dervla Murphy, Oisín Murphy-Lawless, Alison Nuttall, Magdalena Ohaja, Lindsay Reid, Anonymous Reviewers, Staff of *The Practising Midwife*, Raymond De Vries, Nicola White, Bridget Sheeran and Laura Yeates. We are especially grateful to Becky Reed for her constructive comments on the text and for her help with the cover.

I would particularly like to thank Iain Abbot who, in spite of everything, has provided the support on which I have come to depend.

1   Introduction

Homage and legacy

I learned about maternity politics and its significance from a number of midwives whose politicking reached the level of an art form. These midwives honed their political skills in clinical, managerial, policy-making, educational and academic arenas; they manoeuvred and manipulated situations and people with a deft sleight of hand invisible to anyone not looking out for it. Since that initiation, I have come to appreciate others' political dexterity in wider arenas. As well as learning from such experts, there is another source which I am proud to acknowledge. In some ways, this book represents a form of homage to a classic volume, which is familiar to and loved by generations of readers. Because of the dynamism of the subject area, few books on maternity or childbearing politics achieve the status of 'classics'. The book which has indubitably achieved this status is the one edited by Jo Garcia and her colleagues, published in 1990 (see also Chapter 6). Its multidisciplinary scholarship brought a new depth and breadth of academic work to maternity politics. Its continuing use, not to mention its regular disappearance from library shelves, testifies to its ongoing importance and relevance in the rapidly-changing world of maternity scholarship. The legacy of this book, 'The Politics of Maternity Care: Services for Childbearing Women in Twentieth-Century Britain', is apparent in many publications, in addition to virtually every thesis and dissertation, on maternity or midwifery topics. This legacy clearly makes the book by Jo Garcia and her colleagues a hard act to follow.

With this legacy in mind I set out to produce a new book on the politics of maternity. While not an edited book like its eminent predecessor, the present volume seeks to emulate the academic standard set in 1990. There are also other differences. In this book I aim to develop a definition of politics which is relevant to women in addition to the multiplicity of disciplines who practise in maternity, with their even more various agendas. Because 'The Politics of Maternity Care' was an edited volume, developing and applying such a definition would have been difficult. This may have had the effect of making more subtle, or possibly diluting, the focus on politics. Any such effect, however, was more than compensated by the breadth, variety and academic scholarship of the contributed chapters.

While Jo Garcia and her colleagues' book continues to be used and useful, I recognise that the relevance of some of the material has decreased with the passage of time. This is largely due, again, to the dynamic nature of maternity care. It is also necessary to consider whether the changing context of maternity care has reduced the relevance of 'The Politics of Maternity Care'. In order to contextualise the maternity environment, it may be helpful at the outset to reflect on the changes which the maternity services have encountered since Jo Garcia and her colleagues published their ground-breaking book.

Significant developments in the maternity services since 1990

In the decades since 'The Politics of Maternity Care' was published, changes have occurred on all fronts but, for the sake of convenience, I address changes in policy and practice.

Policy developments affecting maternity services

The nature of the National Health Service (NHS) as a 'political football' became most evident during the Thatcher era (UK Prime Minister 1979–90). Partly due to her government's attempts at reorganisation and partly due to longstanding under-funding, the NHS Review was undertaken in 1988. The outcome was the government White Paper *Working for Patients* (1989), which introduced an internal market in health care; this constituted a system of contracting for services between purchasers and providers. This system came into operation in April 1991, making Health Authorities and general practitioners (GPs) responsible for assessing population needs and purchasing services from hospitals and other units of service. At the time of writing, this system has largely been dismantled, but changes in funding and providers are in the forefront of plans by the present coalition government.

Changes in NHS funding are nowhere more apparent since the mid-1990s than in Public Private Partnership (PPP) and Private Finance Initiative (PFI) contracting arrangements (see also Chapter 6). These private sector bodies, in the form of partnerships or consortia, have been used to provide capital investment for both hospital and community developments. A typical PFI project will be owned by a company set up specially to run the scheme and will comprise a consortium of a building firm, bank and facilities management company. While possibly structured differently, PFI projects usually feature four key elements: Design, Finance, Build and Operate. The key difference between PFI and conventional ways of providing public/health services is that the public sector does not actually *own* the asset, ie the property. The health authority effectively leases the property, making an annual payment, like a mortgage, to the private company who provides the building and services. This arrangement continues for the duration of the contract (25–30 years), which may be extended more or less indefinitely through renegotiation. PFI is now used for a large majority of capital schemes, such as hospital building projects (Liebe and Pollock 2009).

Since 1999, the much sought-after political devolution within the United Kingdom has, effectively, given rise to four different NHSs (Connolly et al 2010). Although devolution has, to date, had limited impact in Northern Ireland, people who use the health services in Scotland and Wales are well aware of their relatively privileged position. While there are a number of policy differences, the impact to date on maternity services is more difficult to assess. There are certainly proud reports of exciting developments in the devolved nations (Kirkman and Ferguson 2007; Reid 2011a). It is appropriate to question, though, whether devolution stimulated the development or just the report of the development.

A progressive policy which should have affected the childbearing woman is the increasing focus on client/consumer input into decisions at all levels of health care. This increasing focus is reflected in the document 'Patient Focus Public Involvement' (SEHD 2001). Publications like this seek to operationalise the principle of 'Nothing About Us Without Us', adopted by disability activists in the late twentieth century. The achievement of such lofty ideals, however, requires a change in the culture of health care. This would be facilitated by investment in communication systems, genuine consumer/client information and involvement and universal responsiveness among health care personnel. At the time of writing, it remains to be seen whether sufficient priority is accorded to client input to achieve such an outcome.

The political significance of the inequities and inequalities of the health care system were demonstrated most forcefully, not to say notoriously, by the Black Report (DHSS 1980). Although rates of, for example, life expectancy and infant mortality appear to have improved since 1990, the gap between the most and the least affluent has not; in fact that gap is actually increasing (Mackenbach 2011).

The policy developments envisaged by the Winterton Report (1992) and 'Changing Childbirth' (1993), and their equivalents in the three devolved UK countries, brought seemingly infinite promise for the childbearing woman and her midwifery attendants. Such promise was encapsulated in the cliché 'woman-centred care' (Reid 2011b: 190). By default, though, obstetric and other medical practitioners in the maternity area would be variably affected. These effects, together with the financial implications of such momentous changes, proved insurmountable for managers and policy makers (Rothwell 1996), leaving women's and midwives' aspirations for control, choice and continuity yet to be realised.

Developments affecting practice in maternity

The usual perception of a lack of newly qualified midwives to maintain the workforce had begun to change by 1990; this led to recognition of the difficulty of newly qualified midwives finding employment (Mander 1987). This finding was supported by Penny Curtis and her colleagues, who investigated the midwifery workforce in England (Curtis 2006). These researchers identified the 38.26 per cent of midwives with effective registrations who do not practise, but gave scant attention to the woefully deficient establishments. Thus, the connection failed to be made between perceptions of shortage in clinical areas and budgetary priorities.

The chapter in 'The Politics of Maternity Care' by Rona Campbell and Alison Macfarlane on place of birth was written in the long shadow of the Peel Report, when the homebirth rate was at an all-time low. Since then, perhaps in association with policy developments mentioned already, but also influenced by women's activism, the number of out-of-hospital births has generally risen. As I discuss in Chapter 8, the fledgling midwife-led facilities in freestanding and alongside settings face many challenges (Hatem et al 2008) and the homebirth rate has increased only patchily.

The rise in some areas of the homebirth rate may be linked to enthusiasm for independent midwifery services. Such enthusiasm, however, was not shared by members of the Royal College of Midwives (RCM); when invited in 1993 to ballot on supporting their independent co-professionals, the members voted to withdraw their indemnity insurance (Warren 1994). Since then the statutory regulatory body and the European Union have further threatened independent midwifery (HPC 2009) by requiring exorbitantly-priced professional indemnity insurance as a requirement for practice (see Chapter 7).

The increasing escalation, between 1994 and 2004, of the long-term rise in caesareans has carried serious implications for midwives, childbearing women and maternity services (Mander 2007). The recent levelling off of the caesarean rate in some countries suggests that medical personnel have finally recognised the iatrogenic nature of what they have for too long regarded as the ultimate rescue operation.

The publication of the twin volumes of 'Effective Care in Pregnancy and Childbirth' in 1989 by Iain Chalmers and his co-editors sounded a clarion call to their obstetrician colleagues to put their practice on to a research-based footing. Little did they foresee the Pandora's box of evidence-based practice (EBP) which would be opened on an unwitting world of health care. Not unconnected to the intrusion of EBP is the increasingly litigation-oriented and defensive practice which is currently required of a range of practitioners.

Another innovation which has influenced practice since 'The Politics of Maternity Care' was published is the Baby Friendly Hospital Initiative, launched in 1991. Altruistically, this project's prime focus is on the establishment of breast feeding by preventing interventions which interfere with the physiological initiation of lactation. The extent to which the benefits to babies outweigh the tyranny for mothers and staff is, however, difficult to assess (Mander 2008a).

As well as the possibility of midwives returning to their roots in the form of facilitating breast feeding, a similarly 'radical' approach has emerged through what may be known in this commodified climate as a 'unique selling point' (USP). The concept of 'normality', originally allocated to midwives by medical practitioners for whom such humdrum practice held little lucrative incentive (Donnison 1988), has been grasped avidly. The fact that the concept is poorly defined and equally poorly understood has proved no deterrent. In Scotland, government policy has supported this development in the form of 'Keeping Childbirth Natural and Dynamic' (KCND 2009).

An aspect of maternity attracting less attention is the changing pattern of maternal mortality. While the number of maternal deaths in developed countries such as the United Kingdom is nearing the irreducible minimum, their causes have changed markedly. No longer are the obstetric accidents, such as haemorrhage, major factors. Increasingly significant are the problems of women with complex needs, including lack of basic maternity and psychosocial care. Thus, the medical contribution to the prevention of deaths of women, who for various reasons are alienated from the health care system, is becoming less and less relevant.

A changing picture

This brief overview of some of the developments in maternity care since 'The Politics of Maternity Care' was published has shown that political issues are becoming more, rather than less, significant. Equally, these issues are likely to affect an ever wider range of personnel. These developments demonstrate all too clearly the need for a new book to assist practitioners and others negotiating labyrinthine maternity politics.

Terms and meanings

Jo Garcia and her colleagues gave little attention to the *nature* of politics. Although the contributed chapters in their book addressed issues which were implicitly political, politics was rarely mentioned as such. The exception to this observation is found, perhaps unsurprisingly, rounding off Robert Kilpatrick's interview with Wendy Savage (1990: 340). In this interview Savage's thoughts on the meaning of maternity politics become abundantly clear as a combination of party, medical and gender issues.

Before encountering the complexities of the political maelstrom of maternity care, though, exploring the breadth and limitations of the nature of politics will make this encounter more manageable. My exploration provides, as well as food for thought, an indication of this book's orientation.

Politics

Widely used, with little thought to its meaning beyond negative complexity, politics is a term which deserves to be teased apart.

A definition, which has long been a favourite, comes from my well-thumbed dictionary and emphasises politics' interpersonal and organisational aspects:

> astutely contriving, manoeuvring or intriguing.

> (Macdonald 1977: 1036)

This definition is wide enough to permit an approach sufficiently eclectic to include a number of aspects relevant to clinicians and practitioners. It has been pointed out to me by an anonymous reviewer, though, that this definition neglects crucial aspects of politics, such as power and control. So I undertook a search for a more inclusive definition, which produced helpful additions:

(a)   'the activities involved in getting and using power in public life, and being able to influence decisions that affect a country or a society'
        This definition constitutes 'Party Politics' which, while possibly connected to maternity politics, are subtly different. Party Politics are generally more predictable, with a rigidity of philosophy and infrastructure not found in other forms of politics.
(b)   'a person's political views or beliefs'
        This definition is similarly linked to Party Politics, so is equally limited in its relevance to maternity.
(c)   'a system of political beliefs; a state of political affairs'
        Apart from the possible Party Political dimension, this definition implies a major degree of homogeneity among midwives. While certain shared aspirations and a few commonalities of practice may apply to midwives, this definition is too tightly constraining. This is because midwifery is too closely linked to the cultural environment within which it happens for many global similarities to be identifiable.
(d)   'matters concerned with getting or using power within a particular group or organisation'.

(OALD 2011)

This definition is usefully broader, although Jo Murphy-Lawless opts for a subtly different one (Chapter 6). It succeeds in focusing on the crucial concept of power, while at the same time narrowing the scope to only specified groups of actors or other participants. This definition is clearly a useful adjunct to my original definition; it does, however, beg the question of the meaning of power, which lies at its heart.

Power

In his crucial contribution to the literature on Power, Steven Lukes (2005) draws on the context of Party Political issues in the United States. His original work was undertaken in the middle of the twentieth century and certain aspects of his writing show this, originating from a different generation and less than applicable to the present context. This criticism, however, does not impair the underlying importance of his ideas for a wide range of other fields and times. He argues that power is not the demonstration of absolute authority, as is sometimes assumed but that, given the right conditions, even the relatively disempowered may position themselves to exert power. This power differs qualitatively from that to which they have been subordinated, but this difference makes the exercise no less effective. Lukes' writing on the politics of power serves to operationalise the work of others whose ideas were approximately contemporary. Michel Foucault (1982) and Arthur Berndtson (1970) focus on power as underlying actions bringing change which, in turn, is characterised by novelty and its continuation. The effectiveness of such change is likely to be facilitated or impeded by factors such as consensus or opposition.

Control

As with many terms, control may mean all things to all people. But it has been particularly constrained by ideas about perceptions of societal acceptability in the form of self-control and of the source of control, that is, internality or externality (Rotter 1966; Bandura 1977). The distinction between power and control lies not only in the suitability of the words themselves. As found in a qualitative research project, knowledge is a fundamental factor which is a common requirement for both (Namey and Drapkin Lyerly 2010). These researchers, who examined the concept from the individual's point of view, also identified the crucial role of self-determination, which appears to correspond closely to traditional views of autonomy, as it is perceived as encompassing authority, decision-making and agency.

Practising politics

Whereas the forms of politics outlined here may be too subtle to be subject to scrutiny, the means by which politics are put into practice have attracted attention. The first consideration is how, if politics concerns getting or using power, that power is obtained and manipulated.

Power and practice

As mentioned already, the existence of a power balance or imbalance is not the absolute and negative phenomenon often perceived. Power may be regarded as being more relative, determined by a wide range of factors, of which the various participants may be more or less aware. As well as the existence of this relative (im)balance of power, its exercise is also influenced by the situation in which the actors find themselves. That is, a certain environment may facilitate the display of power by one participant, but under different circumstances another participant may be more competent.

The analysis by Marsden Wagner of the empowerment and disempowerment of different actors in the maternity scenario (Wagner 2007: 35) provides valuable insights into the creation and operation of power differentials. He argues that individuals become powerful not only because of, but sometimes despite, their own efforts. For such power to become established, as Edmund Burke is alleged to have observed ominously (Burke 1909), it is necessary for other participants to remain passive, that is, to *not* oppose this assumption of power. Wagner continues by suggesting that such an assumption of power may begin benignly, even altruistically. But such individuals may develop tunnel vision and become blinkered so that, in the absence of any opposition, their conviction of their own rightness and that they have the only answer passes and escalates unchallenged. These increasingly powerful individuals are then positioned to redefine the situation or territory to their own advantage. This effectively dis-empowers any potential opposition because the powerful individuals are able to present themselves as the solution, albeit to a problem which may not have existed before they created it. The next step in this process is for the powerful individuals to relocate the, now redefined, problem to a place where there is least threat to their sole authority over the outcomes. To achieve this, a certain 'massaging' of information may be necessary. A high level of communication skills and resources are a prerequisite for the dissemination of these fraudulent ideas among the recipient groups and others who are being disempowered. In the unlikely event of any opposition being articulated, small concessions may be offered as a sop to those venturing to display such temerity. Wagner correctly identifies these latter stages of the development of power as the establishment of continuing power through control of the situation. He goes on to suggest that a number of strategies may be employed to ensure that control is established and maintained.

Establishing control

In his supremely relevant analysis, Marsden Wagner indicates that a number of long-term interventions may be applied to consolidate a power base by assuming control of certain aspects (Wagner 2007: 36). This control may initially be through involvement in the education of the disempowered group to further weaken them and to increase the authority of the powerful. A subsequent method of ensuring control is by additionally limiting the activities of the weaker group. This may, first, be achieved by undermining their confidence in their own ability, particularly regarding opposing the powerful. Secondly, control is further strengthened through recourse to other powerful groups, such as legislators, who enact laws to limit the activities of the less powerful group. Control over financial resources may be similarly effective, making the disempowered group relatively impoverished and low status, hence reducing its attraction to new members. Fiscal control over the less powerful group also prevents that group from studying their own situation in order to improve their lot through increasing knowledge. Finally, the powerful group's ultimate control is assured and made unassailable by it making itself autonomously self-regulating. Whereas this powerful group may make inroads into other groups' statutory regulatory systems and influence them, its own position becomes impregnable. In this way questions about the behaviour of members of the elite powerful group are addressed internally. Lack of transparency ensures the continuation of such control.

Without needing to mention the potential for the all-too-familiar corollary in health care, Wagner astutely concludes:

This is absolute power indeed.

(Wagner 2007: 37)

Theory

Having briefly defined some practical aspects of politics, it may be helpful to consider whether and to what extent our understanding may be enhanced by the theoretical literature. In order to do this, I give attention to three crucially important phenomena which I have not mentioned thus far.

Hegemony

Originating with the ancient Greek concept of military alliances between one nation state, or hegemon, and another, the twentieth-century Marxist philosopher Antonio Gramsci applied the idea of hegemony to indirect control of and by different sections of society. Since then the term has been broadened to include cultural and occupational aspects of human life. A useful and very relevant definition was coined by feminist author Nancy Fraser, focusing on the power of certain groups to fashion a society's 'common sense' (Fraser 1989). By this, she meant those facets of everyday life which are too well and widely understood to be worth mentioning. The facets to which Fraser was referring include the power to:

1 create authoritative definitions of social situations and social needs;
2 determine the universe of legitimate disagreement;
3 shape the political agenda.

Thus, the role of certain dominant groups, including social, occupational or special interest groups, becomes clear. The resulting restriction of the environment in which negotiations and discussions about a particular issue begin and end is known as cultural hegemony. The aim of certain groups is to establish mastery, a word which I use deliberately, within this environment. Thus, these groups, agencies or institutions persuade others of their unique ability to define issues and concerns in which they already have a well-recognised interest.

It is apparent that hegemony is qualitatively different from power. The distinction is found in the *level* of the exercise of mastery. Whereas power is exerted at a practical, interpersonal or interorganisational level, hegemony operates at a higher theoretical level by constraining definitions of issues and the thought processes leading to those definitions.

Decision-making

While decision-making has attracted considerable attention, this may have done little to clarify such a complex area. The lack of clarity applies, particularly, to assumptions of the homogeneity of this process. All too often the focus is solely on one level, such as clinical or interpersonal decisions (Jefford et al 2010), and other levels are disregarded. Individuals' input into local organisational, as well as national, policy decisions probably deserve at least as much attention. Appropriate decision-making is intended to ensure that services are responsive to the needs of consumers; it ensures the functional autonomy of the practitioner and increases the woman's control over her experience of childbearing. At the same time, the decisions made by the three major groups (childbearing women, health care providers and policy makers/managers) are likely to impinge on or to influence each other's decisions. Although a number of governmental departments (eg SEHD 2001; DoH 2010a), have endorsed the need for greater and more effective consumer participation, the observation that the public 'role in decision-making remains under-developed' (Callaghan and Wistow 2006: 583) still applies. While the public role continues to be limited, certain occupational groups appear to fare little better (Raynor et al 2005).

Oppression

Just as the concept of power is crucial to political activity, oppression as a converse notion also needs to be recognised and, thus, will manifest itself repeatedly throughout this book. The complexity of oppression has been widely studied, not least by feminist scholars such as Patricia Hill Collins, who has developed others' ideas of intersectionality (Hill Collins 2000). Rather than oppression being a simplistic one-way cause and effect phenomenon, Collins represents it as an interlocking system of oppressive activities. Age, (dis)ability, socioeconomic class, race, gender, sexual orientation and faith are examples of factors which are interwoven to create a web of oppression, which Collins entitles the 'Matrix of domination'. Collins' work has focused mainly on the problems of oppression which African-American women face, making her ideas particularly relevant to the present context.

A brief history of hegemony and power in maternity

The history of power in maternity care reflects to a large extent the place of women in the various cultures and societies. This is partly because it is only recently that, in some countries, men have been permitted to become midwives on a comparable basis with women. There are similarities with women's history generally, including the limited sources, due to history usually having been written by men (Barclay 2008; Cheung 2009).

Power imbalances are demonstrated as far back as the 'handy woman' and the Scottish 'howdie' (Leap and Hunter 1993; Reid 2011b). These women shared an untrained background with the colonial midwife (Jackson and Mander 1995), and her ousting by her formally-educated successor. In the United Kingdom, power relations between the untrained midwife and the usurper were complicated by the perception of threat among 'general practitioners' (GPs) at the arrival of the educated midwife (Reid 2011b).

Feelings of threat among GPs were aggravated by their limited specialist knowledge, even compared to their untrained midwife counterparts. Thus, their ability to establish a practice and a livelihood depended on their creating some competitive advantage over lower-paid occupations, such as midwives and homeopaths (Fahy 2007; Dupree 2011).

While not necessarily benefiting GPs, the prestigious nature of medicine escalated in the nineteenth century, with associated increases in power and financial benefits (Watchorn 1978). This power facilitated the medical control of midwifery through the introduction of legislative midwifery regulation during the opening decades of the twentieth century (Donnison 1988; Reid 2011b; see page 58 and page 141). Such statutory control served to medicalise and further limit midwifery practice into and beyond the late twentieth century (Mein-Smith 1986).

In the United Kingdom, nineteenth-century nurse leaders sought a united front to strive for the common goal of registration. Because midwives considered their need more pressing, they spurned nurses' advances and some, such as Mrs Bedford-Fenwick, reacted by strenuously opposing midwifery legislation (Robinson 1990). A similar rebuff by midwives was encountered by nurses in the 1970s when new legislation, to implement the Briggs Report (Committee on Nursing 1972), was planned. The Royal College of Midwives (RCM) supported the planned legislation (RCM 1986), but the then statutory bodies, the Central Midwives Boards, anticipated that the control of midwifery by medical practitioners would simply be supplanted with nursing control. To further complicate matters, the Association of Radical Midwives (ARM), was formed in response to the threat to the midwife's role. The result of midwives' resistance was that the legislation fervently desired by nurses, eventually enacted as the Nurses, Midwives and Health Visitors Act (1979), was significantly delayed. That midwives are still blamed for this delay and that it continues to rankle is clear from the Nursing and Midwifery Council (NMC) website:

> This was due to the need to take account of ... lack of consensus within the professions [especially from midwives].
>
> (NMC 2010a)

Moving into the present day, the balance of power between medical practitioners erupts only occasionally in the literature. The problematical relationship with midwives, however, as evidenced by the NMC quotation, continues to constitute a running sore for our nursing cousins (Mander 2008b).

The purpose of and rationale for this book

This book is necessary because all midwives currently being educated and beginning to practise need, as stated by Eugene Declercq as long ago as 1994, to be politically aware and active (Declercq 1994: 236). This is partly to ensure that they are able to function effectively as midwives in clinical settings. But at organisational and national levels midwives also need to negotiate cultural and health care systems whose 'changes' impact profoundly on the midwife, her role and function. It is no longer sufficient for midwives and other health personnel to provide safe and effective care for the mother and child. Such an orientation has long since ceased to be adequate, and the need for political astuteness among student and new midwives and other health care personnel has been demonstrated (Savage 1990). This magnificent midwife has been described by Robbie Davis-Floyd as the post-modern midwife, bringing a range of beneficial traditional skills as well as knowing 'the limitations and strengths of the biomedical system' and 'how to subvert the medical system' to ensure that care is woman-centred (Davis-Floyd 2005: 33). For these reasons this book facilitates an awareness of and an ability to manipulate appropriate political strategies.

Many difficulties faced by health care personnel, including student and newly qualified midwives, derive from the mismatch between the ideals which brought them into health care and the reality of the modernist health system within which they learn and practise. This system features hegemonic power being held by certain disciplines to the disadvantage of other occupational groups. The new arrivals on to the maternity stage have needs which are sufficiently important to be addressed openly. This is because students, newly qualified midwives, and others, tend to assume that what they experience is unique. This sad assumption results in feelings of isolation and disengagement, possibly leading to the loss of idealistic practitioners from the profession (Mander et al 2009 and 2010). This book demonstrates the commonality of these systematic challenges as well as remedial strategies. In this way, more constructive approaches to these challenges will be available and may be employed to benefit and retain these new entrants.

Throughout this book I endeavour to present an objective yet balanced portrayal of the phenomena under scrutiny. Such objectivity has, in the past, been criticised as being too condemning of some occupational groups, such as medical practitioners. If this is how my writing is perceived, it is unfortunate. While probably not intentional, such condemnation should be viewed in the context of our obstetric colleagues' sole *raison d'être* being to intervene in what is ordinarily a physiological process. In view of the possibility of iatrogenesis, some censure is excusable.

My focus in writing this book is as far as possible on the individual, whether she be a childbearing women or a midwife. For this reason, I attempt to make the discussion more personal and relevant by using the singular, rather than grouping women and midwives into homogenous masses.

This book and its organisation

The chapters begin with the individuals involved in maternity care, by considering interpersonal issues. Moving on to a larger canvas, occupational or professional groups and the relationships between them are addressed. Because of the significance of the issues for the global majority of childbearing women and their attendants, as well as for more economically advantaged countries, third world matters are explored in Chapter 4. The next chapter scrutinises the differing philosophical approaches to maternity care and their impact for childbearing women. In Chapter 6 Jo Murphy-Lawless contemplates the politics of policy-making in state health systems. Chapters 7 and 8 provide case studies of the deleterious and beneficial effects of political activity, respectively, with a view to the reader being able to learn from others' experiences. The final chapter draws together the major themes emerging in this book, together with some relevant reflection on my own personal experiences of being a midwife, both as a practitioner and as an academic.

2   Interpersonal politics

The extent to which health care in general and maternity care in particular are accessible to the total population varies hugely between different health systems, states, regimes and times. As well as variations in accessibility, the *experience* of those who succeed in accessing health care is similarly variable. A range of phenomena is likely to affect the client's experience, including features of the client, provider and service.

In this chapter, I examine some features of the client group which are associated with differences in their experience of maternity care. This examination focuses on a number of differently powerful client groups who may be particularly disadvantaged, or possibly advantaged, in their experiences of maternity care.

What's in a name?

I have so far avoided using precise terms for those accessing maternity services. The names or titles which we allot to those whom we attend constitute a veritable minefield. The words carry messages extending far beyond simply the fact that this person is accessing a particular service and many reflect the imbalance of power between the provider and the recipient of care. In her well-reasoned argument against 'patient' being used in maternity as long ago as 1986, Ann Thomson reminded readers, that the World Health Organisation (WHO) had defined patienthood in terms of being 'helpless, incapable of understanding and sometimes non-compliant' (WHO 1985). Referring to childbearing women as patients, who are passive and unable to act responsibly, let alone make decisions, is widely thought to be a thing of the past. Such terminology is no anachronism, as I found when I recently tapped 'maternity patient' into a search engine and 42,000 results appeared. Thomson recommended the phrase 'childbearing woman', and that 'patient' should only be used when 'they really do occupy the sick role' (Thomson 1986: 163). Thus, my comfortable position doesn't last; I must bite the bullet, relinquish my seat on the fence and come down on the side of 'the childbearing woman'.

There is no shortage of alternatives to the 'p-word'; contenders include consumer, client, service-user and customer to name but four. A concept which has attracted considerable attention, though, is 'partner' as in 'partnership' (page 105 and 175). As with motherhood and apple pie, it is difficult to argue against this concept, but it deserves to be unpacked beyond obvious feel-good super-ficialities. The term was first applied to midwifery practice in the heady days of the early 1990s, when maternity care in New Zealand was seeking to free itself from the shackles of medical and nursing domination. Partnership emerged as a politically acceptable rallying point for childbirth activists and midwives, who were persuaded that 'Midwifery is the partnership between the woman and the midwife' (Guilliland and Pairman 1994). This message is still articulated loud and clear (Pairman 2006; Gray 2010). Many questions have been asked about the precise meaning of partnership and how such an equally balanced ideal is possible in the real world of midwifery practice (Skinner 1999; Fleming 2000; Mander 2011a). As New Zealand midwifery approaches maturity, these questions have yet to be answered, perhaps by encouraging more flexible inter-pretations or perhaps by a more egalitarian relationship between the professional organisation and its membership. Until that time the term 'part-nership' will probably continue to be applied to a relationship to which it is less than well-fitted.

Asking the service-user

In order to ascertain what title or label the users of health care prefer, the not unpredictable step of asking them has proved popular, particularly in mental health (Deber et al 2005). Canadian researchers suggest that service-users favour the comfortable familiarity of 'patient'. Tracing the roots of alternatives, eg consumer, to their largely commercial origins, Raisa Deber and her colleagues suggest that such terminology is increasingly relevant to health care. Based on a survey of 1,037 people attending community facilities, such as orthopaedics and oncology, they conclude that 'patient' is moderately preferred; but the implication of the imbalance of power which it carries is firmly rejected.

In maternity Mrs N Batra and Richard Lilford undertook a survey to identify a term which would provide childbearing women with an acceptable alter-native to the 'patient' label (Batra and Lilford 1996). But they met with limited success. While 'client' and 'consumer' were unpopular with childbearing women, these obstetricians found that 'mother to be' and 'pregnant woman' were the least unacceptable. More recently, Dominic Byrne and his colleagues (Byrne et al 2000) investigated women's preferences by asking those attending a hospital antenatal clinic to complete a brief questionnaire, and 72.7 per cent (446/613) responded. The term 'patient' was selected by 39 per cent of the respondents as their first choice from a list of possibilities. 'Commercial descriptions' (Byrne et al 2000: 1235) such as 'client' and 'consumer' were preferred by women earlier in pregnancy. Although not mentioned by the authors, this preference probably reflects these women's limited exposure to medical culture.

Systematic effects

Just as Deber and her Canadian colleagues conclude the relevance of 'consumer', Peter Scourfield discusses how 'commercial' labels for the service-user are becoming increasingly apposite (Scourfield 2007). Writing in the context of English personal social services, Scourfield observes that the role of the recipient of care is becoming increasingly entrepreneurial. He argues that the New Right is requiring the service-user to become a 'rational, calculating consumer, able to shop around' (Scourfield 2007: 108) in the market of care for the package appropriate to them. The collectivity and social justice, he states, which have underpinned the long and largely honourable history of the UK National Health Service (NHS), are under threat from this manifestation of individualisation. That such cautionary words are relevant to the maternity services is evident from their increasingly commercial orientation (Mander 2011b), so that 'childbearing woman' may yet prove less appropriate than 'consumer' with the commodification of health.

Against this terminological tangle, I endeavour to refer to the 'childbearing woman' as far as possible. It is occasionally necessary to refer to her as a 'consumer', because that word continues to be used by admirably sensible activists (Beech 2011) and is probably more truthful than alternatives, given the current marketised orientation of the NHS and many other healthcare systems (see Chapter 6).

The childbearing woman as a consumer of care

As the notion of consumerism became implicated in maternity care, it was accompanied by an increased understanding of the idea of woman's autonomy and her role as arbiter in deciding her needs relative to the 'clinical trades'. Originating in a Latin word (*consumere* – to take up completely), 'consumer' has developed the commercial meanings mentioned already. Other definitions of 'consume' include eating or drinking, filling a person's mind or attention, and destroying someone/something completely (Encarta 2011). While a market of consumer goods might co-exist with a free NHS (Klein 2007: 20), the problem is that the poorer and more marginalised socially are unable to 'consume' equally (Bauman 1998), so the term does present genuine problems. Nevertheless, because in authoritative health service research literature (Baggott and Forster 2008; Baggott et al 2005; Leahy et al 2011; Allsop et al 2004) the term 'consumer' tends to be used extensively, I use it here to assist scrutiny of the childbearing woman's experience. This is despite Charlotte Williamson's use of the the p-word as a badge of honour in her manifesto on the 'emancipation of patients' (Williamson 2010).

The implications of medical hegemony for women's autonomy are well-recognised, which has engendered good intentions, but little more (Marshall and Woollett 2000: 352). The history of this power imbalance is long and authoritatively documented (Mander 2004). The woman's position, already weakened by the move of men into providing maternity care, was further threatened during the twentieth century by the move of birth into hospitals. In these institutions the imbalance of power was aggravated by the introduction of 'active management of labour' (Pitt 1997; Moscucci 2003; O'Driscoll and

Meagher 1980). The balance of power appeared to shift momentarily in favour of women with the advent of the well-intentioned but ill-fated 'three Cs', control, choice and continuity (DoH 1993; HOC 1992).

The crucial role of differing knowledges, which arise out of multiple belief systems within one health culture, has since become clear (Edwards 2005a). This means that the dominance or authoritative nature of one set of beliefs serves to limit, threaten or undermine other belief systems which, though equally legitimate, do not carry the kudos or be accepted to the same extent. I have outlined previously some of the methods used to shore up the dominant knowledge system (pages 7–9), which Nadine Edwards identifies as the 'medical model' and the other knowledges as 'midwifery, social or woman-centred' (Edwards 2005a: 23).

Consumer movements in maternity

Through 'Actively working for the rights of citizens in health policy and care' (Leahy et al 2011: 2), activist groups who have seen themselves as 'consumers' seek freedom from hegemonic structures which threaten or restrict those rights. Attempting to link their rights to democratic ideals, consumer movements may endeavour to enlist governmental power, although these authors identify the risks of jeopardising their independence and goals through entering into potentially compromising relationships. These risks have been closely scrutinised in a Dutch context (Van de Bovenkamp and Trappenburg 2010), although the potential benefits, such as participation in policy-making, empowerment and freedom from 'Big Pharma', also emerge clearly. These risks and benefits were cogently summarised in the context of consumers working through pressure groups in B Guy Peters' classic work (Peters 1982) looking at ways in which influence may be exerted on the bureaucracy to establish a *modus vivendi*. Although these bodies may be expected to be in constant conflict, Peters considers that the reason that pressure groups continue to exist is that each needs the other. Pressure groups may provide evidence or ammunition to help bureaucrats with internal arguments. While, obviously, pressure groups feel that they benefit from having the ear of policy-makers both to achieve their ends and maintain the interest and allegiance of their members. This symbiotic relationship sometimes appears too cosy. The forms of interaction helping both parties to achieve their own ends include:

- legitimate interaction, which probably includes MSLC (see page 20) membership;
- 'clientela relationships', when the pressure group makes itself so indispensable that it becomes recognised by bureaucrats as an effectively official consumer representative;
- 'parantela relationships' comprise a particular group exerting influence through their close with the dominant Political Party. Whether the group represents a constituency is less significant than their close 'kinship';
- illegitimate forms of contact are those groups whose activities are outwith the usual legal conventions.

Such consumer activity originated as a by-product of the 1960s' counterculture, combined with a reaction to the increasing medicalisation of western life. That the number of European consumer organisations is continuing to increase reflects how little these aspects of life have improved (Baggott and Forster 2008). Research by Judith Allsop and her colleagues (Allsop et al 2004) shows the extent to which consumer groups in the United Kingdom have moved on since those early days. These researchers suggest that consumer groups may have become more realistic and less altruistic, by focusing solely and more directly on those health conditions of which the groups' founders have personal experience. This study also demonstrated that groups are more prepared, perhaps through necessity, to join together in common cause, rather than dwelling on relatively minor differences in approach. Such alliances are likely to increase groups' effectiveness in applying pressure to governmental bodies on policy development. The groups' relationships with the media were also found to be crucial to their survival, but groups whose members carried a stigma felt that negative stereotypes tended to be reinforced to create a vicious cycle. The ability of some consumer groups to mobilise media support was one of their major strengths, indicating a degree of interdependence between the two parties.

Consumer groups working in the maternity and childbirth area have long had a complex relationship with the feminist movement. That these groups largely arose out of this movement has not always been willingly recognised (Reiger 1999). The groundbreaking role of these consumer groups was identified in Allsop and colleagues' study (Allsop et al 2004), but the narrowly homogeneous characteristics of the members was also noted. Because the various childbirth consumer groups share certain common goals, such as continuing feminist ideals and questioning medicalisation, this allows them to cooperate rather than compete. Collaboration with professional organisations was found to be increasing, albeit variably between different consumer groups. With regard to the media, childbirth groups considered themselves disadvantaged by the popular press disparaging 'earth mother' imagery (Allsop et al 2004: 747). It is necessary to consider whether such views may originate with some journalists needing to work out their own childbearing disappointments through the medium of their column inches.

To illuminate how the consumer is currently positioned in the maternity services, I consider now the functioning of some of the organisations and agencies and the extent to which they support her and strengthen that position.

The National Childbirth Trust

The complicated beginnings of the parenting charity, the Natural Childbirth Association in 1956 have been authoritatively, even perceptively, analysed by Jenny Kitzinger (1990). These beginnings include its evolution into the National Childbirth Trust or NCT; the name change being at the behest of 'doctors who were "offended" by the original wording' (Williams 1997). Subsequently, Ornella Moscucci cast a historian's eye over these developments using 'natural childbirth' as her lens, and found aspects of the relationship with

Grantly Dick-Read cosy to the point of being disconcerting (Dick-Read 1993). The Association, as it was in the 1950s, led by Mrs Prunella Briance, adhered to Dick-Read's dogma of religious morality, eugenic ideals, traditional family life and re-establishment of the British Empire. Such dogma, and the natural childbirth with which Dick-Read linked it, soon lost popularity in the United Kingdom to the psychoprophylactic approach of French obstetrician Ferdinand Lamaze.

Despite such an uncertain start in life, the NCT has continued, flourished and provides a range of services, including 'antenatal classes' (Locke and Horton-Salway 2010). In order to ascertain the role of the childbearing woman as a consumer, the NCT's teaching has been studied by Harriette Marshall and Anne Woollett (2000); texts produced by several organisations were subjected to feminist narrative analysis (Marshall and Woollett 2000; NCT 1996). These researchers found that the childbearing woman was required to exercise considerable self-discipline, so that she would likely find herself removed from her usual social supports and accepting of expert knowledge, rather than family and friends' advice. Any questioning of or challenge to such expertise remained out of bounds. Marshall and Woollett conclude that such antenatal education serves to regulate pregnancy and women who are pregnant. While not necessarily endorsing the medical model, the texts were found to advocate firmly how the childbearing woman should both behave and relate to others.

More recently, Abigail Locke and Mary Horton-Salway studied advice-giving by class leaders, using tape recordings of NCT antenatal classes (Locke and Horton-Salway 2010). Although subject to debate, it remains a crucial tenet of NCT policy that teachers should be mothers (Nolan 2007). These researchers found that teachers relied heavily on 'their personal experience of having children in the past ... to support her advice giving for the institutional role of class leader and baby expert' (Locke and Horton-Salway 2010: 1219). As identified by Marshall and Woollett (2000), these researchers also found that class leaders 'put the onus on women to be responsible for their pregnancies and early parenthood' (Locke and Horton-Salway 2010: 1221). In contrast with the other research, however, Locke and Horton-Salway found that class leaders endorsed an official policy of supporting current medical expertise, rather than previous practices.

These two authoritative studies suggest that the NCT has further evolved from its early consumerist origins. It appears to be developing into part of a powerful, dominating establishment which regulates the activities and relationships of childbearing women.

Association for Improvements in the Maternity Services (AIMS)

Although some of the criticisms levelled at the NCT may also apply to AIMS, its status as a voluntary campaigning pressure group with a more limited remit makes it a less easy target. AIMS originated in 1960, known as 'The Society for the Prevention of Cruelty to Pregnant Women' (Beech 2011), as a result of Sally Willington's experience of maternity care (AIMS 2011); this exemplified, as I have mentioned already, that the experience of one person is a common start for many consumer organisations. AIMS' prime function is to support parents, particularly those encountering difficulties with or having experienced trauma through the health care system. It may also provide help for midwives facing professional problems. Much of AIMS' activity relates to public presentations and to the media and NHS bureaucracy 'seeking the consumers' views' (Editorial 1994: 3). The quarterly journal outlines AIMS' activities and research issues as well as women's experiences.

The radical political function of AIMS should not be underestimated, as demonstrated by its list of campaigns (AIMS 2011; Beech 2011). Political activity on behalf of the childbearing woman is also apparent in its publications, such as Charlotte Williamson's exploration of the emancipation of 'patients' (Williamson 2007). Such emancipation frees people to act according to their own interests, values and responsibilities, without overt or covert coercion. Thus, autonomy is fostered with a view to humanity and justice, giving due regard to civil rights and feminist issues. AIMS utilises not only the experiences of childbearing women, but also the input of relevant academic disciplines.

In her paper, Williamson outlines the possibility of alliances being formed between groups and 'dominant power holders'. The duration of such alliances is determined by other alignments and the nature of the issue in question (Williamson 2007: 7). An admirable example of an alliance was AIMS' cooperation with the NCT on the Charter for Ethical Research in Maternity Care (1997). Another example is when, in 1982, seven prominent women members of childbirth groups and a midwife met in London to discuss the problem of childbearing women's experiences of assault by being given treatment to which they had not consented (Beech 1985). This meeting resulted in the establishment of the Maternity Defence Fund to provide information and support legal action in the event of assault. As well as comings together, schisms may also feature, because of extreme positions or because of a 'too cosy' relationship with a more powerful organisation, which would jeopardise the purpose of the group in advocating for the oppressed individual. More recently, with the support of the Royal College of Midwives (RCM) and the Department of Health, a Maternity Care Working Party comprising a range of organisations and individuals cooperated to the extent of drawing up a maternity wish-list (MCWP 2006).

Groups such as AIMS may be perceived as threatening by some health care professionals who may fear for their autonomy, especially when accused of oppression (Williamson 2010: 48). But Williamson argues that, like the professionals, AIMS' bottom line is high quality services which may be threatened by professional autonomy being undermined by health service managerialism. It is clear that Williamson's line of argument may constitute the opening gambit towards an alliance, as I have mentioned already.

Maternity Services Liaison Committees (MSLCs)

Unlike the NCT and AIMS (see above), MSLCs are established, organised and maintained by local health authorities. These committees originated with the ideals of Changing Childbirth (Smith 2005: 40; Messent 2002; DoH 1993). Nadine Edwards indicates that she attended an MSLC meeting in 1993 (Edwards 1996: 6), but the Department of Health did not get round to publishing its original guidelines until 1995 (DoH 2006: 3). The official remit of MSLCs is to be 'an independent advisory body' which involves commissioners, providers and users in the planning and monitoring of services (Messent 2002). The precise nature of user involvement, however, is open to differing interpretations.

After referring to 'the old medically-dominated Liaison Committees', Edwards pronounces her experience of MSLC involvement to have been 'harrowing' (Edwards 1996: 6), featuring medical manipulation by interference with committee membership, correspondence, papers and agenda. While surveying local women's experiences of maternity services, Peter Messent produced a similarly bleak, but marginally more sympathetic, assessment of MSLCs' functioning:

> it is also quite challenging for the chair of an MSLC to facilitate good and effective working relationships between professional and lay committee members. In the past two years the local MSLC has suffered from a high turnover of both lay and professional members. ... As a consequence, the MSLC did not meet regularly for nearly a year and has struggled to maintain continuity.
>
> (Messent 2002: 629)

A more positive depiction of MSLC activity, however, is found in Kate Smith's description of a Derbyshire committee. Her up-beat account reflects on the necessity of building alliances between childbirth group representatives, as mentioned above. She also raises the perennial problem of retaining members and delegates when their childbearing experiences are receding into the past. Thus, representation of the constituency may be problematical. Smith explains the need for the, unfortunately-named, MUG (Maternity Users Group) which served as an important sub-group of the MSLC but constituted a serious challenge, as it competed for 'volunteer time' (MUG 2005: 40).

Various strategies have been implemented to improve the functioning and effectiveness of MSLCs, with varying degrees of success. Elizabeth Key suggests that a crucial initial step is persuading the Committee that 'maternity units [are] not there just to serve the interests of those working in them' (Key 1999: 11). Perhaps more constructively, Edwards outlines what is necessary if MSLCs are to be anything other than mere talking shops (Edwards 2006). As well as the provision of workshops to prepare and support user-members (Edwards 2005b), she emphasises the need for alliances between user representatives, and possibly midwives, to ensure that they sing to the same hymn sheet. The need to identify and prioritise the concerns of childbearing women is vital and may be achieved by what she terms 'networking' with a range of women of differing backgrounds and orientations (Edwards 2006: 18–19). Edwards outlines the beneficial effect of the existence of a MUG (see above), which is that it ensures that lay members feel sufficiently confident to be able to contribute to the MSLC.

The proper financial reimbursement of MSLC members is crucial for user representatives and any others not paid for attending meetings. A similar recognition of the input of user-members is in the appropriate use of language, which should demystify medical culture and facilitate mutual comprehension.

In order to draw comparisons with UK MSLCs, the situation in the Irish Republic deserves attention. Endeavours to reform a health care system under challenge there have long been progressing. One feature of Ireland's attempts to make maternity care more woman-centred has included the introduction of MSLCs (Kennedy 2010), but the extent of their acceptance and effectiveness has yet to be evaluated.

Groups of consumers

While the consumer movement may consider that it seeks to improve the position of all childbearing women, there are certain groups who, for a variety of reasons, are likely to be particularly vulnerable.

Before addressing the situation of these groups, two interdependent and often-taken-for-granted principles of health care deserve mention. A requirement which underpins any consumer's choice of services is that person's *access* to the range of services available. The usual geographical meaning of this concept may inhibit recognition of the systematic problems of access which are inherent in health care provision. These problems apply to particular services being less easily available to or of a poorer quality for certain populations or sections of the community. On an individual basis, such services may render themselves less accessible through, for example, their ethnic, linguistic or gender bias. Linked with and yet distinct from accessibility is *equity*; while possibly referring only to individuals' access to services, equity needs to be interpreted more broadly to include health outcomes as well as inputs. The right to health is a fundamental ethical principle as expressed by the World Health Organisation (WHO 2008). The inequities inherent in the UK health care system have long been recognised, but remain unresolved.

An example of evidence of such inequity manifests itself in a large and authoritative survey of 26,325 women in England, in which Veena Raleigh and her colleagues identified a complex picture of variably unhealthy experiences of maternity care (Raleigh 2010). These observations were found to apply particularly to ethnic minority, single and less well-educated women. It is necessary to consider where power lies in relation to these groups of childbearing women and whether and how their position is changing or can be changed. In legislative terms, the position of some groups has been strengthened by the recent enactment of the Equality Act (UK Parliament 2010). The new legislation originated in the dying years of the previous Labour administration and superseded, supposedly strengthening, a number of items of anti-discriminatory legislation which have been enacted since the 1960s. The Equality Act introduced the concept of 'protected characteristics' as being in need of special attention, which include: Age, Disability, Gender Reassignment, Marriage and Civil Partnership,

Race, Religion or Belief, Sex and Sexual Orientation. Of particular relevance in the context of the maternity service user are the duties which this legislation places on public institutions to, not just eliminate discrimination, victimisation and harassment, but to go further than that. So that public bodies, including health authorities, are also charged with:

- advancing equality of opportunity between persons who share a relevant characteristic and persons who do not share it;
- fostering good relations between persons who share a relevant characteristic and persons who do not share it (Equality Act 2010, section 149).

Thus, this legislation requires that public bodies should positively promote the rights of vulnerable groups. This public duty, however, does not apply to immigration functions (Hepple 2010), which is probably the very characteristic most likely to apply to the childbearing woman.

It is against the background of this probably well-meaning legislation that I consider the position of certain groups of maternity service users.

The minority ethnic woman

The poor birth outcomes all too often experienced by black and minority ethnic women are sufficiently well-known to not bear repetition here (Earle and Church 2004; Raleigh et al 2010; CMACE 2011). In this section I go beyond these infamous outcomes to consider the power relations which underpin the experiences of ethnic minority women.

The terminology in this context is problematical because of its supremely sensitive nature and seemingly constant updating. At the time of writing, black and minority ethnic (BME) is widely accepted, so this is the term which I will be using:

Black and minority ethnic (BME) – A term used to describe people from minority groups, particularly those who are viewed as having suffered racism or are in the minority because of their skin colour and/or ethnicity. This term has evolved over time becoming more common as the term 'black' has become less all-inclusive of those experiencing racial discrimination. 'BME' was/is an attempt at comprehensive coverage. The term is commonly used in the UK but can be unpopular with those who find it cumbersome or bureaucratic.

(Universities Scotland 2010)

At first sight, regarding the balance of power between the BME childbearing woman and those who provide her care, the relationship is clearly unequal. The care providers may either perceive themselves or be perceived as representing an institution which, irrespective of their good intentions, carries an assumption of authority. This assumption may be based on one or more forms of reasoning; for example, probably because of its origins and organisation, the UK NHS adheres to a 'scientific' model of health care which grew up in western Europe (Raynor and Morgan 2000: 47i/ii). A similar historical rationale is offered by Nicky Ellis; she explains that the institutionalised racism of the NHS is based on its early post-World War II origins, which featured a conviction of white supremacy and resulted in, albeit unintentional, discrimination (Ellis 2004: 240). Drawing on even longer-term concepts, Savita Katbamna considers that the lingering shadow of western imperialism is largely responsible for the 'institutionalised racism and sexism within the national health service' (Katbamna 2000: 32), particularly affecting women of childbearing age.

At an interpersonal or clinical level, individual members of staff may harbour a perception of threat exerted by groups of which they are not a part. In association with multiculturalism's tendency to disregard individual differences and seek simplistic similarities, the result is racial stereotyping (Ellis 2004: 240; Bowler 1993).

Traditionally, the problems attributed to BME clients were linked to language differences which, Ellis maintains, have been advanced as reasons for some groups' worse morbidity and mortality rates, mentioned already (Ellis 2004: 238). It is widely assumed that the increasing availability of interpreting services, like the provision of more appropriate catering, will constitute a panacea to solve any problems faced by BME clients; although Euranis Neile argues that the problem lies in the attitudes of midwives and policy-makers (Neile 1997: 119). The research evidence suggests, however, that interpreting services are limited, even in countries with a high proportion of consumers of different ethnic backgrounds (Lewis 2011a: 50; Bowen 2001; Pardy 1995; Baker 1996). The non-availability or non-use of interpreting services results in family members being asked to interpret, raising culture- and gender-based issues (Earle and Church 2004). The need for more effective use of interpreting services was a major recommendation of the most recent Confidential Enquiries Report:

> An asylum seeker who also spoke no English and whose husband was her interpreter was stabbed by him while pregnant. She had repeatedly failed to attend for care and had had only one antenatal visit. Her nonattendances were not followed up. She had, however, attended the local Emergency Department complaining of constant vaginal irritation and discharge. These are classic signs of abuse.
>
> (Lewis 2011b: 148)

In her study of birth experiences of South Asian Muslim women, though, Ellis found that members of her sample of second generation childbearing women experienced a form of 'muting' or silencing (Ellis 2004: 249) by midwives. This happened through the midwives failing to use their active listening skills and neglecting to provide opportunities for the woman to articulate her concerns.

Writing with a specific focus on the woman with a South Asian background, Katbamna suggests that this woman's situation should be viewed in the context of a male-dominated maternity system (Katbamna 2000: 132). She considers this woman's difficulty in challenging racist attitudes, which are not overt, and of a pressure on the woman to internalise her feelings of distress. It is because of the stress which racism exerts on the South Asian woman that she finds herself having to reject traditional practices with which she is culturally comfortable and to embrace the alien medical model of childbearing. This acceptance is reinforced by fear of disapproval of culturally appropriate practices, such as her need for special foods at certain crucial times in the childbearing cycle.

The BME consumer is likely to find herself at a particular disadvantage compared, especially, with the 'white and middle class' woman (Katbamna 2000: 133). One of the reasons for this is the failure of maternity-oriented consumer organisations (see page 17) to take on board the needs of both the BME woman and her working-class sisters (Baggott et al 2005). Recommendations for the involvement of black and ethnic minority women in developing service standards is one way of overcoming such disadvantage (RCM 2000).

Case Study: The BME childbearing woman in the Irish Republic

It may be due to the cataclysmic social changes experienced in Ireland in the last two decades, that the position of the childbearing woman in the BME community has attracted considerable research and other attention. Because of this much-needed attention, I use Ireland's experience to highlight some of the issues currently prevalent in other economically developed countries. While Suzi Lyons and her colleagues attribute this research attention to Ireland's 'great economic success' (Lyons 2008: 261), it is possible that other factors may also be operating. Ronit Lentin indicates the nature of some of these factors, associating them with, first, the reality of 'Irishness', secondly, the 'otherness' of in-migrants, and, thirdly, the possibility that BME groups may actually be blamed for *causing* racism (Lentin 2001: 2.10). She draws the conclusion, however, that Ireland's ongoing difficulties with the immigrant 'other' are largely attributable to the country's 'unfinished business', left over from the Irish diaspora a century earlier.

Lyons and her colleagues' grounded theory research involved interviewing maternity staff to examine the experience of providing care for ethnic minority women, while views of migrant women were investigated by Patricia Kennedy and Jo Murphy-Lawless (2003; see pages 32–3). Lyons and colleagues considered the impact of 'an unprecedented increase in population' (Lyons et al 2008: 261) on a maternity care system which struggled to cope with even the twentieth century (O'Driscoll et al 1980). This study suggested, probably unsurprisingly, that communication was a major problem despite the availability of inter-preters. The serious implications of such poor communication materialise in the lack of information provided for the woman giving birth in an alien environment; particularly disconcerting is the ethical conundrum of whether the woman's consent to medical and other interventions is truly informed. Perhaps not unrelated to these communication difficulties was the perception that the mothers did not conform to staff expectations inherent in the Irish culture of maternity care, to the extent of becoming non-compliant or even resisting interventions. These well-recognised difficulties were aggravated by widespread staff perceptions of an excessive workload. Together, such perceptions developed into a vicious cycle of stereotyping, similar to the situation reported by Neile, featuring opinions common not only to individuals, but also institutions, structures, organisations and systems (Neile 1997: 120). The staff perception of the homogeneity of the BME women also served to reinforce stereotypes and diminish any possibility of personalised or individualised care. As found by Isobel Bowler in Britain back in 1993, such stereotypes manifested particularly in the use of pharmacological pain control in labour. When women declined such interventions, workload deficiencies were felt to have been further exacerbated. The 'us versus them' approach among staff was found to be characterised by the all too familiar preliminary 'I'm not racist but ... ' (Lyons et al 2008: 272). Overall, Lyons and her colleagues summarise the staff attitude to BME women as requiring them to 'When in Rome – do as the Romans'. This assimilationist approach in Ireland is comparable with the ill-fated attitudes and policies which began in the mid-twentieth century United Kingdom.

Against the background outlined by Lyons and her colleagues, the disconcerting case of Bimbo Onanuga has focused attention in Ireland and further afield on the experience of the BME woman in the maternity system. After a diagnosis of foetal death, for which induction of labour was planned, Bimbo Onanuga was admitted as an emergency to one of the three major maternity units in Dublin (Reilly 2011). The demise of her baby and her complaints of severe abdominal, but not labour, pain are suggestive of an accidental antepartum haemorrhage (placental abruption). A drug, misoprostol, is thought to have been administered to 'ripen' her cervix prior to induction of labour, despite Bimbo Onanuga's poor obstetric history and this drug not being approved for this purpose in Ireland. When Bimbo Onanuga's condition deteriorated, her partner found difficulty persuading staff of the seriousness of her condition. Just as Bowler (1993) and Ellis (2004) had found in Britain, he reported that staff would not take her complaints seriously:

> the nurse who was there with me was telling me she's pretending, that was what she was saying. She didn't use the word pretending actually, but she was telling me it's no problem, that some people exaggerate – I think that was the word she used, 'exaggerate'.
>
> (Reilly 2011)

When a different member of staff eventually raised the alarm, a series of otherwise farcical difficulties ensued. Their nature is apparent from the actions recommended to prevent a recurrence, as reported by the Minister for Health and Children (Deputy James Reilly) in the Dáil Éireann responding to a question about their non-implementation 12 months after this maternal death:

1   The need to identify clinical pathways relating to management of women with an intrauterine death in third trimester to complement existing medical management policy.

2   The Guidelines for Medical Management of Intrauterine Death should be revised in line with a review of the medical literature.

3   Details of all patients for Induction of Labour, regardless of place of induction should be centrally documented.

4   This recommendation cannot be disclosed as it contains personal, private, sensitive and confidential information relating to the individual patient.

5   Develop a brief operational outline of the Gynaecology Department to assist staff who are sent there on an occasional/intermittent basis.

6   Due to the complexity of work, there is a need for an updated training needs analysis of all midwifery and nursing staff on the gynaecology ward.

7   There should be a designated individual with responsibility for coordinating, monitoring and auditing the Basic Life Support attendance and Advanced Life Support Skills attendance, ideally a designated Resuscitation Training Officer.

8   An Obstetric Early Warning System should be introduced and evaluated.

9   Install additional phone lines in the ward.

10   A review of the possibility of emergency call bells or designated phones for emergencies in each room should be carried out and measures taken to address this.

11   Hospital wide analysis of all doorways in clinical areas to establish the feasibility of moving a bed in a critical event.

On the basis of this information, an inquest is being sought into the circumstances of the death of Bimbo Onanuga, but is resisted by the staff of the maternity units involved.

There is no reason why this case study of the situation in the Republic of Ireland should engender complacency among those in other countries, as the Northwick Park Enquiry showed (CQC 2006) and as the most recent UK Confidential Enquiries Report (2011) stated:

> analysis of the English data suggests that for Black African women (P < 0.001) and, to a lesser extent Black Caribbean women (P < 0.001), the mortality rate is significantly higher than that for White women.
>
> (Lewis 2011a: 47)

The international migrant

The challenging situations faced by the childbearing woman in the BME community are thrown into sharp relief by the experiences of one particular group. These are the migrant women, who find themselves in alien lands through either forced or free migration, and they include asylum seekers and refugees (Jentsch et al 2007: 129). Although the difficulties, mentioned above, faced by BME women in Ireland have attracted attention, the antagonism faced by migrants in the United Kingdom has been inadequately recorded. A survey by the Independent Asylum Commission (IAC 2008) recruited a volunteer sample of long-term UK residents which produced 809 responses; the majority 'were critical of the asylum system and felt aggrieved by asylum seekers and the government'. The reasons for such antagonism tended to be rationalised in terms of:

• Britain is a 'soft touch', taking more than its fair share of asylum seekers;
• asylum seekers are here to steal jobs and scrounge on welfare;
• asylum seekers get preferential treatment in housing and public services allocation. (IAC 2008: 14)

That the situation in many parts of the United Kingdom bears comparison with that in Ireland is advanced by Birgit Jentsch and her colleagues due to a common history of not welcoming migrants (Jentsch et al 2007). The sudden and massive change in the traditional picture of emigration out of Ireland, and migration more generally, has been linked to the expansion of the European Union (Kennedy and Murphy-Lawless 2003). Also blamed is the globalisation of human existence in general and women's lives in particular (Helman 2007).

The extent of the appalling childbearing outcomes among migrant women has been reported in the United Kingdom by referring to the risk of maternal death:

> Ten [of the 29 childbearing women who died of sepsis] were from minority ethnic groups, six of whom were asylum seekers or recent immigrants.
>
> (Lewis 2011a: 87)

The real significance of this observation is apparent from the recognition that maternal death is almost four times higher among some groups of women of black African and Caribbean origin than among women of white origin (Lewis 2011a: 47). Alongside these dire maternal outcomes, though, Karen Aroian found that migrant women's babies are less vulnerable than their mothers, demonstrating perinatal and neonatal morbidity and mortality rates comparable with the indigenous population (Aroian 2001).

Jentsch and her colleagues attribute such dreadful maternal outcomes among migrant women to the inaccessibility of maternity services. This is partly due to the women's lack of knowledge about the availability of health care locally, attributable to a lack of information, as observed in the Confidential Enquiries:

> One [recent migrant who subsequently died] was not booked until late in her pregnancy although she had regularly attended the Emergency Department with pregnancy-related problems.
>
> (Harper 2011: 87)

Anxiety and depression associated with a traumatic migration causes contact with unfamiliar health care providers to be particularly challenging. Women who have migrated from a country with a fee-based health care system may be convinced of their inability to pay for health services. Fear of immigration authorities may deter some women from seeking maternity care, as may language or literacy difficulties. Jentsch and her colleagues rehearse the catalogue of cultural barriers in the health services, as well as the possibility that the woman may have come from a culture in which it is customary for the husband to speak for family members (Jentsch 2007). A study of the health care experiences of pregnant asylum seekers identified the serious risks to maternal health endemic in the asylum system; Becky Reynolds and Judy White (2010) found the health problems inherent in the asylum system to be aggravated by asylum seekers being moved at 'very short notice' (Reynolds and White 2010: 21) from initial accommodation (IAC) to distant dispersal centres. While the administrative reasons for such transfers are difficult to question, the failure of health records to be transferred or health care providers to be notified may explain the poor outcomes.

As recognised by Jenny Douglas back in 1992, the exclusion of certain groups of women from contributing the research agenda continues to constrain knowledge and understanding (Jentsch et al 2007: 131). This problem is aggravated by the paucity of research attention to the duration of the woman's stay in her new country.

An attempt, however, has been made to resolve this omission by Shuby Puthussery and her colleagues (Puthussery et al 2008, 2010), in a study focusing on the experience of second generation BME women, ie those born in the United Kingdom. The findings of the study were surprisingly positive regarding issues such as information-giving, differing expectations, interpersonal communication and the limited impact of their ethnicity on their experience of care. On closer scrutiny, though, the reason for such an up-beat picture is found in the methods section; it is reported that midwives were asked to recruit women during their antenatal appointments and, clearly, the midwives selected women who they considered would be good informants. This sampling bias led to an over-representation of women who were older and better-educated, with the median age being 30–39 years and half of the women holding at least a university degree (Puthussery et al 2010: 158). Thus, the researchers identify the need to 'recruit the recruiters' as well as the participants (Twamley et al 2009). It is clear that the conclusions of this study should be treated with caution in view of the overpowering bias towards middle-class women. While this paper appears to conclude that poorer outcomes among BME women result from their being recent migrants, it is possible that many BME women's continuing problems in the maternity services may be more associated with their relatively impoverished status.

Reflections

On the basis of personal observation, there seems to be complacency in the maternity services that everything possible is being done to meet the needs of ethnic minority women. What this means is that interpreters are now widely available, dietary needs are easily addressed and even the extended family's visiting practices are better tolerated (Earle and Church 2004). My observation and my reading, however, lead me to conclude that the idyll comprising the appropriate employment of these facilities has yet to be achieved. In this section, I build on this perception by reflecting on some of the outstanding issues facing the BME woman embarking on childbearing.

The complacency to which I have already referred is found in the prominence attached to the improved childbearing outcomes for Black African women. This is attested by the significant reduction in maternal deaths among this group (Lewis 2011a: 5). Similarly, Aroian has shown that perinatal and neonatal mortality are less serious problems (Aroian 2001). Any complacency, though, is shattered by data on the experiences of migrant, refugee and asylum-seeking women. These women, often needing to access UK maternity services because of civil upheavals in their country of origin, face asylum and health care systems which are ill-prepared to address their needs (Reynolds and White 2010). The result is that health care for such migrant women may be counterproductive.

Complacency is derived from having put in place facilities to deal with aspects traditionally raised by certain groups with obvious or visible physical differences, such as skin colour, hair texture and/or facial structure (Raynor and Morgan 2000: 47). While these aspects still apply and may continue to be less than completely satisfied, attention should also be given to the difficulties of the childbearing woman whose appearance may not differ markedly from that of the host community; but her linguistic, economic, social and experiential background is likely to bear no relation to that of the host population.

As well as complacency based on certain facilities to address particular situations, terminology has developed to the extent of particular assumptions having developed into current shorthand for deprived or impoverished, such as 'BME'. These assumptions manifest themselves in well-intentioned encouragement:

> maternity services must make efforts to make their services accessible to deprived immigrants who do not speak English.
>
> (de Swiet et al 2011: 125)

It is obviously crucial to be aware of the link between poor childbearing outcomes and ethnic background as well as social class and the likelihood that the inverse care law applies (Kirkham 1999a: 94); the health care practitioner, though, must look beyond such generalisations (Barnard and Turner 2011). As Bhikhu Parekh astutely observes, there are widely-held beliefs that all Chinese and East African Asians are highly able; while similar assumptions may be made that the reverse is true of Pakistanis, Bangladeshis and Afro-Caribbeans. He reminds the reader, however:

> Even the high-achieving groups contain pockets of poverty, just as the low-achieving ones include some who have done quite well. The incidence of poverty is certainly higher in ethnic minority groups than in the country at large, but not uniformly so.
>
> (Parekh 2002: 1)

On the basis of Parekh's warning, the urgent requirement for individualisation of the care of the BME woman becomes apparent (Earle and Church 2004). This requirement resonates with the observation by Lyons and her colleagues, based on their research in Ireland of the tendency to regard certain women as 'them' and to focus on differences, rather than looking for aspects in common (Lyons et al 2008: 272). This 'them versus us' orientation results in any behaviours which may be unfamiliar becoming stereotyped in terms of cultural problems, rather than as the individual woman's personal preferences. In this way, the necessity for the ill-fated 'woman-centredness' assumes a whole new meaning and becomes doubly significant.

The prerequisite for woman-centredness in this context constitutes an intervention intended to break a number of cycles which may be operating. The first, and perhaps the most ominous, of these is the cycle reported by Ellis following from her work on south Asian Muslim women (Ellis 2004). She observed that those with a non-English first language and non-majority background were more likely to receive inappropriate care. Such deficiencies result in poorer outcomes and serve to reinforce the staff's low expectations of childbearing ability. A second and more general cycle relates to the social exclusion of some minority ethnic groups which, Ellis maintains, is what leads to a vicious cycle of poverty and the reinforcement of racist ideas about being work-shy (Ellis 2004: 240). In her classic paper, Jenny Douglas argued that stereotyping of black women extends to the research agenda and that the absence of research into black women's issues perpetuates the cycle of ignorance (Douglas 1992: 37). A similar cycle involving stereotyping was recognised in the work of Lyons and her colleagues (Lyons et al 2008), which identified a cycle of staff having a limited understanding of the situation of BME women. Because of the perception of an excessive workload there was thought to be a lack of time to find out about the individual woman – resulting in stereotyping being used rather than extending understanding.

It is possible that these variably vicious cycles may eventually lose momentum. The work of IAC (see page 29), though, suggests that bigoted opposition may thwart this. While education is often regarded as being the answer, Neale's research demonstrates the complacent attitude of educationists to a multicultural curriculum (Neale 1997: 125). On the basis of such evidence it is clear that more active intervention is necessary.

The lesbian woman

In the same way as the minority ethnic woman is vulnerable to stereotyping which may adversely affect her birthing experience, so too is the childbearing woman who is lesbian. While the experiences of the BME woman have long attracted attention in the professional media and in research, the lesbian woman has only relatively recently begun to be recognised as a consumer of maternity services (Wilton 1999; Wilton and Kaufmann 2001). The situation of the LGBT (Lesbian, Gay, Bisexual, Transgender) staff member, though, is different again (Mander and Page 2011) and will be mentioned in Chapter 5. This woman's position is sensitive because of the widely-recognised heteronormative and homophobic attitudes of staff throughout the health care system (Kitzinger 2005; Rose 1993) and the late Tamsin Wilton's ground-breaking work which showed that such attitudes are no less prevalent in the maternity services (Wilton 1999). Antagonism has been attributed to staff fear, arising out of an inability to dissociate sexual orientation from sexual activity (Eliason 1996).

Elaine Lee and her colleagues' study of lesbian women's experience of maternity care demonstrates how they manage to make sense of such a hostile environment (Lee 2011). The informants recognised that homophobic episodes do occur in health care situations, but reported the belief that such experiences applied only to other women and did not recognise or admit to the occurrence of such episodes in their own care. The events which each of the informants reported, and were interpreted by the researchers as homophobically negative, were rationalised and largely attributed to either the personalities of staff members or environmental factors:

> 'I think she was like that with everyone. I think that's just how she was'.
> (Lee 2011: 985)

These researchers contemplate the possibility that these lesbian mothers were in denial about the adverse nature of their contacts. This strategy, together with some degree of rationalisation, was being used by the women to protect themselves from the reality of sub-optimal care. In this way, Lee and her colleagues suggest, the women were able to assume some control over their childbearing experience, rather than having to rely on potentially unsympathetic staff for support which might not be forthcoming. Such a strategy meant that each of these women was able to appreciate her experience of becoming a mother, just as most childbearing women keenly anticipate new motherhood. The authors propose, however, that each of the women using the denial and rationalisation strategies would be likely to find herself empowered by her experience. They conclude with their concern that such naïve and low-key strategies will only perpetuate the homophobic environment in which lesbian women embark on motherhood. It is necessary to question, though, whether it is really the role of the supremely vulnerable new mother to encourage culture change in maternity services, especially as services are supposedly based on equity and woman-centredness, irrespective of the gender orientation or the childbearing woman's other personal characteristics (Spidsberg 2007, 2011).

Women defined by their age

Certain groups of maternity services consumers have attracted attention by virtue of their age. This attention is all too often likely to feature censure or other forms of a 'bad press'.

While the term 'elderly primigravida' has been most frequently used for the first-time mother who is aged 35 years or over, the argument has been advanced that 25 may be more appropriate; this younger age takes account of perceptions of the greater likelihood of health problems (Silverton 1993: 74). Such a derogatory term, irrespective of its precise definition, has fortunately disappeared from use because women, for any number of reasons, choose to and find themselves birthing their babies at increasing age. It may be suggested that medical practitioners no longer regard late childbearing so much as a threat to maternal and infant health, but as more of an opportunity for increasing medical involvement in healthy reproduction, despite a dearth of evidence (Carolan 2003; Lampinen et al 2009). Gender politics impinge on this woman's experience, as well as medical politics, as it has been shown that, irrespective of biological functioning, the woman is subjected to more social disapprobation than her male partner, by the application of premature societal deadlines on the age at which childbearing and parenting is thought acceptable (Billari et al 2011).

On the other hand, the young teenage woman's experience compares seriously unfavourably with that of her more mature sister; her situation has been presented solely as a 'problem' by the popular media and politicians, with the endorsement of powerful transatlantic influences (Macintyre and Cunningham-Burley 1993; Leishman 2007). The precise nature of the 'problem', though, is not invariably or easily apparent. Teenage childbearing has been linked to an 'underclass' (Pearce 1993) trapped in a cycle of deprivation, which has, more recently, been presented as engendering and perpetuating 'social exclusion' (SEU 1999; DoH and DCSF 2010).

The then UK Prime Minister, Tony Blair, exemplified such attitudes when he painted a bleak picture of a treadmill of poverty, educational underachievement, non-existent employment prospects, generations of poor health and a cycle of early motherhood (SEU 1999: 4). In writing this material, though, he was certainly not drawing on the available research evidence (Duncan 2007), making such an adverse picture both inaccurate and incomplete.

Jan Macvarish shows that the experiences of young teenagers who become mothers are neither invariably nor totally negative (Macvarish 2010). A very relevant Swedish example is found in the work of Elizabeth Wahn and her colleagues, who show that young women experienced becoming a teenage mother as being a positive transition into adulthood, despite the psychological and physical challenges (Wahn et al 2005). As with any new mother, each of the young women in their sample emphasised the crucial contribution of good support from family and friends in the early days of assuming her parenting role. Adopting a longer-term view, an authoritative classic research study from the United States indicates that, after early and temporary educational and/or financial and/or career disadvantages, the young teenage mother does catch up (Furstenburg et al 1987).

The debate, such as it is, on young motherhood is ill-served by the agendas and manipulations of the popular media, who present this young woman's situation in terms of a 'moral panic' (Duncan 2007: 309). The limited UK data tend to be compared with Nordic countries, whose health care systems provide far better support, rather than with North American countries, with whose 'teen pregnancy' rates the UK figures compare more favourably. The popular media, as Simon Duncan observes, neglect to remove their rose-tinted spectacles to note that recent figures are equivalent to the supposedly idyllic years of the post-World War II family. In 1956 the birth rate per 1,000 women aged 15–19 years was 27.3 and rising, whereas in 2004 the figure was 26.9 and falling (Duncan 2007: 310).

Thus, although not seeking to endorse views of the teenage mother as any kind of victim, as she has all too frequently been portrayed, she certainly appears to have been used as a pawn in a variety of political disputes.

The disabled woman

The range of disabilities facing childbearing women is extensive, including a range of types of sensory and verbal impairment as well as mobility, intellectual and mental health conditions. In Ireland, the National Disability Survey estimated that approximately 4.3 per cent of women of childbearing age (defined there as 18–44 years) consider themselves to have some kind of disability (NDS 2006: 6b). As with many of the groups of maternity services consumers mentioned here, there is a widespread perception of their problematical nature. Such views of disability as the problem of the affected person and their family have been roundly challenged by disability activists. These 'medical' or 'individual' models of the construction of disability have been or are being replaced by the social model of disability which regards the definition of disability by health and welfare practitioners as being at the root of any problems (Lloyd 2001: 715). This developing emphasis is reflected in the authoritative literature review by Cecily Begley and her colleagues in Dublin, Ireland, which suggests that the source of the problem is not to be found in the woman with a disability. These researchers correctly identify that difficulties for this woman are more likely to originate with 'prejudicial social attitudes and discriminatory and exclusionary practices of individuals, organisations and institutions' (Begley et al 2009: section 2.5.3). Begley and her team go on to argue that childbearing is no more likely to create any further health problems for this woman than it is for her sister who does not have a disability. Thus, the literature suggests that medical intervention to 'prevent' difficulties is likely to be counterproductive and any medical involvement should be on a reactive, rather than proactive, basis (Begley et al 2009: section 2.5.5).

The attitudes inhibiting the likelihood of motherhood for a disabled woman are addressed by Corbett O'Toole in her in-depth analysis of the barriers to sexuality for the disabled woman (O'Toole 2002). She indicates that sexuality and disability are considered mutually exclusive for the woman and services or assistance for the woman to fulfil the sexual facets of her personality are non-existent. The absence of help for the disabled woman reflects attitudes commonly held, particularly among parents and teachers of people with intellectual disability

(Aunos and Feldman 2002). Research undertaken in Canada showed that people with intellectual disabilities tend to be cautious in their attitudes towards sex and homosexuality, but Marjorie Aunos and Maurice Feldman found that intimate contact with familiar and trusted individuals is not problematical. This study suggested that research on disability focusing solely on issues relating to (in)voluntary sterilisation and contraception and on parenting rights may be largely historical; the research agenda is moving forward as attitudes become more humane. Thus, obstacles to sexual relationships, the usual precursor to pregnancy and childbearing, may be being reduced.

The obese woman

While the popular media have been shown to incriminate obese people in general and obese children in particular (Boero 2007), it is only relatively recently that this 'witch hunt' has been extended to childbearing women (Lewis and Macfarlane 2007: 25; Cnattingius et al 1998). The introduction of the concept of 'size zero' has been generally deplored, but such thinness continues to be highly desirable. The associations between obesity and potentially fatal childbearing conditions, such as thromboembolic disease, infectious states and cardiac disorders, has led to ill-founded assertions of causation (Mander 2011c). Obesity tends to be linked to lifestyle factors, such as difficulty with exercise and inappropriate diet, but it has also been associated by some with more negative characteristics, such as 'gluttony and sloth' (Ashton 2003). In this way unsubstantiated assumptions, victim-blaming and value judgements are likely to affect the care of the woman with what is euphemistically being termed a 'high BMI'.

Conclusion

In this chapter I have discussed whether and how certain groups of women may be affected by the interpersonal politics of the maternity care system. Despite the activities of a number of consumer groups which I have outlined, maternity services have difficulty providing care for women with certain personality characteristics or lifestyles. The result is that the woman's care is negatively affected and adverse health consequences ensue.

The crucially important personal characteristic which I have not raised specifically in this chapter is the one that is shared by all consumers of the maternity services. This is gender; I would argue that all maternity service users are women, albeit many with male partners and babies who may be boys. As Tricia Anderson observed, the oppression of childbearing women is a longstanding feature of maternity care in the United Kingdom and, probably, elsewhere (Anderson 2004: 262). The most disconcerting feature of this form of oppression is found in the conspiratorial involvement of the person who claims to be 'with woman', that is the midwife. The effects of this gender-related oppression on women's care by a male-dominated and fundamentally patriarchal maternity system will emerge in the following chapters.

3 Interoccupational politics

Introduction

The dynamism characteristic of maternity care is largely due to the regular reinvention of care providers' ideals and ideas. Such regular renaissance or metamorphosis is seen not least in the activities, roles and titles which the various maternity-related disciplines undertake and assume. These reinventions are further compounded by the entrée into the birthing room of previously disregarded, unknown or newly-created care providers. These developments, being intimately associated with practice and care, clearly carry momentous political implications; not only for the childbearing woman, but also for other contiguous and otherwise associated occupational groups.

In this chapter I contemplate these implications for those who may be involved and/or affected. First, though, I need to consider the health care environment in which such developments and interactions happen. This consideration will lead into my deconstruction of patriarchy, a concept which underpins the functioning of many of the groups involved and which re-emerges throughout this book.

Occupational environment

The socio-cultural setting in which health care in general, and maternity care in particular, occur inevitably influences the form of that care. This setting will be affected by many factors, including historical, occupational, political, economic and gender-related issues. Writing from her North American viewpoint, Robbie Davis-Floyd argues the prevalence of the 'technocratic' approach to maternity care (Davis-Floyd 2001: S5). She attributes the widespread acceptance of such an approach to the capitalist, male-oriented institutions of health care, which are predisposed to improving their supposedly 'scientific' credentials. Similarly, Cecilia Benoit and her colleagues (Benoit 2005: 725), adopting a multinational approach, emphasise the importance of male-centred power in the organisation of health care occupations. It is factors like these which have interacted to fashion the health system in which maternity services are offered and which Jo Murphy-Lawless addresses in Chapter 6. These factors contribute significantly to the theoretical concept underpinning the relationships between occupational groups and between members of those groups practising in maternity. This theory is the all too familiar concept of patriarchy.

Patriarchy

As this is one of those terms likely to mean different things to different people, Karen Warren has usefully condensed Adrienne Rich's well-known definition of patriarchy (Rich 1977: 57) into 'the systematic domination by men' (Warren 1987: 14). Adopting a radical feminist perspective, Mary Stewart develops this definition in a particularly relevant direction, by stating that such sex-specific oppression of women is implemented through male control of the female body (Stewart 2004: 32). Thus, patriarchy defines women as having the primary functions of either the bearing and/or raising of children or the satisfaction of men's sexual desires.

The origins of the term 'patriarchy' are found, according to Liz Stephens, in the Victorian domestic ideal of the head of the household and bread-winner being the father (Stephens 2004: 43). Such an apparently natural and, hence, barely visible model has been widely accepted, albeit subliminally, in working relationships between nursing and medical staff in the UK NHS; this may be due to the model having been unambiguously articulated, fervently endorsed and widely implemented by Florence Nightingale (Gamarnikow 1978). Even more disconcertingly, though, this model of female submissiveness and male domination has recently been identified as typifying relationships between midwifery and medical personnel in the maternity care system (Gould 2002).

In a qualitative research project focusing on 'normal birth', Annette Keating and Valerie Fleming (2009) identified four key features of patriarchy, which resonated strongly with Karen Warren's ground-breaking work (Warren 1994). Keating and Fleming interviewed midwives in a birthing environment and identified the predominance of:

- *Power and prestige* – comprising behaviours and agencies allotting higher status and valuing prestige to mete out power over power.
- *Hierarchical thinking* – the fundamentally important role of levels of decision-making and autonomy. The medical practitioner at the hierarchy's pinnacle, with midwives at differing levels depending on experience, and the supposedly compliant and passive childbearing woman ranking lowest.
- *Dualistic or 'either/or' thinking* – consisting of the dichotomous or binary system of reasoning, dwelling on essentialism, rather than relative realities which are more true to life. These are 'fixed oppositional categories' mentioned by Denis Walsh (2004: 67), which fail to allow for the 'grey areas', complexities, fluidity and dynamism of the real world.
- *Logic of domination* – power and prestige being rewarded with superiority. Thus, domination's corollary is justified as the subordination of those perceived as lower status.

Radical feminists regard patriarchy as the template from which all other power-based systems developed (Kaufmann 2004: 6). Underpinning the second wave of feminism, radical feminists claimed a huge impact on childbearing and other aspects of women's health. In support, Tara Kaufmann argues radical feminism's responsibility for women's greater consciousness of their bodily functioning and the avoidable nature of rape, sexual harassment, intimate partner (domestic) violence and male-dominated health services.

Outlining the impact of patriarchy on midwives over the centuries and their struggle against pervasive medical hegemony, Carol Bates indicates effects of late twentieth-century changes within the health care and legal systems, which served to further fortify men's position (Bates 2004: 132). These salutary developments have been aggravated by naïve educational and professional aspirations pursued by some midwives, leading them to seek advancement through ill-advised strategies aligning themselves with medical practitioners. Bates exemplifies audit as one such strategy, to which evidence-based practice (EBP; page 56) should also be added.

Occupations and professions in maternity

Although the words 'occupation' and 'profession' are often used interchangeably, because of the latter's very precise sociological meaning and other connotations, it is better employed sparingly. Sam Porter and his colleagues differentiate the two terms by defining a profession as more than just an occupation displaying 'skills, service and altruism' (Porter 2007: 526). In addition to high social status and commensurate income, a profession is essentially imbued with power, a crucial component of which is the capacity to control its own functioning (Freidson 1970: 71). While medicine is regarded in sociological terms as the archetypical profession, the limited extent to which midwifery can claim power to control its own functioning renders the title 'semi-profession' more appropriate (van Teijlingen and Hulst 1994). The high degree of occupational self-determination exerted by certain occupations enables them to regard themselves as 'classical' professions (Porter et al 2007). Porter and colleagues proceed to define the 'new' professions as those in which professional and client share control. Thus, it is the new professions to which midwives aspire, according to these researchers; the concept of shared control has certainly been espoused in some midwifery settings, as discussed in the material on partnership (see pages 14, 75, 105).

Debates about professional status have been dismissed on the grounds of their limited relevance to women's occupations (Davies 1990; Wilkins 2000), but they still attract serious consideration (Porter et al 2007; Sandall 1996). It is likely, however, that the debate has progressed from crude discussion of relative levels of occupational status. In her analysis of 'professional' developments, Jane Sandall shows how late twentieth-century midwives employed political strategies comparable with those used by midwifery pioneers at the time of the first midwifery legislation in England (Sandall 1996: 221). Such exclusionary tactics were initially employed to ensure a middle class, female occupation (Witz 1990). While exclusion by gender is no longer feasible, high educational standards, low domestic responsibilities and autonomous practice contribute to the current midwifery professionalisation project. The much sought-after professional status, though, is a mixed blessing. Although the perceived high status which being a profession carries is desirable, the paradoxical disciplinary control of members' behaviour and practice is distinctly less attractive (Abbott and Meerabeau 1998).

The complexity of the relationships between occupational groups in maternity was skirted by Jan Williams's analysis of controlling power in childbirth (Williams 1997). Although she identified a struggle between the childbearing woman and health professionals to exercise power, she barely mentioned any tensions between disciplines. Even less did she indicate any friction between individual members of discrete occupational groups. Williams exemplifies the widely-held view that what are all too often termed 'medical professionals' are part of one homogeneous occupation with shared aims and values. It is more likely, though, that relations between midwifery and medicine are vulnerable to some degree of conflict. As well as conflict existing between these two occupational groups, it also features within the groups, demonstrating the need to address here both *intra*occupational as well as *inter*occupational politics. Among midwives differences in woman-centredness have resulted in some being derided as 'with institution' (Hunter 2004: 266) rather than 'with woman', and the even more medically-oriented being ridiculed as 'medwives' (Davis-Floyd et al 2009). Among medical personnel, ideological differences between obstetricians at least contributed to Wendy Savage's suspension (see page 162). Clearly, these differences represent a continuum rather than a dichotomy, with overlapping ideals both shared by and distinguishing occupations and their sub-groups (Pitt 1997). Miranda Page (2010) explains this continuum in terms of it stretching between the medical model and the social/midwifery model of care and quotes from Raymond DeVries to illustrate the extent of these discrepancies:

> If we organized (sic) midwives along a continuum, with those who use all the tools of modern technology at one end and those who are non-technological in orientation at the other, those on the extreme ends of the continuum would not recognize each other as members of the same occupation.
>
> DeVries (1993: 132)

New occupational groups

It is generally accepted that the trappings of professional status appeal strongly to occupational groups. Claims to such status feature more among groups undergoing development, which is likely to be associated with the evolution of new knowledge and attitudes and the creation and application of new techniques. The search for a status which is perceived as being so desirable carries political implications for consumers as well as existing disciplines. To illustrate these implications, I scrutinise four examples of occupational groups seeking or undergoing professionalisation in maternity.

Maternity care assistant

Although known by various titles, such as maternity support worker (MSW), maternity care assistant (MCA), maternity health care assistant, health care assistant, auxiliary nurse or maternity aid (Hussain and Marshall 2011; Browne 2005; Jones and Jenkins 2004: 60; Davies 2009; van Teijlingen 1994; CNOs 2010), this occupational group is well-nigh ubiquitous.

Long-term UK position

Within living memory the UK midwife was required to follow a strict schedule of visits to a woman after a homebirth (CMB 1952: 105). Twice daily visits for three days and daily visits until at least day ten facilitated good support and early identification of problems. Now the homebirth rate is lower and hospital stays are shorter, so that each woman admitted to a postnatal ward has an infinitely greater need for care, support and education. At the same time, though, the widespread perception of a shortage of midwives means that women believe that midwives have insufficient time to attend to their psychosocial needs. While there have traditionally been auxiliary staff in maternity units to assist generally with 'hospitality' and cleanliness, a new breed of staff member is being introduced to solve the shortage of and pressure on midwives by supporting midwifery practice (RCM 2009). The introduction of support staff resonates strongly with the situation in other countries, for which reason the international picture now deserves attention.

International comparisons

The duration of hospital stay for the woman giving birth in hospital varies markedly between countries, due largely to the method of financing health care. In 2009 in an insurance-financed healthcare system such as Switzerland, the average postnatal stay (5.9 days) was almost three times longer than in the tax-based Icelandic NHS (2.2 days) (OECD 2009). The benefits of the hospital stay are affected by whether there is any follow up in the form of home visits after discharge and by what category of staff. In the United Kingdom in 2003 women who had had a spontaneous birth in hospital spent on average 1 day in hospital postnatally; following instrumental births and caesareans the stay was 1 or 2 days and 3 or 4 days respectively (DoH 2007a). The decreasing hospital stay means that community midwives provide care for larger numbers of women at an earlier postnatal stage. Thus, UK community midwives also experience a more demanding work load, but staffing may not be increased proportionately.

Dutch situation

The organisation of maternity care in the Netherlands is often viewed with rose-tinted spectacles by those unfamiliar with the issues, resulting in recommendations for imitation (Wiegers 2006; Mearns 2009). The reality of transferring such a system from one culture to another would be infinitely, if not impossibly, complex (van Teijlingen 1990; Mander 1995). As Edwin van Teijlingen reports, the system is prized by Dutch bureaucrats because costs are lower than neighbouring states' (van Teijlingen 1994). He explains that the Dutch maternity home care assistant (MHCA) provides most postnatal care as well as some childcare and housework. This popular arrangement means that the new mother has relatively intensive support when most needed. Additionally, the midwife is free to increase her income by attending more births. Thus the maternity home care assistant raises the midwife's status by allowing her greater professional autonomy.

My own observation is that the Dutch midwife most often considers herself a 'medical' practitioner. This is a title to which few other European midwives would wish to lay claim, leading to suspicions that the Dutch midwife is a decidedly different being from her European namesakes, as she is an entrepreneur with high social status. Part of this status derives from, although the Dutch midwife attends and carries responsibility for the birth, the MCHA providing much hands-on intrapartum and postnatal care. The obvious interpretation is that it is the maternity home care assistant who is genuinely 'with women' and who is more comparable, in practice terms, with the UK midwife.

Thus, as well as the Dutch system of maternity care not being comparable in the sense of transferability, the roles of the major care providers appear to bear no comparison either. A vital debate is developing about this amongst Dutch midwives as they endeavour to adjust to changing pressures and the fact that home birth is losing ground (Visser 2012; De Jonge 2012).

The United Kingdom – a developing picture

The 'knock-on' effect of the European Working Time Directive (EWTD, DoH 1998) has resulted in reallocation of tasks in the maternity area (Hussain and Marshall 2011). Because midwives have been required to substitute for junior medical staff, more health care assistants have been employed to take over tasks previously considered the midwife's province. Reports of the education of this new grade of assistant seek to reassure about the adequacy of her preparation, while simultaneously avoiding raising any concerns about threats to the midwife's role.

In Wales the 'maternity care assistant' represents a contributor to quality maternity care (Davies 2009). Such a statement *per se* is relatively benign; but claims that the MCA plays a part in addressing media criticisms of 'midwife shortages' (Davies 2009: 20) is more disconcerting.

In Scotland the education of the 'maternity care assistant' (Rennie et al 2009) is also said to produce a practitioner who will impact positively on the quality of care. Without explaining how, these authors go on to assert that this new occupational group will benefit the retention of midwives in midwifery practice (Rennie et al 2009: 19). Protestations, though, that 'MCAs are here to stay' and 'midwives need to embrace them' (Rennie et al 2009: 19) imply that MCAs' acceptance is incomplete.

The future – a word to the wise

Reports of innovative programmes to prepare MCAs go to considerable lengths to reassure that the MCA will only work under a midwife's supervision and undertake only delegated tasks (Hussain and Marshall 2011; Rennie et al 2009). Although such guidance sounds simple, Catriona Hussain and Jayne Marshall report confusion about the precise nature of the MCA's roles. Such confusion, these authors maintain, raises concerns about further erosion of the midwife's role and whether she is able to remain accountable for fulfilling her statutory responsibilities. Hussain and Marshall post a timely warning to midwives of their need to 'be advocates for the midwifery profession by questioning current practice and challenging new developments in the workplace' (Hussain and Marshall 2011: 340). Thus, the welcome extended to the MCA clearly arouses anxiety about the politics of professional relationships among other midwives.

Obstetric anaesthetist

Now an all too familiar presence in the birthing room, the political implications of the obstetric anaesthetist's creation and professionalisation deserve attention.

Origins

Those of us with long memories recall the days before the advent of the obstetric anaesthetist. Then, if a woman needed an emergency anaesthetic, for example for a surgical birth or manual removal of the placenta, the duty anaesthetist, known as the 'gasman' (Barter 2011: 39), from the general hospital operating theatres was called to administer general anaesthesia (GA). In the late twentieth century, though, the introduction, acceptance and ubiquitous availability of epidural analgesia and anaesthesia changed maternity care utterly. Simultaneously the obstetric anaesthetist became established.

When first introduced, epidural analgesia in labour was used to provide effective pain control in well-defined potentially pathological situations, such as a woman with incoordinate uterine action or dystocia (Moir 1973). The cataclysmic change in the use of epidural *analgesia* occurred when its potential to become epidural *anaesthesia* was realised; this followed the recognition of the abysmal contribution of GA to maternal mortality (Morgan 1987). While the *number* of maternal deaths associated with or due to anaesthesia peaked between 1964 and 1969 (during which time period there were 100 such deaths), of greater significance was the escalating *proportion* of such maternal deaths. In spite of the birth rate rising in the late 1960s, maternal deaths attributable to haemorrhage and abortion fell significantly. But while the number and proportion of maternal deaths due to other causes was declining, the proportion of direct maternal deaths due to anaesthesia approximately quadrupled, from a stable level of about 3 per cent between 1952 and 1963, to 13 per cent between 1982 and 1984 (Cloake 1991).

The majority of maternal deaths associated with or due to anaesthesia were attributed to the regurgitation and aspiration of acid stomach contents into the mother's respiratory tract (Mendelson's syndrome) during the intrapartum induction of GA (Morgan 1987). Epidural analgesia gained acceptance in obstetrics when the contribution of anaesthesia to maternal mortality was greatest by eliminating the need for this hazardous induction (Doughty 1987). Thus, the increasing acceptance of epidural analgesia happened most opportunely, and enabled anaesthetists in obstetrics to gain, initially, approval of their practice. Later professional credibility for obstetric anaesthetists was sought. Originally regarded as merely relieving labour pain, epidural analgesia eventually, through removing the need for GA, reduced anaesthesia-related maternal deaths. Favourable experiences with women with epidurals soon convinced obstetricians that intervention in labour could be conveniently and relatively safely managed using epidural analgesia to reduce pain and then, when it almost inevitably became necessary, to remove sensation. The mother's acceptance of epidurals was probably equally willing, having been 'fostered directly or indirectly by the professionals' (Hibbard and Scott 1990), resulting in anaesthetic services developing into a growth industry. Sheila Kitzinger, though, endorsed these anaesthetists' comments by arguing that encouragement to take advantage of epidural services was perceived by some mothers as 'coercion' (Kitzinger 1987). Such attitude change persists, with examples of recommendations of 'marketing' in the writing of John Crowhurst and Felicity Plaat (2000: 165).

Professionalisation

The classical process of professionalisation, by which an occupational group detaches itself from a majority occupation or profession, is clearly apparent in the obstetric anaesthetist's break from general medicine. The essential characteristics of an occupational group aspiring to professional status begin with prolonged and specialised training to become a professional (Carr-Saunders and Wilson 1933), clearly relevant in the present context. Probably even more relevant is Alexander Carr-Saunders and Paul Wilson's account of the acquisition of expertise in a specific 'technique' over which the occupation has a monopoly during this training. For the obstetric anaesthetist this unique selling point (USP) is the siting of an epidural catheter.

A further essential characteristic of an occupational group striving for professional status is the need for a relevant association; which serves to promote both the interests of its individual members and the profession as a whole, and possibly to enforce standards. In the present example this body is the Obstetric

Anaesthetists' Association (OAA) which came into being in 1969 with the aims of providing:

- the highest standards of anaesthetic practice in the care of mother and baby;
- education and training for anaesthetists and other practitioners in the United Kingdom and overseas;
- a resource for women seeking information about pain relief in labour and anaesthesia for Caesarean section (sic).

(OAA 2011)

To Carr-Saunders and Wilson's list of criteria, Andrew Abbott adds the development of a professional culture, including professional trappings; examples are a logo, journal, annual conference and identifiable clothing, such as neck ties (Abbott 1988). Abbott also mentions the need for ethical codes and jurisdiction as indicators of having achieved professional status.

Issues of professionalisation

The extent to which obstetric anaesthetists' professionalisation has progressed and its political implications for other disciplines has become apparent.

INVOLVEMENT DURING PREGNANCY

As mentioned already, it has been argued that professional status is closely allied to the assumption of power by the relevant occupational group. A very pertinent example of this is obstetric anaesthetists, having secured a foothold in the birthing room, seeking to extend their role forward into the pre/antenatal period. Clearly, such a role would present opportunities to increase their share of the 'market' during labour.

It is widely accepted that it is appropriate for the anaesthetist to consult during pregnancy with those women with long-term health problems, eg diabetes mellitus, who may need intrapartum anaesthetic services (Plaat and Wray 2008). The contribution of obstetric anaesthetists to childbirth education for 'low risk' women, however, is very different. This antenatal involvement has been reported as extending to teaching about labour pain, pain control and epidural analgesia. To facilitate teaching, anaesthetists prepare educational resource materials and presentations using a variety of media (du Plessis and Johnstone 2007; Paech 1999). The involvement of anaesthetists in childbirth education has reached the point of approximately half of maternity units in the United States offering classes by them (Saunders et al 2006). These authors urge that obstetric anaesthetists 'should be more proactive about educating pregnant women' (Saunders et al 2006: 102). Countless questions arise from the involvement of obstetric anaesthetists in healthy childbirth education, such as:

- How was the decision made for what is effectively a sales pitch to be provided?
- How did childbirth educators allow their role to be usurped?
- How is the balance, in terms of research on woman-centredness, of anaesthetists' material monitored?

This last question is crucial because anaesthetists can hardly be expected *not* to take advantage of such a golden opportunity to endorse their own USP. Such an expectation would be naïve, especially when there are examples of anaesthetists taking full advantage of marketing opportunities for such endorsement. One such example is found in the materials in the OAA website, where a booklet on 'Pain Relief in Labour' offers seven pages of epidural-related material, while all other methods are collectively addressed in merely four pages.

INFORMATION-GIVING

It may not be surprising that the information provided for childbearing women by obstetric anaesthetists is less than well-balanced. This imbalance reflects, according to Ulla Waldenström, the vast research literature on epidural techniques, which inexplicably disregards the experience of the childbearing woman receiving the epidural (Waldenström 2007).

Simultaneously, there is little data about women's limited knowledge of epidural analgesia and its side-effects, as I have often found when informing women seeking epidural analgesia that an intravenous infusion is necessary. It was down to a US study, by Eugene Declercq and his colleagues, to identify that, although an overwhelming majority (75 per cent) of women knew of the *effectiveness* of epidural analgesia, only a small minority (26 to 41 per cent) were aware of any side-effects (Declercq et al 2002: 22). It is disappointing, but unsurprising, that obstetric anaesthetists' partial information-giving results in such a deficit in crucial understanding among clients.

DRUG ADMINISTRATION ERRORS

I have mentioned above that the acceptance of regional analgesia originated in the appalling mortality rates resulting from GA. Paradoxically, this original *raison d'être* may be manifesting itself again. Perhaps victims of their own success, over-familiarity with regional anaesthetic medications may have led to relaxed practices resulting in maternal death (Jones et al 2008).

OBSTETRIC ANAESTHESIA AND MATERNAL DEATH

As well as the dismal prospect of maternal deaths being attributable to drug errors, obstetric anaesthetists continue to feature in Confidential Enquiry reports for other reasons. Anaesthesia is currently a factor in approximately half of maternal deaths (McClure and Cooper 2011).

PREDISPOSING FACTORS

The death of a mother in association with anaesthesia is likely to be blamed, at least partly, on her obesity (McClure and Cooper 2011: 105). According to Mark Stacey, obesity causes death by impeding ventilation (Stacey 2007: 19). Such technical difficulties have been shown to lead to tragedies, sometimes disconcertingly ascribed to the anaesthetist's 'trainee' status (McClure and Cooper 2011: 105).

WORKLOAD AND STAFFING

Limited experience may lead to blame by other disciplines, as in the death of a woman due to failure to secure endotracheal intubation (McClure and Cooper 2011: 103), which was blamed on an 'inexperienced anaesthetist' by an Emergency Department specialist (Hulbert 2011). The implications of an anaesthetic service being provided by trainees, or anyone not fully proficient, does not bear thinking about. While it is clear that trainee anaesthetists need sufficient experience and 'hours of work' to make them competent in an area as challenging as obstetric anaesthesia, ensuring suitable supervision raises staffing problems.

Additionally, the high demand which has been created for anaesthetic services clearly causes concerns about safety. This happens when midwifery, obstetric and anaesthetic personnel are already fully committed at peaks of activity in the normal workload. Difficulties arise if a woman with an acute, severe illness is admitted and requires high-dependency care. When staffing is calculated on the basis of *average* activity, there needs to be well thought through contingency planning for all disciplines to guarantee further skilled assistance in such circumstances (McClure and Cooper 2011: 108).

NON-INVOLVEMENT OF OBSTETRIC ANAESTHETISTS

The professionalisation of obstetric anaesthetists has been examined largely from the viewpoint of women and non-medical disciplines. Their acceptance, however, by other medical practitioners may leave something to be desired. The result is the anaesthetist demanding to be involved with seriously ill women at an earlier stage:

> the assessors considered that senior advice or assistance from an anaesthetic or critical-care specialist was requested too late.
>
> (McClure and Cooper 2011: 105)

A not dissimilar plea has been made for the earlier recognition by managers of the potentially beneficial contribution of obstetric anaesthetists to hospital enquiries relating to maternal deaths and 'near misses':

> These reports are still of variable quality and clearly completed in-house and therefore open to bias. Hospital managers are again asked to consider

whether unbiased external input would assist in this process and ensure greater objectivity.

(McClure and Cooper 2011: 108)

PATRIARCHY AND PATERNALISM

Paternalistic approaches to consumers of care in the maternity area are still found among obstetric anaesthetists. While the 'patient' has generally largely been replaced by the 'woman' or 'mother', she still re-emerges occasionally, demonstrating persisting underlying patriarchal attitudes. The Confidential Enquiries have managed to dispense with the 'patient' but the obstetric anaesthetists still refer to the 'obstetric patient' (eg McClure and Cooper 2011: 104). Similarly, Hanlie du Plessis and Chris Johnstone in what ought to be a forward-thinking paper on ethical and medico-legal issues, insist that the maternity consumer is still a patient (du Plessis and Johnstone 2007). An equally anachronistic paternalistic approach is found in these authors' recommendation of the need for 'reassuring patients' about safety issues. It is no surprise that woman-centred information-giving is so seriously neglected when patriarchy is clearly alive and well among those offering obstetric analgesia and anaesthesia.

Doula

The title 'doula' is a term whose origins are shrouded in mists of myth. Its original meaning has been revisited and revised *ad nauseam*. With each revision the meaning has moved further from the original 'female slave' and closer to the current 'labour supporter' (Mander 2001: 113–14). In examining the doula literature, the reader soon realises that the modern doula's North American origins serve to confound rather than illuminate. The literature relies heavily, for endorsement of the doula, on the RCTs on psychosocial support in labour. When an author states 'Subsequent research found that women who had labour support by doulas … ' (Gilliland 2002: 763), it is clear that she has not actually read the material. This is because the labour support RCTs focus on a mixed bag of supporters, with few approximating to the doula as she currently presents (Mander 2001: 102).

The entrance of the doula into the birthing room raises issues which are politically sensitive, particularly for occupational groups already practising in maternity.

Professional status

The professional status of new arrivals on the birthing scene has been a recurring theme thus far and is of no less significance in the doula's case. Writing as a 'disenchanted' midwife who has become a very vocal and admirably articulate doula, Adela Stockton emphasises the reasons why it is not in the doula's interests to seek professionalisation (Stockton 2010a: 28).

Stockton's argument states, first, the irrelevance and possible disadvantages of the doula's professionalisation. This argument is based on the benefits to all of the doula being an unqualified or lay practitioner with whom the woman can identify (Stockton 2010b). Stockton's statement contrasts with the findings of a Swedish study in a health system ordinarily comparable with the United Kingdom's (Lundgren 2010). In her qualitative research project, Ingela Lundgren identified the doula as occupying a betwixt and between position which, I suggest, resonates with the concept of semi-professions (Etzioni 1969). The childbearing women who were interviewed were unable to accept the doula's lay status due to their contact with the doula being strictly scheduled. Additionally, the doula was reported to possess far more specialist knowledge than any lay person possibly could. Thus, Lundgren considers that the doula inhabits a 'borderland' (2008: 178) between non-interventive and professional care. In this study the midwife's engagement with the woman in labour was disappointing – to the extent of the midwife being described as 'distant' (Lundgren 2010: 178). The reason for this unfortunate assessment of the midwife deserves attention and it is necessary to question how it happened. On the one hand, it is possible that the doula's presence may have impeded the midwife's ability to form a supportive relationship with the woman. On the other hand, it may be that it was the system of care, which involved each midwife caring for a number of women in labour, that prevented engagement (Lundgren 2010: 174). Thus it may be the case that the role and acceptance of the doula is a reflection, not simply of the needs of the childbearing woman, but of a healthcare system which has ceased to be 'woman-friendly'. That such a situation also pertains in the United Kingdom has been suggested elsewhere (Mander 2001: 169; Chakladar 2009).

The differences in healthcare systems affecting acceptance of the doula was the second strand of Stockton's anti-professionalisation argument (Stockton 2010a: 28). In what is, effectively, a tirade against the US doula, Stockton condemns the professionalisation of the North American doula. She links this changed status with a role which has become very different from the UK equivalent, in that the North American doula undertakes clinical interventions, eg vaginal examination, which would be the province of the UK midwife or medical practitioner. This transatlantic difference may be due to the scarcity of midwives in the United States, where most intrapartum care is by LDR (labor/delivery room) nurses (Mander 1997) with the OB/GYN attending the birth. Thus exporting the US model of disempowering the midwife and supplanting her with a doula, may explain Lundgren's Swedish findings.

Organisational issues

Having considered the implications of the environment or healthcare system for the professional status of the doula, we should examine the developments within the doula industry to advance her status. Just as the obstetric anaesthetist, in the early days of his professionalisation, needed an association (page 43), the doula has become similarly organised. Doulas of North America International (DONA 2011) was founded in 1992, followed in 2001 by Doula UK (DUK 2011). As well as establishing a website, a philosophy and a code of conduct, these organisations offer a complaints procedure and assistance with locating a doula. Doula UK requires any would-be members to go through a 'Recognition Process' and to have completed an approved preparation course. While not explicitly necessary for 'Recognition', both aspects involve educational standards.

Analysing the position of the doula, Stockton is wary of the educational opportunities available to, even required of, the UK doula. Her caution is partly due to concerns about who will do the teaching and, consequently, what will be taught. Her concerns imply that the student doula will be taught by midwifery and medical personnel, resulting in a doula poorly-differentiated from midwives and hospital medical staff. Stockton's wariness is also associated with the effect of such education on the occupational development or pro-fessionalisation of the doula. To Stockton the spectre looms of a higher grade of doula with academic qualifications, casting doubt on and belittling the practice of less well-educated doulas. The educational programmes to which Stockton refers include those accredited by 'Middlesex University In London' (sic; Doula Consultancy 2011); also included would be the programme for the 'maternity support therapist' (Holistic Community 2011).

Just as the doula's education raises concerns, so does her regulation. The doula may have observed the repercussions of statutory regulation on, particularly, the independent midwife and become wary (see Chapter 7). While statutory regulation might advance the doula's professional status, it would simulta-neously reduce the significance of her USPs, such as her individuality and independence from the healthcare system.

Tensions

In view of the discussion up to this point, it is not surprising that some conflicts have arisen from the doula's arrival in the birthing room. The implications of these conflicts, particularly for other maternity practitioners, make them highly political.

FINANCIAL COSTS

The discussion around the costs of a doula all too often focuses on the ability of the childbearing woman/couple to pay her fee. This may be interpreted as meaning that the less affluent may be unable to afford her services. The question of costs, though, is less straightforward, as we should consider the costs *to whom?*

Doula costs are linked to her education. While the costs of the three-year midwifery programmes common to European Union countries are, in the United Kingdom, largely state funded, doula programmes are self-funded. Such programmes are, however, invariably shorter.

After her education, the costs of employing a doula fall largely on the childbearing woman/couple, unless the doula works on a voluntary basis (Stockton 2012). This contrasts with the midwife who, in the United Kingdom, is ordinarily an NHS employee. Thus, a doula represents no financial outlay for the NHS. However, were the doula to become an NHS employee, as she is employed by maternity units in some countries, her employment costs would be lower (Stockton 2010a: 39), due to her shorter education and more limited role.

CONTINUITY

A further aspect of the doula's practice, which is likely to be one of her main selling points, is her continuity of attendance. This continuity is rarely available to the NHS-employed midwife. The relationship between the birth doula and the woman begins during the final trimester of pregnancy; it involves a one-to-one rapport (Stockton 2010a: 40), which extends through labour, birth and beyond. The doula remains with the woman for her labour, irrespective of its duration or complexity. Unlike most midwives, the doula is invulnerable to shift changes or, due to managerial expediency, needing to attend more than one woman in labour (Lundgren 2010).

RELATIONSHIPS WITH OTHER PERSONNEL

Working relationships between the doula and staff in the birthing room have attracted considerable attention because of the potential for territorial conflict. It is unfortunate that much of this attention has featured the North American situation where the role of the LDR nurse differs from that of the UK midwife. Writing as a doula, Amy Gilliland explains the role of the LDR nurse as fundamentally technical, comprising clinical assessments and administrative responsibilities (Gilliland 2002: 764). Perhaps appropriately, Gilliland refers to North American research showing the limited contact during labour between the nurse and the childbearing women and, hence, the restricted emotional support which the nurse offers. Gilliland discusses the conflict which sometimes develops between the nurse and the doula due to the doula's 'challenging' (Gilliland 2002: 765) behaviour or the nurse's frustration that she is prevented, by the system, from providing the doula's standard of care (Stevens et al 2011). The Australian situation, where midwives report conflict due to the doula practising outwith her role (Stevens et al 2011: 510), resonates strongly with that in North America. Ballen and Fulcher's report, that nurses perceive that the doula tries to 'run the labour' (Ballen and Fulcher 2006: 308), endorses the Australian findings, summarising the potential for inter-professional conflict as down to 'territorialism and turf' (Ballen and Fulcher 2006: 308).

A NOT UNCOMMON FINDING

Disconcerting findings arose out of a focus group study examining midwives' and doulas' perceptions of the Australian doula role (Stevens et al 2011).

These researchers identified a 'broken' system of maternity care (Stevens et al 2011: 512), the details of which resonate powerfully with the UK situation. While Jeni Stevens and her colleagues identify a number of potential 'flash points' between the midwife and doula, their conclusion is surprisingly, perhaps inconsistently, positive. They suggest that better collaboration, to benefit the childbearing woman, is the answer to these systematic and situational problems.

For these researchers and other observers of the functioning of the doula, her contribution has not been entirely welcomed. Her presence has been perceived more as being a necessity to improve the functioning of a failing or 'broken' system of maternity care in the interests of the childbearing woman (Akhavan and Lundgren 2012; Stevens et al 2011; Stockton 2010a: 50; Chakladar 2009). Such a solution, I venture to suggest, compares with applying a sticking plaster to control a haemorrhage.

Consultant midwife

Since the closing years of the twentieth century, the consultant midwife has featured prominently in publications and presentations. The basis of this high profile, though, is not entirely clear. Her sudden prominence and uncertain credentials mean that her position in childbearing politics deserves scrutiny.

Origins

Midwife consultant posts, along with equivalents for nurses and health visitors, were established throughout the United Kingdom in 2000. Their initial *raison d'être* was to kick-start progress for patient outcomes, with associated benefits for practitioners:

> Establishing nurse, midwife and health visitor consultant posts is intended to help provide better outcomes for patients by improving services and quality, to strengthen leadership and to provide a new career opportunity to help retain experienced and expert nurses, midwives and health visitors in practice.
>
> (DoH 1999: 5)

These lofty ideals were intended to be achieved through senior personnel becoming expert practitioners, rather than assuming purely managerial roles. In this way, the post-holders would exhibit leadership and act as consultants to other grades, while also initiating staff and service developments. The circular announcing these posts sought to emphasise that this multiplicity of functions would be integral and integrated, rather than discrete (DoH 1999: 6).

The initial focus on the aims, though, soon changed to give more attention to the means by which the consultant midwife would achieve them. Thus, the 'leadership' panacea came to feature alongside the inevitable management jargon:

> The term consultant midwife is the one which has replaced that of clinical midwife lead and more accurately fulfils the clinical leadership role without managerial responsibilities. The role provides clinical leadership in conjunction with the lead consultant obstetrician and complements the role of head of midwifery. Consultant midwives contribute to effective leadership, training and mentoring, as well as having specific responsibilities such as promoting normal childbirth or reducing inequalities. Consultant midwives are able to drive service improvement through working with colleagues in health and other agencies to develop effective care pathways or specific services for specific client groups.
>
> (DoH 2007b: 43)

Reception of the consultant midwife

Despite their overwhelmingly positive welcome by the midwifery media (Rogers and Weavers 2005; Rogers and Cunningham 2007; Dunkley-Bent 2004; Cooke 2004), some disquiet has emerged, as articulated to the Select Committee on Health (2003):

> Since the development of the consultant midwife role (2000) there have been a significant number of such posts advertised, a number of which remain unfilled. The reason for this is multifactorial but one issue is the lack of preparation for the role.

Thus, the consultant midwife's warm reception was not well-supported with a secure educational infrastructure. A similar observation emerged out of another infrastructural shortcoming. More support being needed for nurse consultants was one of the findings of a nursing research project (McIntosh and Tolson 2009), which lacks any midwifery equivalent. While there is no shortage of authoritative generic research projects focusing on the consultant practitioner (Coster et al 2006; Sidebotham 2001; Booth et al 2006), research into the unique situation of the consultant midwife is notable by its absence. Thus, unlike her nursing equivalent, the evidence base about what the consultant midwife does and does not do is weak, meaning that her effectiveness remains uncertain.

Leadership

The birth of the consultant practitioner, as mentioned above, was heralded with a powerful remit to adopt the leadership role (DoH 1999: 5; DoH 2007b: 43), which has long been sought in the 'caring professions' (Burdett Trust 2006). The need for a role to be introduced to provide such leadership reflects disappointingly on the functioning of managers in these occupational groups. If the twin concepts of leadership and management are not actually synonymous, being a leader has long been a crucial aspect of the manager's role (Drucker 1974: 325).

The widespread perception of a need for more and better leadership in health care is discussed by McIntosh and Tolson (2009) in their preparation for a qualitative study of the nurse consultant's leadership role. These researchers identified some degree of confusion about what the leadership component of this role comprised. For example, activities described by some respondents as leadership morphed into service development for others. Some consistency, however, was identified in the nurse consultants' enthusiasm to employ trans-formational leadership, in preference to the more traditional and hierarchical transactional leadership. McIntosh and Tolson, not unlike the evidence to the Select Committee mentioned above, regret the lack of infrastructural support for consultant nurses in demonstrating leadership, which is highly demanding in personal terms.

A *déjà vu* feeling of 'mission creep' arises with the extension of the consultant nurses' leadership role into other related areas. While attempting culture change by the consultant midwife is appropriate in the form of a new approach to antenatal care (Rogers and Cunningham 2007), seeking to change the health service culture is a very different matter. The requirement to change the local NHS culture to one of research activity and evidence-based practice (Chummun and Tiran 2008) may be the last straw for what is already an over-burdened role.

Role

On the basis of this analysis it appears that, when introduced, the consultant role was sufficiently ill-defined to allow a range of personnel to anticipate the possibility of off-loading unwanted aspects of their work on to this newly-created individual. As has been shown by what little research there has been, this off-loading has further problematised a particularly challenging role, which from the outset featured a distinct deficit in infrastructural support.

Learning from new occupational groups

This analysis of the arrival of these four occupational or professional groups on the maternity stage shows that their advancement stems from different sources. Whereas the doula and obstetric anaesthetist appear to be keen to present themselves and their activities as the, possibly complementary, answer to the childbearing woman's needs, the MCA and the consultant midwife seem to be being shoe-horned into their new roles with varying degrees of preparation and support. This analysis has shown, however, that the arrival of these practitioners has wide-ranging implications for pre-existing occupational groups. Some of these implications are largely positive whereas others, more disconcertingly, benefit one participant at the expense of another. If members of staff are thus disadvantaged, it is necessary to contemplate the implications for the childbearing woman and her baby.

Strategies

As well as the introduction into maternity of new occupational and professional groups, together with their characteristic agendas, certain strategies have been espoused by more established disciplines, with repercussions for others. The espousal of these strategies, and their repercussions, amounts to political activity.

Medicalisation of childbearing

Medicalisation is another of those terms often used unthinkingly, thus discrediting its significance as a 'process of social change' (van Teijlingen 2005). With the medical model forming part of a theoretical framework, medicalisation may be seen to operate differently at conceptual, institutional and clinical levels (Conrad and Schneider 1980). Adopting a sociological orientation, Wendy Christiaens and Edwin van Teijlingen have teased out the development of the meanings of medicalisation and applied them to childbearing (Christiaens and van Teijlingen 2009). The term's original use in the 1960s is associated, first, with Eliot Freidson's early work on the sociology of the professions and, later, with Ivan Illich's work on iatrogenesis (Freidson 1970). Christiaens and van Teijlingen trace the meaning of medicalisation from the widespread application of medical terminology to good health, through the ensuing increasing medical influence over human life to the potential for harm resulting from medical involvement. These authors consider that medicalisation's most recent meaning reflects the problematisation of healthy life events, such as childbearing and the menopause. According to Christiaens and van Teijlingen, this process has enhanced medical status by generating a market of consumers dependent on medical expertise.

Medicalisation of birth has been defined in terms of 'medical intervention' during childbearing (Cairoli 2010), but such a limited definition is unnecessarily restrictive. Continuing his sociological orientation, Edwin van Teijlingen regards medicalisation of birth as operating in different ways at technological, conceptual, interactional, controlling and gender status levels (Lowis and McCaffery 1999). At the interactional level in clinical practice, medicalisation indicates the change in the culture of childbearing from a domestic and social phenomenon to a potentially pathological event.

While Cairoli has attributed it to the hospitalisation of birth (Cairoli 2010), medicalisation of childbirth actually predated the move of physiological childbearing into hospital by approximately three centuries (Mander 2004). The link with hospital birth, though, cannot be ignored in a UK context; the changing place of birth certainly accelerated medicalisation, by providing medical practitioners with a 'captive population' for the epidemic of interventions into physiological childbearing which ensued.

As well as the more obviously medical interventions, such as induction of labour, birth assisted with forceps and caesarean, medicalisation has brought a range of other interventions, which have become so ubiquitous as to verge on being regarded as 'normal'. These interventions, which are often considered 'routine', include the partograph, continuous electronic foetal monitoring, regional analgesia, augmentation/acceleration of labour, dorsal position for labour/birth, episiotomy and third stage oxytocics (Johanson et al 2002).

Active management of labour

The level of medicalisation mentioned above has reached its virtually 'routine' status due to the widespread acceptance and implementation of the plethora of interventions collectively known as 'active management of labour' (AML). Active management needs to be differentiated from active birth and was the brainchild of a series of 'Masters' of the National Maternity Hospital in Dublin, Ireland (O'Driscoll et al 1973). The original rationale was said to be the Masters' pity for the suffering of women enduring prolonged labour (O'Driscoll and Meagher 1980); a country with limited health resources struggling to cope with a disconcertingly high birth rate or 'throughput' has been suggested as another possible reason (Murphy-Lawless 2011c: 448).

Active management is characterised first and foremost by close monitoring of the progress of the woman's labour by frequent, ie up to quarter-hourly, vaginal examinations recorded on the partogram. Such monitoring is inevitably associated with more active intervention, such as the onset of labour being diagnosed only by vaginal examination, at which point artificial rupture of membranes is advocated. If the rate of cervical dilatation then drops below one centimetre per hour or fails to stay above the 'action line' on the partograph, further intervention becomes obligatory, in the form of an intravenous infusion of oxytocin (Bohra et al 2003).

The Dublin 'dogma' presents a picture of a form of intrapartum management which verges on 'military efficiency' (O'Driscoll and Meagher 1980: 89). One much-praised feature of active management is the continuous 'support' for the woman in labour, which sounds ideal until it is realised that it is often by an unqualified learner, such as a nursing or medical student.

While originally alleged to reduce the duration of women's suffering, active management has serendipitously been credited with reducing the number of caesareans. This has further increased its attraction to other cash-strapped healthcare systems under threat from escalating caesarean rates. A systematic review, though, provides surprisingly feeble endorsement of this beneficial effect (Brown et al 2008).

Just as the spectre of the Dublin dogma seemed to be receding and common sense was at risk of breaking out, the baton of O'Driscoll and colleagues' ideology appears to have been taken up by other, most unlikely, torch-bearers (Montagu 2009). Paul Reuwer and his colleagues in the Netherlands have entered the active management affray with a veritable fusillade of pseudo-physiology

(Reuwer et al 2009). These authors endeavour to persuade the reader of their woman-friendly credentials and their enthusiasm to ensure good understanding and support of physiological labour. This recognition of physiological labour, though, together with prophylactic intervention to make certain that labour remains physiological, resonates powerfully with the Dublin dogma with which we are all too familiar.

While recognising the parasympathetic control of physiological labour (Reuwer et al 2009: 56), Reuwer and his colleagues claim that such endocrine activity is facilitated by the recommended continuous one-to-one support. Despite this recognition, though, they steadfastly require O'Driscoll's intensive monitoring of progress by frequent vaginal examination. Such discomforting and anxiety-provoking monitoring is hardly likely to facilitate effective parasympathetic functioning.

Particularly surprising is these authors' insistence on pregnancy not being permitted to extend beyond 42 weeks. Despite the well-known poor outcomes of induction of labour before the woman's body is ready to give birth, Reuwer and his colleagues impose an absolute veto on pregnancy lasting beyond that long-revered date (Reuwer et al 2009: 206).

This dominance of the calendar is matched by the dominance of an unholy alliance between the partogram and the clock. Just as the Dublin masters did over 30 years earlier, Reuwer and his colleagues choose to ignore that physiological labour does not invariably progress at a steady and predetermined rate. Both groups of authors require intervention with oxytocic drugs in the event of cervical dilatation not maintaining the fallacious line first drawn up, on the basis of seriously questionable data, by Friedmann in 1954.

The condescendingly patriarchal approach which pervaded the Dublin dogma is also alive and well in its Dutch successor. O'Driscoll originally demanded constant eye contact between the childbearing woman and the support person in order to control the woman's behaviour. As previously, Reuwer and his colleagues decline to credit the childbearing woman with sufficient intelligence to recognise the onset of her own labour. For this reason, irrespective of the nature and duration of the woman's labour prior to her first vaginal examination, her labour is deemed only to have started *after* that assessment. Thus, despite rhetoric about childbirth being 'empowering and ultimately satisfying' (Reuwer et al 2009: 11), what emerges are the usual paternalistic assumptions and women being fobbed off with platitudinous promises of time-limited labours.

Evidence-based practice

The virtually ubiquitous acceptance, and subsequent imposition, of evidence-based practice (EBP) arose out of Archie Cochrane's observation of the lack of scientific rigour in medical clinical decision-making (Cochrane 1972). He went on to single out obstetricians for merciless criticism for their want of such rigour. The knee-jerk response among obstetricians was to put their house in order, a task which was undertaken with the fervour of converts under the leadership of Iain

Chalmers (Chalmers et al 1989). By the time a reasonable definition of EBP was forthcoming (Sackett et al 1996), that fervour had cooled. But during this 'cooling-off period' concerns had begun to be articulated about the relevance of RCT-based evidence to the care decisions made by, for example, midwives (Page 1996; Clarke 1999). Such criticism peaked with the possibility of EBP constituting a threat to midwifery through its inherent medicalisation agenda (Bogdan-Lovis and Sousa 2006). The relevance of EBP to midwifery continues to be questioned, in view of the need for the active participation of the child-bearing woman in any decisions (Munro and Spiby 2010). That evidence which is RCT-based may be less than appropriate to midwifery practice has also cast doubt on the EBP agenda (McCourt 2005).

These concerns about the questionable relevance of EBP to midwifery have raised the possibility of a more woman-friendly version (Wickham 1999). This compromise position, known as evidence-informed practice (EIP), seeks to take advantage of the strengths of EBP while avoiding dogma. Interventions based only on superstition or prejudice are excluded, but the judgement and knowledge of the midwife practitioner and the childbearing woman form an equal triad with research-based evidence (Nevo and Slonim-Nevo 2011). The dynamic relationship between the woman and the midwife is clearly crucial in EIP, and the dialogue into which they enter when care is accessed and provided becomes constructively transparent.

The pressure on midwives to adhere to the EBP agenda has been profound and enduring, as shown by the early efforts by medical practitioners to direct midwives along the EBP route. Such direction carried with it an element of medical hypocrisy in the form of 'do as I say, not as I do', an example of which would be continuing medical reliance on routine ultrasound in pregnancy (Bricker et al 2008). Direction of midwives towards EBP came from authorities such as Iain Chalmers in his requirement that midwives use only 'strong research' (Chalmers 1993: 3). If the introduction of EBP bears comparison with evangelical movements (Traynor 2002), it would appear that Chalmers has undergone a Damascean conversion to reach his recent recommendation of evidence-informed practice (Chalmers 2005).

Systems

The processes and interventions which I have addressed in this section are clearly political in their consequences for others, such as midwives and childbearing women. While such strategies are operationalised by individuals, it is the *systems* of healthcare which allow and perhaps encourage these individuals to take advantage of the position in which they find themselves. In this way, influence to the detriment of others is able to be exerted.

Regulatory processes

The limited effectiveness of the ecclesiastical regulation of midwives from the sixteenth century led to a number of attempts to improve midwifery's standing

(Witz 1992). As briefly mentioned in the Introduction (page 10), these attempts peaked in the late nineteenth century with a battle royal between, among others, medical practitioners. On one side, the newly-arrived general practitioners were concerned that the birth, their source of clients and remuneration, would be usurped. On the other side, members of, for example, the Obstetrical Society of London (Nuttall 2011) sought a pliable occupational group who would not threaten their status as experts in interventive practice. These factions sought either an unthreatening handmaiden or a minimally skilled practitioner to relieve medical men of less lucrative work (Kirkham 1999a).

The latter agenda held sway in England in the form of the Midwives Act (HMSO 1902), resulting in minimally educated midwives who were controlled by a statutory body dominated by male medical practitioners. Jane Sandall summarised the professional effects of the 1902 legislation:

> The doctors' demarcationary strategy was to police the boundaries between midwifery and medical practices.
>
> (Sandall 1996: 216)

A roll of practising midwives was drawn up to regulate those with a recognised certificate together with unqualified midwives, known as *bona fides*. On the ground, midwives' practice was required to be closely supervised, a task which was delegated to county councils/boroughs. Supervision sought to address the maintenance of standards, such as cleanliness and infection control, and ensuring appropriate education (see Chapter 5). According to Robert Dingwall and colleagues, these supervisory activities could be used to advance general practitioners' interests by unnecessarily suspending a midwife from practice (Dingwall et al 1988: 160). Pamela Dale and Kate Fisher (2009), though, indicate that any such tensions have been over-emphasised.

As I have mentioned already (page 54), the medicalisation of childbearing progressed apace during the twentieth century. This process, though, was in inverse proportion to medical regulatory power. The decline in medical regulation was most obvious in the implementation of on the Briggs Report (Committee on Nursing 1972). The resulting legislation took the form of the Nurses, Midwives and Health Visitors Act, which was eventually passed in 1979 (Robinson 1990) and brought into being a single statutory regulatory body for the three occupational groups, the UKCC (United Kingdom Central Council for Nursing, Midwifery and Health Visiting) followed by the NMC (Nursing and Midwifery Council). During planning, the proposed legislation was supported by the Royal College of Midwives (1986). On the other hand the then statutory body, the Central Midwives Board (CMB), correctly anticipated that the current, albeit declining, medical control of midwifery would merely be replaced with control by nurses (Sandall 1996). To further complicate matters, the Association of Radical Midwives was formed in response to the threat to the midwife's role (Hughes 1995). The result of midwives' resistance was that the legislation which was much sought after by nurses and health visitors was seriously delayed, to the chagrin of those two groups. That midwives continue to be blamed for this delay and that it continues to rankle is clearly apparent from the NMC website:

> This was due to the need to take account of … lack of consensus within the professions [especially from midwives].
>
> (NMC 2010a)

There are other aspects of the control of midwives which are not precisely related to their statutory regulation; these include their relationship with the current statutory regulatory body (NMC) and are addressed in Chapters 5 and 7.

Resource allocation and staffing

As well as the rather obvious influence over others' activities through statutory regulation, more surreptitious political manoeuvring may also be applied systematically. The medical domination of midwifery through the CMBs was clearly apparent through the membership of these Boards and nursing domination through the NMC is similarly obvious. The control of midwives' activities through, for example, financial constraints may not become evident without scrutiny of budgets.

The UK healthcare system

The UK and other systems of maternity care have, at least anecdotally, attracted critical scrutiny for their limited woman-centredness (Svensson et al 2007: 14). It may be argued that the finite nature of health services' resources has required that their business culture should take precedence over the culture of care. This sorry state has resulted in fundamental problems which manifested themselves in response to criticisms of uncaring midwives. Sarah Davies reports that midwives are not being recruited to fill vacancies (Davies 2011a) and that those in post feel overwhelmed by the demands placed on them; this means that the post holders are at risk of becoming 'uncaring and therefore dangerous' (Davies 2011a: 45). Davies goes on to observe that 'blaming individuals for failing to care is no solution when the whole system is wrong' (Davies 2011a: 45). This problem of staffing has been summarised by Charlotte Philby as:

> Nationwide, more than one-third of heads of midwifery have been told to cut staffing levels; two-thirds say they haven't enough people to cope with current pressure.
>
> (Philby 2011)

In response, Cathy Warwick of the Royal College of Midwives is reported to have replied: 'It's about to get worse'. It may be that it was a comparatively fortunate midwife who was able to state: 'I can offer you safe care' and who went on to qualify 'but it's inhumane care; I can look after you without letting you die, but I can't make it a nice experience' (Philby 2011).

These problems of maternity care systems are examined in more suitable detail by Jo Murphy-Lawless in Chapter 6.

The Canadian experience

Because midwifery in Canada has recently enjoyed a renaissance from its previous 'alegal' status (Burtch 1994: 4; Relyea 1992), its systematic challenges and interoccupational tensions have attracted more publicity than in countries with longer or more consistent midwifery traditions (see Chapter 8). Although the Canadian experience is complicated by significant differences associated with provincial autonomy on health matters, Wendy Peterson and her nurse-colleagues demonstrated country-wide issues (Peterson et al 2007). Collecting data from the four provinces in which midwifery care is publicly funded, these researchers identified significant barriers to the acceptance of midwifery. The most important barrier was fee structures favouring medical practitioners, closely followed by 'turf wars' and interdisciplinary disdain.

ONTARIO

The influential paper by M Joyce Relyea (1992), reflecting on the resurgence of Canadian midwifery, carried in its discussion of professionalisation an aura of foreboding that midwives risked becoming alienated from their grass-roots support. Such premonitions have been shown to be well-founded by researchers such as Stephanie Paterson (2010). In order to obtain the recognition of the medically-dominated legislature and health care system in 1994, midwives in Ontario were required to forego their woman-centred credentials. This sacrifice has resulted in these midwives taking on board medical concepts, such as 'risk' and 'normality', which are alien to their constituency of childbearing women. The legitimacy thus obtained is viewed as resulting in a hierarchical relationship between midwives (together with their clients) and medical practitioners. This hierarchy is apparent in the consultation/transfer obligations built into the legislation, which require midwives, under specified circumstances, to consult a medical practitioner. But, as Paterson observes, there is no reciprocal requirement of physicians. Thus, it is apparent that the women who supported the regeneration of midwifery in Canada perceive themselves to have been short-changed by the legislation, through the creation of a maternity system which retains the long-familiar patriarchal medical dominance.

ALBERTA

The legalisation of midwifery in Alberta in 1992, recounted by Rachael McKendry and Tom Langford (2001), occurred concurrently with some other provinces enacting similarly enlightened policies (Relyea 1992). Close on the heels of midwifery's legalisation, though, Albertan politics took a sharp lurch to the right; the administration was 'vacillating between moral conservatism and a centrist position on social issues' (McKendry and Langford 2001: 538). The death knell of Albertan midwifery was sounded with the withdrawal of funding for care, the cancellation of the midwifery education programme and the withholding of hospital admission privileges for midwives. Thus, by the end of the century, Albertan midwifery was little better positioned than its previous 'alegal' status, as the resurgence in midwife numbers had dwindled and fallen below pre-legalisation figures. An across-the-board reduction in health care spending affected midwives particularly badly because they would have been forced to share funding with medical practitioners; thus midwife-medical antagonism fuelled Albertan midwifery's decline.

SUPPORTING REVIVAL

It is apparent from reports of the Canadian midwifery 'revival' that support from clients is crucial to initiating, but insufficient to ensure the success of a culture of midwifery. Political astuteness, which was less well-developed in Canada, is a further prerequisite if longstanding systematic anomalies associated with medical domination are to be terminated.

Conclusion

This chapter has addressed the political dimensions of interoccupational political developments in the maternity area. The implications of the recent arrival of certain occupational groups have been scrutinised together with the strategies and systems employed by and on behalf of these groups.

4   The politics of maternity beyond the western world

In order to highlight certain political issues which are present in, but not unique to, low income states, I seek now to examine third world maternity politics. My reason is that the influence of politics, including gender issues, on childbearing experiences and outcomes is more clearly illustrated by the various power differentials in the 'developing' countries. I am in no way seeking to demonstrate western superiority, having argued elsewhere that the experiences of some women in developed countries differs little from what happens in less developed areas (Mander 2010).

As well as this rationale for scrutinising low income countries' maternity politics, I need to add another proviso. This is the dynamism of the international environment, which is particularly pertinent at the time of writing, as the frantic financial climate causes difficulty in anticipating the future economic situation. Thus, countries such as India and China which, until recently, have been regarded as 'third world' are developing disconcertingly rapidly into first world states (Wolf-Phillips 1987). So, yet again, scrutiny of the political environment is complicated by its dynamism (Jeffery et al 2002).

To address these issues it is necessary, first, to consider by way of context the status of women; this involves whether and to what extent the woman can exert autonomy over her life in general and her childbearing in particular. Her status is further illuminated by looking at certain phenomena which illustrate her position. After this general contextualisation, I focus on the woman's experience of health, health care and maternity care by drawing on relevant examples. This chapter concludes with reflection on maternal morbidity/mortality, which are the ultimate discriminatory outcomes, together with political issues influencing them.

The woman's status

The woman's place in society is brought into sharp focus by childbearing issues. As Mavis Kirkham astutely observes 'cultural change and different social powerholders' (1999b: 78) have redefined women's experiences. Despite this redefinition, though, Lesley Doyal's bleak assessment still pertains:

there are no societies in which women are treated as equals with men, and this inevitably affects women's health.

(Doyal 2001: 1061)

While an improvement in women's status might be expected to increase their safety and be associated with better health outcomes, such an expectation may be unfounded (Mogford 2011).

A dynamic situation?

As mentioned already, the dynamics of cultural and political systems mean that observations and reports become less reliable. The assumption tends to be made, however, that economic development brings across-the-board better living standards. That this assumption is far from safe emerges in observation of rural life in North India (Jeffery et al 2002: 104); in such a hierarchical society, those who have least input into public affairs, such as women, benefit least. This means that prospects for young women have been adversely affected by rising expectations among *nouveau riche* families in India as manifested, for example, by escalation of demands for dowry payments; thus the already negative value of daughters has further deteriorated.

Women's disadvantage starts even earlier, though, in foetal life and during infancy. Although generally improved, the mortality rates for girls remain 16 per cent higher than boys' (Croll 2000). Alongside such limited improvement, sex-selective abortion means that the sex ratio is continuing to worsen, resulting in only 850 girls being born for every 1,000 boys (page 69).

Gender politics

For certain groups of women, their husbands' control over what they do and do not do is strict, as emerged from a highly relevant literature review of access to maternity services (Gabrysch and Campbell 2009). Focusing on sociocultural factors influencing maternity care use, these researchers consider women's concerns about formal care, which features discriminatory attitudes among staff; such discrimination involves religious or ethnic prejudice, manifested as antagonism about, for example, family size. Similarly, there is fear of being prevented from fulfilling culturally-determined precautions against 'pollution' (page 70). That women's concerns are justified was demonstrated by a study in Yemen, which found that staff with higher biomedical education were perceived to show less consideration for the childbearing woman (Kempe et al 2010).

Sabine Gabrysch and Oona Campbell consider whether factors such as maternal education are associated with 'greater decision-making power, increased self-worth and self-confidence' (Gabrysch and Campbell 2009: 7). They go on to show the significance of the woman's autonomy which, if limited, diminishes her control over material resources, personal activity and even mobility/transport decisions. Autonomy affects a range of personal issues, having been defined by Tim Dyson and Mick Moore as 'the capacity to manipulate one's personal environment ... in order to make decisions about oneself or family members' (Dyson and Moore 1983: 45); lack of autonomy, however, may be mitigated by the woman's informal position within the household. Unlike autonomy, women's status operates at a communal or societal level, yet it still influences her autonomy; both are vulnerable, however, to the male-dominated political vagaries of poverty and under-development (Gabrysch and Campbell 2009: 8).

Concluding their literature review, Gabrysch and Campbell condemn views of education as a panacea to resolve women's limited access to maternity and other services, on the grounds that it constitutes 'victim blaming' (Gabrysch and Campbell 2009: 16). These researchers maintain that the absence of adequate infrastructure for services in many rural areas prevents educational strategies being effective. This direct link is probably accurate, but the researchers neglect the likelihood of indirect benefits of women's education. The impact of more educated women on the personal and political systems in which they participate should not be underestimated (Grosse and Auffrey 1989).

The financial dependence of the woman on her husband for survival, particularly in economic terms, has, like illiteracy, been blamed for disempowerment, low status and reduced autonomy (Sharma et al 2007). The picture is not straightforward, as research by Sharad Kumar Sharma and his colleagues in Nepal has shown; this is because some women are sent to work in order to ameliorate dire poverty, and derive no personal benefit from their employment. Such women would be in jeopardy due to their poverty, as well as their low-status employment.

The examples mentioned already demonstrating women's vulnerably unequal position are further developed by work in India by Alaka Malwade Basu and Gayatri Brij Koolwal (2005). These researchers sought the meaning to women of 'freedom', 'autonomy' and 'empowerment'. Basu and Koolwal identified that the husband's permission was needed by a large majority of women to visit their own friends and birth family (84.4 per cent) or go shopping in the market (78.2 per cent). The woman's limited autonomy was clearly apparent in decisions about her accessing health care. For a majority (51.4 per cent) of women this decision was made, without the woman's input, by the husband and/or others, such as the mother-in-law. For women who enjoyed freedom to make decisions such as these, the researchers indicated the possibility of penalties being applied, should the correct decision not be made.

In mainland China, while some areas forge ahead in health and sociocultural development (Qiu et al 2010), there remain provinces where such changes are negligible, if present at all (Tian et al 2007). In the impoverished Yunnan province in south west China, Lichun Tian and her colleagues identified the woman's restricted contribution to decision-making in general and to childbearing decisions in particular. The husband and male family members would decide about a second or even third pregnancy, in the event of daughters being born, turning the woman into a mere 'childbearing machine' (Tian et al 2007: 287).

Son preference persists strongly for economic and/or cultural-religious reasons (Jeffery et al 2002: 103), resulting in a Chinese woman without a son being regarded as a 'dog without a tail' (Tian et al 2007: 288). Tian and her colleagues argue that political activity, through governmental action, will be necessary if women's status is to be raised in less-developed parts of China. As discussed by Gabrysch and Campbell (2009) in a global context, Tian and colleagues propose that a crucial first step is to reduce female illiteracy which is 37.6 per cent, compared with 15.9 per cent in men, in Yunnan (Tian et al 2007: 294). These authors argue that, with suitable financial incentives, such a momentous step would be successful; they go on to, perhaps disingenuously, make comparisons with the success of 'China's family planning policy' (Tian et al 2007: 295).

Writing in the context of a range of low-income settings, Bregje de Kok and her colleagues demonstrate the particular vulnerability of women experiencing childbearing loss (de Kok et al 2010). Because children are regarded as a 'source of identity, status, power and economic survival' (de Kok et al 2010: 1706), the husband may abandon a wife who does not produce a live child; leading to assertions of a childless wife being condemned to a 'living death' (de Kok et al 2010: 1706).

These issues of gender politics are further illuminated by certain childbearing-related practices which constitute problems.

Intimate partner violence

To navigate this terminological minefield, I avoid the implied cosiness of abuse being 'domestic'; I also assume that readers realise that 'violence' takes many forms, not only physical trauma (DoH 2005). Hence, I prefer the term 'intimate partner violence' (IPV), while recognising this term's imperfections, because 'the perpetrator is most often the woman's partner, [but] it may also be other family members' (Lewis 2011c: 146). IPV in childbearing exemplifies crucial aspects of gender politics, because pregnancy has long been acknowledged as a predisposing factor or trigger (Stark et al 1981).

In low-income countries, antenatal care is less well established or routinised and so IPV during pregnancy is even less likely to be recognised. Following a daughter's birth IPV is widely-reported, in association with the son preference mentioned already (page 65; Croll 2000: 79–80). This issue was brought home to me most forcibly when I attempted to arrange the discharge from the postnatal ward of a woman recently arrived in the United Kingdom and her newborn daughter. She was petrified of leaving the hospital to go home to her in-laws, but a charity for ethnic minority women helped.

Writing about India, Huma Ahmed-Ghosh observes that some low-income states constitute patriarchal societies in which the woman's status is too low to matter (Ahmed-Ghosh 2005). Her childhood is spent amid concerns about the sufficiency of her dowry. After marriage and departure to her husband's family home, she is subordinate to his relatives, particularly his mother. It is only possible for her status to improve if and when she gives birth to a son. Thus, the young woman is disciplined by the family into which she has married; this disciplining takes various forms including 'physical beatings, marital rape, mental torture, withdrawal of money, abandonment, starvation, threats to kill ... ' (Ahmed-Ghosh 2005: 110). The complex relationship between the woman's status and her vulnerability to IPV is unpicked by Elizabeth Mogford (2011); on the one hand IPV indicates low status, while also a result of that status. Mogford differentiates status as depending on the woman's location; women with a high status within the home, as demonstrated by mobility and autonomy, are less vulnerable to IPV. The woman whose low status reflects her income, education and employment, though, is more vulnerable.

Disciplining by the husband's family was reported to Michelle Hindin while researching the relationship between food shortages and women's autonomy in southern Africa (Hindin 2005). Autonomy was investigated by looking at the circumstances under which a woman considered that her husband was right to physically chastise her. By way of a population profile, this research showed that 41.9 per cent of women in Zambia reported having been beaten by their husbands (Hindin 2005: 100). Women were asked about the circumstances under which a woman should expect to be chastised and were given examples such as 'going out without permission', 'refusing sex' and 'burning the food'. Compared with Zimbabweans or Malawians, Zambian women were consistently more likely to expect punishment, with 82.4 per cent expecting chastisement for 'going out without permission' (Hindin 2005: 101).

One basis of IPV emerges from the work of Simeen Mahmud and colleagues working in Bangladesh (Mahmud et al 2011). These researchers report that women's increased visibility and mobility together with their greater input into family decision-making renders the woman more vulnerable to IPV. This observation resonates with the 'resource theory of power' (Goode 1971), through which the threat to the man's self-esteem or even his dominance (Mogford 2011) cause him to become violent. This threat may take the form of pregnancy, which he fears will change the couple's relationship, ie his supremacy (Mezey 1997; Dobash et al 2000); or it may take the form of women's status changing, leading a woman to expect to contribute to family decision-making.

To show circumstances in which a woman may consider that beating is 'justified', Ahmed-Ghosh reports a survey by the Delhi-based Lawyers Collective (Dobash et al 2000). It is not clear, though, whether such 'justification' increases the likelihood of IPV by encouraging it or teaching women to accept it (Mogford 2011). The Lawyers Collective survey found that a majority of women felt that neglecting the house or children merited punishment. Similarly, 'talking disrespectfully to the husband or to the in-laws, complaining about the in-laws' would attract retribution thought justifiable (Ahmed-Ghosh 2005: 110). Noteworthy among these 'offences' perceived as punishable was the woman's 'infertility or inability to bear sons' (Ahmed-Ghosh 2005: 110).

Bangladesh-based research by Sidney Ruth Schuler and her colleagues sought to ascertain why and how women could condone, and possibly participate in, such patriarchal violence (Schuler et al 2011). These researchers found that wife

beating was a fact of life in their society and that such punishment was condoned if the woman was considered to be at fault. Thus, in a society which
believes that the sex of the baby is determined by the mother, she would be
held responsible and blamed if the baby was not the preferred sex.

Female genital mutilation/cuttings (FGM/FGCs) or female circumcision

This issue, like the various uses and meanings of the terminology, is both
confused and confusing. Referring to cuttings and refashionings, altering the
woman's external genitalia to varying extents, the terminology is partially clarified
by reflecting the speaker's views. These viewpoints are inherently political and
operate on at least two distinct levels.

First, at a personal and clinical level, female genital mutilation (FGM) has long
been condemned by women's health specialists because, at best, it is unnecessary
and, at worst, a cause of acute and chronic physical and psychological pathology
(Rushwan 2000). This school of thought reports four rationales for FGM:

> maintaining group identity
> maintaining cleanliness and health
> preserving virginity and family honour by preventing immorality
> furthering marriage goals by enhancing the man's sexual pleasure
> (Lundberg and Gerezgiher 2008: 216)

Women who perform this procedure, or encourage or force their daughters to
undergo it, increase their standing in their community.

Secondly, more globally and theoretically, female genital cuttings (FGCs) or
circumcision have met a relatively sympathetic reception by feminist writers
and other critics of western cultural imperialism (Irvine 2011; Wade 2011).
Research by Bettina Shell-Duncan and her colleagues seeks to demonstrate the
extent to which women who have been 'cut' feel themselves to belong to a superior
sisterhood, much admired by the community of which they form an elite.
These researchers give little attention to the women in 'Senegambia' who choose
to remain 'uncut', dismissing them as a marginalised and unclean minority
(Shell-Duncan et al 2011). This multimethod study gives the impression of parallel
universes inhabited by 'cut' and 'uncut' women; each has its own distinct adherents and supporters within shared communities, with the former regarding the
latter as lesser beings.

Neither advocates nor opponents consider the implications of FGM/FGCs
on childbearing, although Shell-Duncan reports the perception that the pain of
the procedure is suitable preparation for childbirth. Such limited attention has
begun to be addressed by European researchers in countries where immigration
has made FGM/FGCs a significant health issue. In Sweden, for example,
Pranee Lundberg and Alganesh Gerezgiher undertook an in-depth qualitative
study of childbearing-related issues arising for Eritrean women migrants
who had undergone FGM (Lundberg and Gerezgiher 2008). These researchers

identified issues of pain relating to the procedure and to childbirth, fear of the birth and giving birth in an alien culture. Knowledge of such matters among health care providers was variable, so the women's informal support became crucial. Lundberg and Gerezgiher also report the women's plans to have the procedure reversed, to be made 'open', and prevent their daughters being similarly mutilated.

Both advocates and opponents of FGM/FGCs, because of personal and cultural sensitivities, rely on women reflecting the dominant cultural views. Thus, Shell-Duncan and colleagues report only the views of 'cut' women who are happily so in a society where 78 per cent of women are 'cut' (Shell-Duncan et al 2011: 1277). Similarly, Lundberg and Gerezgiher articulate only the views of 'cut' women in Sweden who are unhappy with their state. While recognising the near-impossibility of obtaining views from minority populations on such a sensitive topic, it is necessary to realise that such views are likely to exist and need to be considered if this matter is to generate more light than heat.

Daughter discrimination

The obverse of son preference (page 65), daughter discrimination, takes several forms, varying with gestation/age and severity or fatality (Croll 2000: 10). The literature relates largely to Asian contexts, with most research looking at India and mainland China. I address three forms here in chronological order.

AMNIOCENTESIS AND SEX-SELECTIVE ABORTION

Since the advent of amniocentesis and ultrasound, daughter discrimination has been applied to the girl before birth, resulting in her even earlier demise. After amniocentesis was introduced in India in 1974, and with gynaecologists' enthusiastic involvement, it was commercialised and developed into an industry (Croll 2000: 60). Amartya Sen observes that amniocentesis and sex-selective abortion are not ubiquitous throughout India, demonstrating less impact in the south and east, whereas the north and west are seriously affected (Sen 2003). Sen finds himself unable to establish any correlation with any of the usual indicators, like poverty, political allegiance or religious orientation. So he pleads for more research to identify the rationale underpinning the incidence of this appalling phenomenon.

Responding to an earlier paper by Sen, Elisabeth Croll outlined the situation in mainland China (Croll 2001). Due to daughter discrimination combined with a precarious administrative system, not all female births are notified, so, Croll states, sex-selective abortion is quite universal. She reports its practice in not only rural, but also urban areas and in wealthy as well as deprived provinces (Croll 2001: 229). Additionally, since the 1980s many Chinese have, because a fervently patrilineal culture has implemented the 'one child' policy, been keen that ultrasound be used to facilitate sex-selective abortion (Peng 2010: 789).

FEMALE INFANTICIDE

The widespread twentieth-century assumption that infanticide was historical has been countered by Elisabeth Croll, showing that in India the practice is increasing in northern and western provinces, as well as discrete southern areas (Croll 2001: 227). She indicates that infanticide is spreading through faith groups and castes previously unaffected (Jeffery et al 1984). Second or subsequent daughters are most vulnerable. While newborn daughters are reported as 'stillborn', older girls succumb to neglect through lack of health care and poor or lethal food-stuffs. In China, Croll identifies that the introduction of the 'one child' policy was associated with a 'sharp increase' in female infanticide (Croll 2001: 229).

MISSING WOMEN

Barbara Miller's ground-breaking, if possibly inconsistent, work on the 'Endangered Sex' first illuminated Indian son-preference leading to daughter neglect and demise (Miller 1981; Jeffery et al 1984). Subsequently, Amartya Sen's demographic research identified the sex ratio disparities in China and India as being due to neglect through poor health care and nutrition (Sen 1992). He observed that such neglect was especially, but not exclusively, practised during childhood. Reviewing the situation later, he reported that the situation was marginally improved in south Asia, but had deteriorated in China (Sen 2003). While older girls and women might be less vulnerable, any improvement in their prospects was more than counterbalanced by discrimination prior to birth in the form of sex-selective abortion (page 68).

We should consider the benefits of development and the possibility of young women's better education (page 65) and employment improving their status and, hence, survival. Better education has been shown to improve status and lower fertility, but has not influenced son preference (Croll 2001: 231). Thus, the fact remains that women's mortality rates continue to exceed men's until the age of 35, and mothers' education 'actually exacerbates excess female child mortality' (Sabarwal 2007).

GENDERCIDE

Variably helpful to those of us who are numerically challenged, sex ratios demonstrate the extent of daughter discrimination leading to gendercide. Amartya Sen outlined the principles behind the calculations, beginning with the usual proportion of about 5 per cent more boys than girls being born (Sen 1992). This imbalance evens out because 'women are hardier than men and ... survive better at all ages – including in utero [sic]' (Sen 1992: 587). Any imbalance is further evened out by men being more vulnerable through armed conflict, risky life-styles and social friction. These effects result in marginally more women in the population and Sen's original paper argued that any reversal of this situation is attributable to gender inequality, associated with the interventions outlined above.

As mentioned already, collecting data on newborns' gender is not a priority in some societies, so figures may be unreliable. The existence of son preference, however, is supported by Asian countries' figures. An extreme example is found in Yunnan Province, a particularly deprived region of the People's Republic of China. Tian and her colleagues report that, in 2001, 123.4 boys were born there for every 100 girls (Tian 2007: 288). In India, Croll observes, the ratio of females to males has fallen as low as 930 females to 1,000 males. In 1991, sex ratios for Chinese children were below 900 girls to 1,000 boys in many districts (Croll 2001: 227).

While recognising the huge variations existing in countries as large as China and India, the problem of the 'missing women' is clearly immeasurable. The significance of the demise of the babies, girls and women affected by these practices, though, is regarded by some as less than the inevitable forthcoming demographic catastrophe of 'marriage squeeze' (Peng 2010: 789). In response to such criticism, I argue that it is daughter discrimination which matters, because these girls and women are subject to gendercide *now*, rather than at some future point in time.

The challenge of daughter discrimination has been approached by Non-Governmental Organisations (NGOs), regional initiatives and national legislation; China and India have outlawed infanticide and ultrasound for sex identification (Croll 2001). Such developments, though, have proved ineffective because of girls' 'invisibility', as they and their problems tend to be subsumed under women's and children's initiatives. As Croll astutely observes, the admirable efforts to resolve issues such as street children, child labourers, child soldiers and child trafficking/prostitution rarely provide gender details. Thus, the invisibility of gendercide persists.

The political nature of these activities and their deplorable outcomes has been clarified by Cheryl Bernard, who has proposed that the perpetrators consider such activities constitute:

> an acceptable exercise of male prerogative, a legitimate and appropriate way to relieve their own tension in conditions of stress, to sanction female behaviour ... or just to enjoy a feeling of supremacy.
>
> (cited by Heise et al 1994: 29)

The deeply engrained nature of daughter discrimination was brought home to me when visiting a maternity unit in a major Chinese city. I observed several situations demonstrating the standard of care provided, including baby swimming and baby massage, as well as post-natal wards. In none of these situations did I see a baby girl. On mentioning my observation to my hosts, I was informed that it was 'coincidence'.

Pollution

Another way in which patriarchal societies are able to exercise male prerogative is found in the concept of pollution. Probably more widespread than the interventions mentioned above, pollution's outcomes may be less dire. Crucial to pollution is the relationship between society and the individuals making up that society. In the perceptions, manifestations and control of pollution the actions and behaviours of the society and its members have powerful implications for each other.

The concept of pollution exists more or less explicitly in many cultures. Because of the differing contexts, although it invariably features certain characteristics, pollution is known by several alternative names. While the term 'pollution' featured in the title of Mary Douglas' groundbreaking book (1966), 'impurity' was used by Santi Rozario (1992) to focus on society, rather than individual members. Margaret Mead and Niles Newton (1967), concentrating on the pathologically negative aspects of this concept, chose to refer to its 'defiling' nature.

The meaning of this concept was brought home to me when working with an articulate and devout South-Asian woman. Grieving the death of her newborn daughter with cardiac problems, she lamented that her grief was aggravated by being unable to find solace in her Koran or attending her baby's funeral. Both were forbidden due to her 'unclean' state. Like me, my midwife colleagues found difficulty accepting this grieving mother's predicament.

RATIONALE

Relating the experience of Chinese women, Emily Ahern observes that any fluid or substance released from the bodily orifices is automatically assumed to be powerfully unclean, irrespective of the person's state of health (Ahern 1978: 271). Particularly symbolically polluting, according to Rozario writing about southern Asia (Rozario 1992: 99), are fluids associated with sexual intercourse, menstruation, childbirth and breastfeeding. Differential fluid production is the crucial disparity in the relative purity of women and men, as man is perceived as purer because male pollution is controllable by celibacy. Further, Douglas (1966: 3) emphasises how each sex's reproductive fluids are perceived as particularly dangerous to the other; despite which, men's vulnerability to women's sexual fluids is considered more hazardous. So, although symbolic balance or symmetry between the sexes may be possible, this is not so. A fearful hierarchy exists due to men's greater vulnerability and women being more dangerous (Katbamna 2000: 131). Together with fluids representing different levels of impurity, their release also renders women more dangerous, partly because female pollution is uncontrollable by celibacy, as in blood shed during menstruation. Additionally, that women produce fluids associated with four bodily processes, rather than just one like men, aggravates women's impure state (Rozario 1992: 99).

Women are considered uniquely polluting due to blood lost during menstruation and childbirth (Callaghan 2007). Blood carries multiple levels of significance, being essentially good and beneficent while in the circulation. When lost vaginally, however, it becomes utterly evil and dirty (Ahern 1978: 271).

The dangerousness of blood prevents women from functioning, due to invented detrimental effects on eg wine, meat, bread, preserves and infants (Shorter 1983: 287).

During menstruation and childbearing the woman's polluting nature reduces her status to the lowest level of society – becoming 'untouchable' (Jeffery et al 2002). Menstrual blood and lochia (shed vaginally after birth) are construed as identical, because menstrual blood supposedly collects in the womb during pregnancy. Birth fluids are considered dirtiest of all, due to their nature, quantity and duration of production (Ram 2009: 108).

SIGNIFICANCE OF POLLUTION

Pollution's significance varies between different groups. Rozario (1992: 98) suggests that Islamic beliefs are less extreme than Hindus'. While pollution is recognised in 'primitive' religions, Mary Douglas found that such beliefs are not unique to them, as early Christians objected strongly to pollution by blood (Douglas 1966: 1). Rozario develops the Christian interpretation of pollution by showing its close correspondence to the concept of sin (Rozario 1992: 98). Patricia Jeffery and her colleagues emphasise the universality of the concept of childbirth pollution (Jeffery et al 1989: 124), likening pollution to power in that, unless used wisely, power has the potential to become evil.

A significant issue is the problem of marginal states, applied to people not included in the patterning of society and considered liminal or 'placeless' (Douglas 1966: 95). This applies most importantly to the foetus, being regarded as both vulnerable and dangerous. To ensure its growth and survival the foetus is dangerously demanding and the pregnant woman, satisfier of those demands, also becomes dangerous.

The group among whom pollution achieves its major significance is the family. Rozario maintains that the purity of women determines the honour and status of men and, hence, family (Rozario 1992: 98). She shows how anxiety about women's pollution or purity engenders men's preoccupation with control over women. This preoccupation results in child marriage and widow burning (*sati*), as the woman's purity can only be ensured by her being married. Thus, direct connections appear between sexuality, pollution, purity of the family (as represented by the blood line) and masculine control over women. Rozario continues that, if impure, the woman is thought powerful, whereas purity is associated with disempowerment and needing protection. Thus, patriarchal power is enhanced.

SYMBOLISM

The symbolic meanings of pollution only augment its political significance, being linked with crucial transitions in the life cycle, and their associated threats to composure and integrity of the individual. A healthy body is viewed symbolically as representing orderly society, in this way pollution's significance becomes obvious (Bharj 2007: 61; Douglas 1996: 114). On this basis, it is logical that lochia, with exposure to the associated risk of death during the transition to motherhood, should be regarded as supremely dangerous (King 1983: 121).

The symbolic role of women is to act as keeper of the gate by which entry is gained into the family. This is an immense responsibility as the effectiveness of this role determines the continuing purity or otherwise of the patrilineal family line. If the woman is thought relaxed in her sexual behaviour or in her observance of ritual, the threat is to far more than those who are in direct contact with her; the orderliness of society may be at stake through the agency of women and the fluids released during and following the birth.

Through its symbolism, the balance of power between men and women in the extended family, and society, underpins the concept of pollution.

IMPLICATIONS

The social function of the concept of pollution is indubitably more significant than its health function. One of the ways in which this operates is through the ordering of the social group with well-defined structures. Crucial to pollution is the concept of 'dirt', which Douglas defines as simply being 'matter out of place' (Douglas 1966: 35); a definition expanded to recount how, symbolically, dirt offends against orderliness in society. Efforts to remove or control dirt through pollution precautions constitute attempts to organise the social environment. Douglas indicates, however, that it is not just the reality of dirt which threatens social order. It is also disobedience to the rules and rituals which control the perception of dirt and, thus, maintain a pure or unpolluted environment. Ahern builds on Douglas's argument by emphasising that it is the patriarchal social order which is perceived as under threat (Ahern 1978: 277). Disobedience to conventions take the form of deliberately or inadvertently ignoring certain rituals, causing impurity to develop. The orderliness of the *status quo* may be interpreted in two, possibly linked, ways. The first, more obvious, aspect relates to individuals' wealth. Rozario (1992) contends that purity is more easily achieved by the wealthy, presumably due to their vested interest in maintaining a stable, orderly society.

Links between purity and social status lead to the second aspect, which is the different roles of women and men. In a society in which decisions are made by the eldest male in the family, a young woman is likely to be blamed for causing social disorder or 'disharmony' if and when she decides not to follow those decisions (Ahern 1978: 276). In more general terms, assumptions are made by a patriarchal society that the woman is impure and the man is pure (Rozario 1992: 102). Although more explicit in some societies, female sexual purity is crucial to all of the major religions and, as mentioned already, the need for such purity may be traced back to the honour, status and reputation of a patrilineal elite. In this debate women are inevitably inferior, less powerful and, therefore, oppressed. Thus, the concept of pollution is used to maintain the *status quo* by reinforcing longstanding social pressures.

In summary, the literature shows that the concept of pollution is employed to maintain a balance of power between women and men, indisputably advantaging the latter. This concept is based on assumptions of the dangerously evil nature of women both at certain well-defined times and more generally.

While the literature reflects an overpoweringly persuasive picture of the oppression of women in many societies, other views have been expressed. Quoting a workshop presentation by Alaka Basu, Roger Jeffery and his colleagues suggest that the domination of women may not be socio-cultural, but rather economic and political. Basu's presentation made reference to the 'very strong reasons' (Jeffery et al 2007: 287) for protecting childbearing women and to the lack of other services where maternity provision is deficient. That 'not all workshop participants agreed' (Jeffery et al 2007: 287) suggests an ongoing debate on the nature of pollution and that the meanings of this many-layered concept are being extended into the fiscal sphere.

Health systems (see Chapter 6)

Healthcare is all too often treated as a political football, but in this section I consider the politics of what happens to women users of healthcare systems in developing countries. Many of these phenomena, as astutely noted by Iain Chalmers, are associated with globalisation:

> The links between technological and other developments in the wealthier countries and what happens in the low- and middle-income countries may not always be obvious. The nature of the interrelationship in the context of perinatal health care is due to globalisation.
>
> (Chalmers 2004)

Despite Chalmers's characteristically profound observation, 'globalisation' is becoming a cliché – a decline aggravated by it being a word which is frequently, and frequently wrongly, used. So globalisation deserves discussion. Rather than an internationalist approach or regionalisation, globalisation refers to those processes which purportedly convert the world into one single entity. This may be no bad thing *per se*, but these processes erode and destroy national, cultural and linguistic boundaries while absorbing poorer countries into the adverse consequences of globalised consumer capital developments (Hirst and Thompson 1996; Klein 2007). Thus, globalisation's potentially dire implications, for a matter as culturally sensitive as childbearing, emerge (Bettcher and Lee 2002). In the context of healthcare provision, as well as other 'industries', these implications have been foretold.

A major instrument of globalisation has been the World Trade Organisation (WTO) which, in conjunction with transnational corporations (TNCs), has brought about the demise of public funding streams (Pollock and Price 2000). In healthcare, the reduction and obliteration of public funding has led to the discontinuation of many services and the introduction of funding systems like

PFI (private finance initiative) and PPP (public private partnership; see Chapter 6 and page 2). The increasing influence of international agencies like the WTO, supposedly regulating world trade, and the World Bank is disconcerting (Walt 1998). Not only does the power of international organisations threaten the welfare of low- and middle-income countries, it also threatens the potential benefits of other more specialised agencies such as the WHO.

Commercialisation and medicalisation of health care

Economic and social development is associated with many low-income states' health care systems having been changed with or, more likely, without governmental or popular input. The new model all too often emulates a system such as that found in the United States, where medicalisation, competition and market forces feature prominently, with minimal 'safety net' provision for the seriously impoverished (Harris et al 2007; Global Health Watch 2011). For similar reasons a culture of self-regulation and individuals' personal responsibility is encouraged, resulting in the state assuming less responsibility for even basic or emergency services (Jeffery and Jeffery 2008). Privatisation has been encouraged without any corresponding external scrutiny or accountability. The lack of state regulation means that families are vulnerable to exorbitant charges demanded by under- or unqualified 'medical' practitioners, who administer ineffective and inappropriate interventions and jeopardise the life and health of the woman and baby (see Iatrogenesis page 76). This situation is aggravated by women's appropriate mistrust of services available, probably at lower cost, in publicly funded maternity units. The suspicion that practitioners' recommendations are founded purely on their own financial interests fuels this mistrust and delays healthcare-seeking when professional input becomes a matter of life or death (Jeffery and Jeffery 2010: 1714).

While advice to 'shop around' the medical market is relevant to remedy chronic health problems, an emergency occurring during a prolonged or complicated labour prevents such luxury. Thus, input by women into or control over the maternity care market is negligible. The debts which individuals and families accrue from accessing such exorbitantly priced emergency services reach figures greatly exceeding the family income and plunge families into a never-ending cycle of debt.

This situation barely impacts on more privileged and articulate members of the community and, for this reason, the situation is unlikely to be changed, even less improved. The effectiveness of the market in ensuring quality, or even safe, health care has proved, yet again, to be illusory. As Patricia and Roger Jeffery dishearteningly observe of North India:

> rural women experiencing obstetric emergencies remain caught between a moribund state and a rapacious market that is readily accessible only to those who can pay.
>
> (Jeffery and Jeffery 2008: 85)

Male domination

As well as a range of environmental and institutional barriers, a woman's access to health care is all too frequently controlled by her menfolk (Ojanuga and Gilbert 1992). This control may be fuelled by financial considerations (Jeffery and Jeffery 2010) which, in turn, reflect the woman's status or the value attached to her life and health. Control of the woman's use of health care is equally likely to be determined by the patriarchal issues already raised in the discussion of 'pollution' (page 70). In this situation the menfolk fear that the woman will be attended by male health care providers, thus jeopardising the family 'honour'. An extreme form of such control is reported by Durrenda Nash Ojanuga and Cathy Gilbert in countries where the husband's legal consent is needed for her to obtain treatment (Ojanuga and Gilbert 1992: 616). These authors go on to establish the link between such patriarchal decision-making and maternal mortality (page 82). Jeffery and Jeffery illustrate this issue clearly in their case study of a maternal death in Uttar Pradesh caused by the husband's delay in giving permission for attendance for maternity care (Jeffrey and Jeffrey 2010: 1713).

The significance of this manifestation of male power was brought home to me by a colleague's experience of midwifery in rural Pakistan (Brims 20011). Before being permitted to teach women about family planning, she was required almost farcically to show the material to the menfolk. This was despite the men having no understanding of the techniques or issues. Their concern, though, was that they needed to control what the women were being taught.

Iatrogenesis

The concept of harm in the course of treatment has long been familiar to health care providers, but only relatively recently has it been named. Ivan Illich explains that 'iatrogenesis' is derived from the Greek words *iatros*, meaning physician, and *genesis*, meaning origin (Illich 1976: 11). This word emerged out of his analysis of a number of institutions, including medicine and education, which proved counter-productive in reaching their stated goals (Illich 1995). In his analysis of the consequences of medical interventions, Illich identified three major concerns:

- 'clinical iatrogenesis' (Illich 1976: 21) – harm caused by supposedly therapeutic interventions, eg infections;
- 'social iatrogenesis' – the various forms of harm that result from the 'socio-economic transformations which have been made attractive, possible or necessary' by health services developing professional and institutional structures and systems (Illich 1976: 49). This is the removal from communities of the ability to care for their own;
- 'cultural iatrogenesis' – changing attitudes of an entire society, eg to disability, infirmity and old age.

For obvious reasons, Illich and his ideas have been vilified, largely on the grounds that his case is seriously overstated. I venture to suggest, though, that there is more than a little resonance between Illich's three forms of iatrogenesis and the changing practice of maternity care in both less and more developed countries.

Important examples of iatrogenesis, as mentioned already, are the reproductive tract infections (RTIs), which frequently follow family planning interventions, causing women's debility and social exclusion in many third world countries (Wasserheit 1989). This author, reflecting the time of writing, recommends prophylactic antibiotic cover to address the problem, little knowing the pitfalls of indiscriminate antibiotic administration.

Approaching the problem of third world iatrogenesis more systematically, Vincent De Brouwere and Wim Van Lerberghe address clinical problems by blaming 'doctors and hospitals' for their reluctance to apply scientific standards and be accountable for patient outcomes (De Brouwere and Van Lerberghe 2001: 18). These researchers recognise that institutionalisation of birth is unlikely to be the universal answer, not only because of the resource implications, but also because of the increased likelihood of 'over-intervention' and the resulting 'iatrogenicity' (De Brouwere and Van Lerberghe 2001: 106); this point is supported by data indicating that maternal mortality rates (page 82) are higher where women give birth in maternity units attended by 'professionals' (De Brouwere and Van Lerberghe 2001: 116). The technological imperative is held responsible in the form of more frequent use of diagnostic techniques.

At an even higher systematic level, De Brouwere and Van Lerberghe's econometric analysis shows the contribution of supply-induced demand. This is closely associated with the commercialisation and medicalisation of health care in low-income countries (page 75). These authors reflect on the widespread assumption that PFP (private for profit) providers invariably deliver more effective health care than public services, using the caesarean epidemic (page 80) as an illustration. The iatrogenic nature of the increasing caesarean rate is evidenced by the 'not insignificant proportion of maternal morbidity and mortality' (De Brouwere and Van Lerberghe 2001: 351). This point is supported by the classic paper by Xavier De Muylder, which demonstrates the unspeakably small majority (53 per cent) of women having caesareans in developing countries who did *not* suffer post-operative complications or need a blood transfusion (De Muylder 1993: 102).

The cascade of intervention

A widely recognised phenomenon, at least in higher income countries, and corresponding closely to the definition of iatrogenesis (page 76) is the cascade of intervention. This is the escalating situation developing when administration of medication to reduce labour pain also reduces the strength and frequency of uterine contractions, constituting iatrogenic dystocia. Drugs administered to augment or accelerate contractions, such as oxytocics (page 78), are over-effective; excessive contractions reduce the baby's oxygen supply, presenting as foetal distress and requiring emergency intervention, probably by caesarean, to remove the baby from its hostile environment (Varney Burst 1983). I have been unable to locate material on the cascade of intervention *per se* in third world countries, but the inexorable advance of medicalisation leads to the suspicion that it may become unavoidable.

The partograph/partogram

The contribution of the partograph to iatrogenesis is through its fundamental links with active management of labour (AML page 55; O'Driscoll et al 1973) and the cascade of intervention. The partograph originated as the 'cervicograph' in Zimbabwe (Philpott 1972), where this visual representation of labour progress was intended to indicate the need for higher levels of healthcare. The research basis of the introduction of the partograph has been shown to be gravely defective (Lavender 2003). Authoritative systematic evaluation was delayed until 1994 and a study of the WHO partograph in SE Asia (WHO 1994). As with the original, this partograph's evaluation was 'deeply flawed' (Rosser 1994), because failure to implement an RCT and the introduction of a 'package' of confounding interventions rendered it seriously defective. So the evaluation which was undertaken by Tina Lavender and her colleagues in England focusing on women's satisfaction was the first reliable study (Lavender et al 1998).

The political implications of the partograph are found in its potential to initiate the cascade of intervention, ultimately leading to caesarean. This potential danger manifested itself in an Australian study, where the partograph 'increased action, rather than assessment' (Groeschel and Glover 2001: 26).

Some researchers have found the partograph to be used less widely than they thought appropriate (Fawole et al 2010; Neal and Lowe 2012). It is necessary, however, to question whether a potentially iatrogenic intervention lacking a strong evidence base should be advocated for use in any clinical setting, irrespective of its level of development.

Uterine stimulants

The likely *raison d'être* and outcome of active management and the partograph is the administration of drugs to increase uterine contractions. This administration is intended to accelerate labour, thus boosting the cascade of intervention. As a group, because their main effect is to hasten birth, these drugs are known as 'oxytocics'. Their iatrogenic side-effects, in addition to those dangers mentioned above (page 77), include uterine rupture, haemorrhage and maternal death. For these reasons, assessment prior to and ongoing monitoring of mother and foetus during administration are essential, in a properly equipped and staffed clinical environment (Flandermeyer et al 2010). While the use of oxytocics in low-income settings has been neglected, there are two significant exceptions.

OXYTOCICS IN CHINA

The recent burgeoning economic advances in China have affected urban areas, with immeasurable swathes of this immense country remaining underdeveloped.

In the same way, health care has been variably westernised. While preparing for an innovative research project, midwifery practice was observed and was frequently found to feature the acceleration of labour using oxytocics (Mander et al 2010; Cheung et al 2009). Routine oxytocic administration to hasten labour caused concern to the Chinese midwives, perceiving their limited choice:

> Because staffing levels are low at night, [women] whose labours will extend into the night are likely to be administered syntocinon (a synthetic oxytocic) to speed up the labour in the hope of an earlier birth.
>
> (Mander et al 2010: 524)

The routinised administration of these drugs was a source of anxiety, especially in view of the shaky indications for their use:

> routine pharmacological induction and augmentation of labour [is] for the convenience of the staff.
>
> (Cheung et al 2009: 104)

OXYTOCIN IN THE SUBCONTINENT

The administration of oxytocin in India has been more thoroughly investigated and published. Unlike China where homebirth is strongly discouraged, in South Asia a significant proportion of babies are born at home. All too often, though, this will be in a rural village or urban slum (Moran et al 2010). In the absence of appropriate assessment and monitoring, the unguarded administration during labour of oxytocin by under- or unqualified 'medical' practitioners threatens the mother's life for two reasons. First and foremost is the likelihood that intramuscular (IM) injection of oxytocin will cause one massive, tonic uterine contraction leading to foetal demise, uterine rupture and uncontrollable maternal haemorrhage (Holmes 1955). For this reason warnings are published against oxytocin being administered by IM injection (WHO 1996), although Petra Brhlikova and her colleagues report that 'oxytocin is usually administered' IM in rural home deliveries (Brhlikova et al 2009: 43). The second, possibly linked, reason is the instability of the drug if stored for too long or not refrigerated (Flandermeyer 2010).

The extent of the problem should not be underestimated, as there are many accounts of the ubiquity of the hazardous administration of oxytocin. In a Bangladeshi context, Allisyn Moran and her colleagues report that 48 per cent of women giving birth at home received oxytocin (Moran 2010: 1609). The practice in India, however, appears to be even worse and deteriorating markedly, with rates of up to 75 per cent being reported in 2005 by Patricia Jeffery and her colleagues (Jeffery et al 2007: 174). These researchers observed that the women most likely to be administered IM oxytocin are those of higher socio-economic status and/or better education, suggesting that this intervention carries kudos. Perhaps surprisingly, Jeffery and her colleagues found that maternal mortality has not been affected by the increasing administration of oxytocin, but perinatal death and neonatal morbidity rates have risen.

Caesarean

As well as the threat which it exerts over the culture of childbirth, caesarean carries more risks in developing countries than in developed ones (Mander 2007), a point clearly made by José Villar and his colleagues:

> a medical intervention ... effective when applied to sick individuals in emergency situations can do more harm than good when applied to healthy populations.
>
> (Villar et al 2006: 1827)

The reflections by Xavier De Muylder conclude that increased post-caesarean mortality is likely to be due to infection, as well as anaesthetic problems and technical problems during surgery. The risk of mortality is exacerbated by the mother possibly having been undernourished or in poor health during pregnancy and then enduring prolonged labour. De Muylder contemplates the risk for the woman in any future pregnancy due to scar dehiscence and uterine rupture, which are a death sentence in under-resourced settings. While recognising the significant post-caesarean reduction in fertility, this author omits to mention the likelihood and dangers of abnormal placental situation and development in future (Jackson and Paterson-Brown 2001).

The WHO realised that the 'caesarean epidemic' carries greater risks for women in lower-income countries and sought to prevent this impending tragedy by convening a meeting in Brazil to identify the appropriate caesarean rate (Beech 2004). Despite agreement that the evidence established that a rate above 10 per cent cannot be justified on health grounds, commercial interests prevailed and the Fortaleza fudge concluded:

> Countries with some of the lowest perinatal mortality rates in the world have caesarean section rates of less than 10%. There is no justification for any region to have a rate higher than 10–15%.
>
> (Lancet 1985: 437)

Inevitably, 15 per cent has become the much-quoted and much-flouted figure. Such flouting has been particularly evident in developing countries, such as China and Brazil, where birth by caesarean has become a status symbol. In some areas the vast majority of babies are born by caesarean (Cheung et al 2006; Harris et al 2007).

Due the high prevalence of HIV in many low-income countries, vaginal birth carries risks of mother-to-child transmission. Elective caesarean effectively reduces the neonatal risk (Read and Newell 2005), but the balance between costs and benefits to mother and baby makes the caesarean decision difficult.

Health personnel

The association between the status of health care providers and childbearing outcomes is not always easily apparent. It is necessary to consider the political implications of attendants' status for the woman's birth experience.

The midwife

In considering the international background of the 'caesarean epidemic', the impact of the near-absence of the midwife in some countries deserves attention. In China, the decline and fall of the midwife has been well-documented, and her title has been assumed by labour ward nurses (Cheung et al 2005). In Brazil, the midwife is too low status to be employable (Nuttall 2000). In Greece, only nurses are mentioned in the available literature (Mossialos et al 2005). In all of these countries caesarean rates are spiralling exponentially and the midwife features only to be excluded from the equation. In the literature on the low-income countries, where the caesarean situation is complicated, the midwife appears in neither research nor statistical literature.

Why does it matter that there is no reference to the midwife in these countries where caesarean is a major public health issue? This is because the country in which the midwife is most powerful, the Netherlands, boasts one of the lowest caesarean rates (Declercq and Viisainen 2001). This view is supported by findings in a country seriously concerned about its caesarean rate. American data clearly show that 'non-obstetrician care' (Mahoney and Malcoe 2005: 177) is fundamentally important to address the caesarean problem. Further, Marsden Wagner's observation that the extent to which midwives lower the caesarean rate is related to their autonomy in their practice (Wagner 2002), may be as true of lower as of higher income countries.

The person most likely to resolve these challenges has been dubbed the 'post-modern midwife' (Davis-Floyd 2005). Combining the strengths of both the traditional, community-based midwife with those of the professionally educated midwife, the post-modern midwife is questioning of her own as well as others' practice. This midwife moves between differing systems of maternity care while constantly maintaining her woman-centred orientation.

The Traditional Birth Attendant (TBA) and the dai

The decline of the Indian state health system and the appearance/expansion of certain practitioners is outlined by Jeffery and Jeffery (2008). Largely unqualified practitioners offer advice from roadside booths, during home visits and in nursing homes, often administering medications by injection (page 79) and selling drugs. This effective privatisation of health care coincided with the government's espousal of a more commercial, market-oriented approach to health. Simultaneously, Traditional Birth Attendants (TBAs), known locally as *dais*, were trained to provide safer care, aiming to lower maternal mortality rates. Encouragement from the World Bank introduced a new practitioner – the Auxiliary Nurse-Midwife (ANM) – who, as part of the corrupt governmental health system, encourages costly private practice and tends to be avoided. This means that most women in rural areas must rely on the services of trained or untrained dais from their own or nearby villages (Jeffery and Jeffery 2008). The picture presented of the *dai* is that she is low caste and poorly trained (Jeffery et al 2002) but, most importantly to her clients, she is affordable.

Attempts to improve the practice of the *dai* or TBA have been evaluated (Sibley et al 2007), but the evaluations have been too small and lacking in rigour for conclusions about her or her training to be drawn. As the work of Patricia Jeffery and her colleagues indicates, though, this practitioner may be no worse than the alternatives and brings the advantage of being marginally less unacceptable.

Maternal outcomes

Unlike evaluations of maternity services in more developed countries, which tend to focus on measures of satisfaction, low income countries measure outcomes in terms of morbidity and, all too frequently, mortality.

Maternal mortality

Perhaps because maternal mortality is still a 'silent tragedy', solutions, such as the Safe Motherhood Initiative, have met with limited success (Baraté and Temmerman 2009). In order to address this problem, in 1987 a group of international NGOs with differing agendas organised a Safe Motherhood Conference in Nairobi, Kenya (Ohaja 2012). The measurable aim was to reduce pregnancy-related deaths and complications by 50 per cent by 2000. In view of poor progress the United Nations took up the baton when drawing up the Millennium Development Goals (MDGs) at a New York summit (UN 2000). Of eight goals, MDG Five focuses on maternal health, with the target of reducing the 'maternal mortality ratio by three quarters' between 1990 and 2015 (UN 2000). Disappointingly, the UK Department for International Development reports limited inroads being made internationally to achieve this goal (DFID 2010). Eastern Asia appears to be the only region likely to reach MDG Five, with its 5.5 per cent annual reduction in the maternal mortality rate (MMR). Of 87 countries with an MMR equal to or greater than 100 in 1990, nine countries are 'on track'. Those reported to be 'making progress' total only 47, with another 22 not making 'sufficient progress'; while eight countries have made 'no progress'. This contemptible response to the UN's well-meant but possibly naïve initiative speaks volumes about decision-making in the 30 under-responding countries. Politicians' decisions frequently seek a 'quick fix' to demonstrate visible change for minimal cost by focusing their efforts on major centres of population (Baraté and Temmerman 2009: 234). So less easily identifiable areas or problems remain unaddressed.

A basic problem, which has yet to be resolved, is counting the number of maternal deaths (Mander 2010). Keeping accurate statistics may not be a priority in under-resourced health care settings and in rural and remote areas the death of a childbearing woman may not be attended by a person sufficiently knowledgeable to report it. This means that MMR figures depend on, for example, population-based estimates (Bick and Sandall 2010; Baraté and Temmerman 2009). It is not impossible that a government seeking to impress potential funders may disguise or 'massage' statistics to present figures more conducive to their political purposes.

Similarly, the role of funding agencies may be less benign than would be hoped. Bob Baulch used aid concentration curves and the Suits index to investigate the equity of aid distribution (Baulch 2006). While some agencies, such as the World Bank and those in the United Kingdom, distribute the majority of their aid to low-income countries, others, such as the United States and the European Commission, allocate a similar majority to middle-income states. Thus, political posturing further deprives those already most deprived.

Funding problems are exacerbated, as Pascale Baraté and Marleen Temmerman identify, by the problem of competition between, for example, NGOs operating in the same field (Baraté and Temmerman 2009). Such competitive activity is counterproductive due to available funding being spread too thinly to be effective. These authors indicate that NGOs' 'vested interests, sensitivities and their own agendas' (Baraté and Temmerman 2009: 433) inhibit collaboration and creativity and impede significant change. The situation in India is spelled out even more clearly by Roger Jeffery and his colleagues:

> action … seems to be stymied by a lack of political will, no new ideas, a preoccupation with population control, and an apparent lack of awareness of the key issues.
>
> (Jeffery et al 2007: 286)

Thus political activity is needed for all involved to 'clean up their act' (Baraté and Temmerman 2009: 234).

Example

Exemplifying the association between political (in)activity and maternal death, eclampsia is a condition peculiar to childbearing, featuring potentially fatal maternal convulsions. In the United Kingdom the number of deaths due to eclampsia or pre-eclampsia has been stable for two decades with 19 women having died between 2005 and 2008 (Lewis 2011a). Of the 50,000 women dying worldwide every year from eclampsia, 99 per cent die in low- and middle-income countries (Aaserud et al 2005). The Magpie trial (2002), however, established that magnesium sulphate is the appropriate treatment, in preference to anticonvulsants (Duley et al 2008). Although this information has been widely disseminated, the efficacy of this safe and disconcertingly cheap remedy has yet to impact on maternal mortality in low-income countries. The study of this problem recognised explicitly the crucial role of politics and politicians (Aaserud et al 2005). The authors reached the heartrending conclusion that policy-makers need more than information if practice is to change. Morten Aaserud and his colleagues argued that international organisations must become advocates by encouraging colleagues to implement research findings. The response was tragically unsurprising:

> efforts made ... to persuade the President of the International Federation of Obstetricians and Gynaecologists that he and the organisation had potentially important roles in promoting the uptake of magnesium sulphate met with reluctance for himself or his organisation to interfere in the clinical freedom of individual clinicians.
>
> (Chalmers, personal communication 2005)

Attempted remedies

As well as the relatively ineffective MDG Five (page 82), other initiatives have been introduced to address the plague of maternal mortality. The Safe Motherhood Initiative builds on the work of the Safe Motherhood Inter-Agency Group (IAG 2010). While the rhetoric is comprehensive, including equity, poverty reduction and human rights, the reality seeks to address more detailed and mundane activities.

The White Ribbon Alliance is a US-based organisation claiming to be a global movement for whom Sarah Brown is global patron. The website emphasises a health or even medical orientation, focusing on complications and family planning, without mentioning safe abortion (WRA 2012). This organisation presents maternal mortality figures, but the dire US figures, a rate wedged between Moldova's and Bahrain's, are difficult to locate.

Summary

Maternal mortality has for far too long been regarded as a women's health issue and attempts to remedy the predicament have featured only medical treatments. Maternal mortality needs to be recognised as a political issue requiring political solutions. This observation is endorsed by the comments of Mahmoud Fathalla who stated that women 'are dying because the societies in which they live did not see fit to invest what is needed to save their lives' (Fathalla 2006: 414).

Morbidity

While maternal mortality, despite being an absolute, is not easily quantified (page 82), morbidity is even more difficult to measure. But some conditions, such as vesico-vaginal or obstetric fistula, have attracted considerable attention (Hamlin 2009). This physically debilitating condition follows obstructed labour and constitutes a social death sentence, due to constant dribbling incontinence of urine.

The repair of obstetric fistula is developing into a growth industry in countries such as Tanzania, as evidenced by the finding of 8,830 hits when 'obstetric fistula repair' was put into a search engine. While surgical repair of fistula is relatively cheap and successful, the woman's social rehabilitation is more challenging. Maggie Bangser and her colleagues report that fistula repair services are being developed widely, but are less sanguine about the prevention of fistula (Bangser 2011). Like maternal mortality, fistula prevention requires political action to ensure accessible maternity care.

Neonatal politics

Of particular significance in low-income countries, infant feeding has become a universal political issue. This was originally due to marketing activities of formula manufacturers, such as Nestlé (Rundall 1996: 63), resulting in 'commerciogenic malnutrition' (Jelliffe 1972). The formula industry, unsurprisingly, resisted threats to its profits from exposure of its unethical marketing practices (Palmer 1993). In 1981 the International code of Marketing of Breast-milk Substitutes was drawn up, with the only opposing country being the United States (WHO 1981). National codes and legislation were developed to operationalise the International Code, although new products and marketing techniques have been introduced to circumvent regulations which are widely regarded as irrelevant (Watson and Mander 1995).

Another initiative, which may not have alienated breastfeeding promotion among some, is the Baby Friendly Initiative (BFI). Conceived in 1992 as the Baby Friendly Hospital Initiative, the BFI aims to remove or reduce systematic interventions likely to impede the establishment of breastfeeding (UNICEF 2012). While it is my observation that women interpret 'baby friendliness' as a panacea, the reality of this initiative may deliver somewhat less than the rhetoric (Ogunlesi et al 2005). The implementation of the BFI has tended to be somewhat less than woman-friendly (Mander 2008a). The 'traditional top-down' approaches (Thomson et al 2011) are proving less than completely effective and Gill Thomson and her colleagues are endeavouring to identify more appropriate strategies. While the BFI is potentially hugely significant in low-income countries because of the limited possibility of even a relatively safe alternative to breastfeeding, its relevance to more developed countries is questionable.

Conclusion

In this chapter I have discussed the many wide-ranging political issues which impinge on childbearing women in low-income countries. It is crucial to bear in mind, though, that these issues are in no way peculiar to the third world. For various reasons, many of these issues emerge as significant in more economically developed countries as well.

5   Politics of practice philosophies

Midwifery is but one of many occupational groups which regards itself as a practice-based discipline. Far from being demeaning, such a claim is more a badge of honour, as this means that practitioners firmly grounded in the real world share it with those for whom they provide care. Particularly significantly, such firm grounding constitutes an outstandingly strong basis for the theoretical knowledge on which care may be based. This point is emphasised in the crucial distinction which Ros Bryar and Marlene Sinclair make between theory which midwives actually use and that which is merely 'espoused' (Bryar and Sinclair 2011: 38).

The question which inevitably arises, though, out of such respect for theory, is the relationship between practice and knowledge. While knowledge must precede practice, the relationship develops as a virtuous and escalating cycle; the factors affecting that escalation, however, deserve attention. This is because out of practice, not just knowledge but *knowledges* are enhanced. These differing knowledges (page 16) give rise to tension and conflict between different disciplines, practitioners and the childbearing woman. Such disharmony may be comparable with the 'astutely contriving, manoeuvring or intriguing' characteristics of politics (Macdonald 1977: 1036; page 5), which emerge through the discussion in this chapter.

These various knowledges are likely to manifest themselves in the variety of practice philosophies, and their theoretical origins demand consideration. This is because some knowledge or approaches to the care of the childbearing woman have been accepted, implemented and even enforced by more powerful groups, on the basis of what all too often proves to be flimsy or non-existent foundations. Other approaches to care, which tend to be less interventive, have been less successful in their acceptance and implementation.

In this chapter, I begin by considering some of the factors which influence the acceptance of practice philosophies. I then move on to examine those which prove to be closely inter-related and which have achieved wider acceptance, followed by those philosophies which have been less widely and less favourably welcomed.

Factors influencing acceptability and acceptance

The extent to which a philosophy encounters a positive reception is affected by a range of more or less substantial factors, as well as a degree of serendipity or timeliness.

Intangible factors

Intangible factors include the general system of beliefs or specific culture into which the ideology is introduced (Gaines and Davis-Floyd 2004) and whether the new approach accords with the existing *milieu*. Clearly the *status quo* is not easily quantified, being affected by perceptions of traditional ways of doing things (Gaines and Davis-Floyd 2004) and ideas about quality (Christiaens et al 2008); although the latter are far from static, being dynamically linked to rising expectations. Traditional activities, verging on the routine or ritual, lend security in an uncertain environment; these, in turn, may lead to questionable practices, eg routine hospital admission, being perpetuated (Gaines and Davis-Floyd 2004).

Such intangible factors may be associated with deeply- and firmly-held beliefs, which give rise to impressions of integration, wholeness and wholesomeness. Approximating to 'gut feelings' and similar to intuition, these impressions have been shown to feature in assessments which are commonly used, and which may incorporate the objectification of the 'subject', as opposed to the more human, humane and person-friendly 'sensing' of what is happening (Blaaka and Eri 2008).

Aspirational factors

Aspirational factors influencing the approval of new ideas include their association with sought-after phenomena, such as progress (Blaaka and Eri 2008), to which the advent and increasing reliance on technology may be attributable. Similarly, science, which Atwood Gaines and Robbie Davis-Floyd define as 'a cultural construct' (Gaines and Davis-Floyd 2004: 97), is regarded as highly desirable. Biomedicine, however, may be little more than '"just another ethno-medical" system, one that, like all others, reflects the values and norms of its creators' (Gaines and Davis-Floyd 2004: 96). Not unrelated are the interventions intended to improve the efficacy of care. Aspirations to control bodily functions, normally outwith human control, may be perceived as solutions to problems inherent in female physiology, regarding it as less than perfect to the point of defectiveness (Walsh 2010). Such interventions have overstepped the mark, by moving on from the person-friendliness of nearness or proximity into the realm of invasiveness (Blaaka and Eri 2008).

Interactional factors

Interactional factors relate to the location of agency in introducing a philosophy through vested interests taking advantage of social conditions to increase their individual or organisational control; although the recognition of social structures may lead to these notions of control being presented in guises such as 'informed choice' (Walsh 2010). Such control-related concepts are derived from Michel Foucault's ideas on 'the gaze' or surveillance and have produced hierarchical relationships featuring conformity, docility and compliance (Foucault 1973). Ideologies to control practitioners are likely to take the form of guidelines or rules for action (Gaines and Davis-Floyd 2004). Considered helpful and beneficial by some, these imperatives inevitably relocate control and power with the rule-making, rather than the rule-following, group. This ideological domination serves to negate any concept of equality, democracy or balance in collegial or clinical interactions (Blaaka and Eri 2008).

Status–related factors

Status-related factors occur in hierarchical situations in which the position of users, clients or patients renders them less powerful, eg people with mental health problems, those whose behaviour is considered deviant, children and women. The effects of these factors is only exacerbated by the gender, or gendered approach, of practitioners (Gaines and Davis-Floyd 2004). A construct which has been created to enhance these factors, and which I discuss below, is risk (Blaaka and Eri 2008). For these status-related factors to affect the acceptance of ideas, though, a certain level of sensitivity and perceptiveness is necessary. If the ideas are introduced in the absence of such human understanding, the acceptance of new ideologies will be enforced, irrespective of conflict arising (Blaaka and Eri 2008). Thus, once again, the role of power in introducing initiatives and innovations becomes clearly apparent (Gaines and Davis-Floyd 2004).

Status has also been shown to have less direct effects on the acceptance of ideas. Status may be enhanced by the development and exploitation of fear of dire consequences arising out of failure to comply (DeVries 1996). Drawing on the classical professions as examples, Raymond De Vries recounts how they have historically legitimated their authority by instilling fear of the results of non-compliance. De Vries then reflects on the implications for the midwife's professional status of her failure to employ such tactics.

Widely-accepted practice philosophies

For a variety of reasons, some of which I have discussed already, certain philosophies of practice have gained broad recognition and acceptance.

Evidence-based practice

Ulla Waldenström, being uncharacteristically Pollyannaish, has asserted that evidence-based practice (EBP) carries the potential to increase the occurrence of normal birth (Waldenström 2007). Despite this assertion, EBP is most fervently espoused by those with least, if any, interest in normality (see below).

The emergence of EBP was stimulated by Archie Cochrane's observations, of the lack of scientific rigour in medical clinical decision-making (Cochrane 1972). He singled out obstetricians for withering criticism as the worst offenders. A group of obstetricians, with other maternity practitioners, reacted to Cochrane's scathing condemnation by attempting to redress the situation (Chalmers et al 1989). In order to create an evidence base for practitioners lacking opportunity, ability or inclination to search and evaluate the literature, this Collaboration began reviewing research systematically, resulting in the development of the Cochrane Database. Characterised as a 'mode of thought' (Wall 2008: 37), EBP has become regarded as a philosophy; from its earliest days it was intended to provide a theoretical basis for decisions, being defined as:

> the conscientious, explicit and judicious use of current best evidence in making decisions about the care of individual patients.
>
> (Sackett et al 1996: 71)

The ready acceptance of EBP has been criticised as due to occupational groups being 'unable or unwilling to question the assumptions behind the EBP movement' (Wall 2008: 38); although there may also be an element of avoiding exclusion, reminiscent of tents and urinary function. This inability or reluctance to question has been overcome to some extent, particularly admirably by nurses (Mitchell 1997) who have reacted against EBP's 'medical origins' (Chapman 2012: 36). Midwifery has responded disappointingly variably. Some researchers have encouraged practitioners to more actively accept EBP, after establishing midwives' limited understanding and uninformed reluctance to follow guidelines (Bogdan-Lovis and Sousa 2006). Other researchers have recommended practitioners to reinvent EBP in a more woman-friendly format (Munro and Spiby 2010). Lesley Page has condemned what she perceived to be a midwifery 'backlash' against all the benefits of 'evidence-based care' (Page 1996: 191), emphasising that midwives should, as always, focus on their contribution at the start of 'family life' (Page 1996: 192). Such encouragement, recommendation and condemnation reflect the top-down imposition of EBP ideology on midwives, with little consideration of how EBP conforms to their longstanding knowledge-base.

The knowledge on which midwives have long drawn differs in many ways from EBP and from obstetricians' knowledge. It is, for example, broader than EBP, not being confined to evidence produced by RCTs (Edwards 2005a: 154). It is further different in its origins, not seeking the 'scientific' or 'objective' credentials, so prized by EBP devotees. Mary Belenky and her colleagues proudly hail this form of knowledge as 'subjective' (Belenky et al 1997: 88), being founded not on relying on what others have said, written or found, but on women's personal experience and deeply-held convictions. Obviously, because of its fundamental humanity, such knowledge is more significant in midwifery than other 'caring professions'. It is likely, though, that such knowledge has been devalued by the high status often attached to 'scientific' knowledge in general and to EBP in particular. Thus, a hierarchy of knowledges is operating, with the most highly esteemed being determined by the orientation of the viewer, and others being discounted or disregarded.

The limited congruence between women's and midwives' ways of knowing and EBP has given rise to suspicions of 'exclusionary organizational behaviour' (Wall 2008: 43); this comprises a game of constantly changing rules in which complex human encounters are changed on the whim of a systematic reviewer. In this way the EBP movement seeks to proselytise by marginalising any non-evidence based forms of knowledge and ensure medicine and medical knowledge remain supreme in the health knowledge hierarchy. Adherence to the EBP regime is policed by surveillance techniques (Denny 1999: 254) which, in mid-wifery, are monitored by devices such as the partograph and cardiotocograph. The institutionalisation of care is taken for granted, in the same way as hospital birth has become the cultural norm in developed countries.

Thus, the introduction and widespread enforcement of EBP demonstrates the all too familiar link between power and knowledge. The provision of health care has become systematically organised according to rules drawn up and patrolled by the dominant occupational group; this preserves the superiority of their knowledge and, hence, their powerful position. In this way other occupational groups find themselves marginalised, and their care reduced to the level of Tayloristic automatons, slavishly succumbing to the EBP diktat (Chapman 2012: 39).

Example: Continuous Electronic Fetal Monitoring (CEFM)

Introduced shortly before EBP, CEFM constitutes an excellent example of its relevance and application. The enthusiasm with which CEFM was implemented is demonstrated by Jo Garcia and Sally Garforth (1989), whose authoritative data established that almost 40 per cent of maternity units had policies of 'more than half' of labouring women being monitored using CEFM (Garcia and Garforth 1989: 158). Identifying the variability of policies, Garcia and Garforth went on to show the large majority of consultant-led units with policies requiring all women in labour to be subjected to CEFM (Garcia and Garforth 1989: 160). The implications of these policies emerge in the work of Robbie Davis-Floyd, who has argued the role of CEFM in transforming the culture of birth into one of not trusting the woman's body to function without the cardiotocograph (CTG; Davis-Floyd 1990: 184). Similarly, women have come to believe that, without the 'support' of the CTG, the baby's heart might actually stop beating (Davis-Floyd 1990: 180).

These policies and beliefs have happened despite longstanding persuasive research showing that CEFM improves outcomes for neither woman nor baby (Haverkamp et al 1976). These outcomes included maternal pain, caesarean birth, neonatal well-being and neonatal convulsions. Twelve subsequent randomised controlled trials have endorsed these original findings (Alfirevic et al 2006). Despite this accumulation of authoritative research, CEFM has become 'a routine part of care during labour' (Alfirevic et al 2006: 2).

This observation clearly shows that research evidence is not being used as the basis of practice. Midwives believe that they are using EBP when they perceive that they are more likely to employ intermittent monitoring by Pinnards or a hand-held electronic device; this perception is not supported by survey data (Mead 2004: 75). This means that midwives regard themselves as rejecting the medically-imposed requirement to implement CEFM. But Marianne Mead suggests that midwives are both neglecting midwifery skills and following medical preference for non-evidence based practice.

Medicalisation

Having already addressed the professional issues associated with the medicalisation of childbearing (page 54) and the way that organised medicine seized power from midwives, I now concentrate on the philosophy of medicalisation and its implications for practice. Eliot Freidson's classic work focused on medicalisation as the mission of medical professionals to assume control over many aspects of society (Freidson 1970). The medical fraternity was shown to be assuming power by redefining health and illness and taking control of any condition considered to justify the 'ill health' label. It may be that this process constitutes part of a general change, resulting in 'bureaucratisation' and 'technicalisation' of life. These processes have augmented the power of the specialist, as lesser mortals become dependent on experts. George Lowis and Peter McCaffery outline the escalation of specialists' power, of which medicine is a supreme example (Lowis and McCaffery 1999: 26). The process of medicalisation of childbearing has been facilitated by technological developments, use of an elite language or jargon, problematisation of healthy childbearing, assumption of control of all aspects of childbearing and masculinisation of obstetrics. These processes not only enhance medical practitioners' status, but they also persuade people in general and childbearing women in particular of the need for the input of these self-styled experts.

The philosophy of medicalisation has built on the concept of control, with the assistance of technological developments, such as instruments, monitoring devices and drugs. Perceptions that success in childbearing was attributable to such interventions not only improved the image of the experts who relied on them, it also demeaned the standing of other practitioners, such as midwives, who were prohibited from using them (Lowis and McCaffery 1999: 26). Medicalisation as a philosophy has taken advantage, in the United Kingdom, of the introduction of the NHS to transfer childbirth from the domestic sphere, with its social orientation, to the disease-focused hospital. This transfer confirmed the developing idea that childbirth is, if not an illness, at least risky. Robert Percival's aphorism that birth is 'only normal in retrospect' (Percival 1970) reflected this development and was employed to justify a panoply of medical interventions. The concept of 'risk' (page 96) was introduced and used to further vindicate the philosophy of medicalisation.

The transformation of birth into a mechanical process by medicalisation has brought with it the requirement for control by monitoring and new technologies (Lee and Kirkman 2008: 458). This transformation follows the pathologisation of the childbearing body. Medicalisation has been enhanced by views of the childbearing woman as merely a collection of parts, each requiring attention from a different specialist, to whom the concept of holism is an anathema. Feminists argue that such dismemberment results from the medical perception of the male body as ideal, making the female body deviant and the pregnant body potentially pathologically substandard (Lee and Kirkman 2008: 459).

By transferring birth into institutions and, thereby, redefining it as an 'illness', medicalisation has also transferred control over birthing from the female midwife to the male, or male-oriented, obstetrician. This 'displacement' of the midwife brought an entirely different view of childbearing, which was claimed to be 'scientific', and was probably responsible for medicalisation being accepted not unwillingly by consumers (Lowis and McCaffery 1999: 29).

Reports, issuing forth since the 1970s (Fox 1977), of the decline of medicalisation appear to be greatly exaggerated. The excesses of medicalisation have persisted and may be increasing (see 'caesarean' below). UK authors have related medicalisation to a 'name and blame' culture (Johanson et al 2002: 894) and suggested reversal of the process by changing the philosophy of the NHS. These authors' suggestion that team working will halt medicalisation reflects naïve wishful thinking, bearing no relation to the real world of healthcare politics.

Example 1: Active management of labour

I have considered professional aspects of active management previously (page 55), but the concept is being used here to exemplify certain features of the philosophy of medicalisation. Originating in Dublin, allegedly to remedy the woman's experience of prolonged labour, active management included three essential elements (see below; O'Driscoll et al 1969). These elements comprise interventions to actively control the woman's labour, as opposed to the more traditional caring watchfulness. While Fredric Frigoletto regards such conventional care as 'passive' (Frigoletto 2007), in active management the woman must be passively compliant; this is indicated by childbirth education ensuring that 'women will understand the process that awaits them once labor begins' (Frigoletto 2007). Active management may not remain true to its original tenets but, regardless of how these interventions have evolved, they continue to be known by the original name.

Criticisms of active management, as of the medicalisation which it represents, are legion and its defenders have worked long and hard to counter them. A significant criticism, which applies to many aspects of medicalisation, as well as of health care in general, is that it fails to address fundamental problems, focusing instead on symptoms. This critique is explained in Nadine Edwards's astute observation that the problems of childbearing, such as prolonged labour, are more appropriately approached by addressing 'material and social poverty' (Edwards 2005a: 82) than by employing active management and similar obstetric technological interventions.

Although not one of the original three elements, the *continuing presence* of one formal carer has assumed particular significance in marketing active management as a panacea for the caesarean 'epidemic' (Mander 2007). While Neil Pembroke and Janelle Pembroke consider the spiritual value of the presence of the midwife to the woman in labour as having the potential to contribute significantly to a positive birth experience, they also note that an absent midwife has the reverse effect. Similarly, but on a more practical level, good support is well-known to reduce the woman's need for pharmacological analgesia (Mander 2001).

The presence entailed in active management, though, is qualitatively different. The attendant, who is required to be a continuing presence during labour, is likely to be a student, rather than a qualified staff member. This, probably unqualified, attendant is obliged to not only provide emotional support and complete clinical observations and care, but also maintain constant eye contact. The originators believed that the woman closing her eyes is of profound significance, indicating, they maintained, a tendency to introspection, the onset of panic and 'the first step along the road to total disintegration' (O'Driscoll et al 1993: 93). The required continuing attention thus aims to prevent such a downward spiral. The availability of sufficient personnel to guarantee such presence in Dublin is facilitated by the unit policy of active, possibly aggressive, management of labour.

Thus, in active management, rather than offering social support, the presence of the attendant aims to control the woman's behaviour, as a guard or prison officer would monitor a criminal to prevent, for example, self-harm. Nadine Edwards elucidates this aspect of 'support', when she avers that it is continuous in order to ensure that the woman complies with what is being done to her. The constant presence of the attendant aims to retain control of the woman to enhance her self-control. Edwards goes on to discuss how this level of control over the woman is exercised at the cost to the woman of her being in touch with her own knowledge, her own body and its functioning. Thus, active management alienates the childbearing woman from her longstanding resources and coping strategies, leaving her particularly vulnerable to any trauma which may befall her.

Active management, as directly and indirectly indicated already, comprises *control* of the woman's labour being removed from her or her body and being assumed by those attending her (Frigoletto 2007). Such control begins with accurately diagnosing labour together with time of onset, which is not permitted to precede admission. Control continues with constant monitoring of the maternal and foetal condition and, particularly, progress of the labour as recorded on the partograph. The third and possibly most contentious element of control is the prompt intervention, using oxytocin and/or amniotomy, to augment or accelerate a labour in which progress is deemed sub-optimal (Frigoletto 2007). This confiscation of control from the woman contrasts with a conventional labour, when a woman chooses, first, how much control she will exercise and, secondly, if and when she wishes to relinquish it (Larkin et al 2009).

The diminution or removal of the childbearing woman's control through the imposition of active management has downgraded her to a passenger in the birthing process (Baker et al 2005). The prevailing philosophy of medicalisation has been combined with an obsession with pathology by paternalistic obstetricians whose technology fuels fetocentrism. Sarah Baker and her colleagues found that the woman's lack of control during labour was associated with poor communication by staff relative, mainly, to the 'minor' interventions, such as induction or episiotomy (Baker 2005: 332). Baker and her colleagues argue that the woman's fears and anxieties about what is being done to her are aggravated by the absence of discussion or explanation and these, in turn, compound her feelings of being in an uncontrollable downward spiral. The continuation of such negative feelings has been explored by Nordic researchers who interviewed women two to 20 years later; Ingela Lundgren and her colleagues identified some women's recollections of empowerment, but others reported continuing feelings of 'failure and mistrust' (Lundgren et al 2009: 125) demonstrated in their vivid accounts of their birthing experiences.

Example 2: The caesarean

As an unwelcome but illuminating example of the philosophy of medicalisation, caesarean requires further attention after I considered its third world role (page 80). Characterised as the 'ultimate rescue operation' (Mander 2007: 8), the caesarean debate has focused on the disadvantages of emergency caesarean compared with elective surgery. Data now suggest, however, that even the advantages of elective caesarean have been overstated due to, for example, neonatal morbidity from iatrogenic prematurity (Davis-Floyd et al 2009) and maternal mortality/morbidity due to subsequent abnormal placental development (Hemminki and Merilainen 1996).

Feminists attribute the links between medicalisation and caesarean to medical men's perception of the female body's imperfect nature and functioning (Lee and Kirkman 2008: 460); a perception which constituted the *raison d'être* for obstetrics' existence. Professional power has been demonstrated and reinforced by interventions, such as caesarean, serving as 'ritual acts used to de-sex birth and turn it into a medical process' (Sheila Kitzinger 2005: 2). Unsurprisingly, feminists have argued the treacherous nature of medicine (Lee and Kirkman 2008: 450), and the control exerted by medicalisation being more associated with ideological claims than any benefit to the childbearing woman. Such arguments are only supported by caesarean's morbidity and mortality rates (Mander 2007).

Globally, caesarean exemplifies medicalisation in the way that the operation is *endorsed* or 'sold' by medical practitioners to childbearing women. The effects of such endorsement on caesarean decision-making are clearly apparent in the 'caesarean epidemic' (Teakle 2004). Perhaps based on their own limited experience of uncomplicated birth, medical practitioners represent childbirth as unpredictable, hazardous and risky. To medical people this sad scenario requires them to take control, by performing more caesareans. Amy Lee and Maggie

Kirkman, rehearsing this discourse, show its use to justify the medicalisation of *all* birth, not just medical involvement in 'complicated' births (Lee and Kirkman 2008: 454).

At the same time as arguing this justification, Lee and Kirkman show that women's choice of caesarean is portrayed by medical practitioners as being 'in spite of medical advice' (Lee and Kirkman 2008: 454–55). The medical rhetoric portrays women as foolish, in that they give trivial reasons for choosing caesarean, rather than accepting that medical advisers know best. The medical argument continues by suggesting that women have become 'consumers', rather than patients, positioning them more strongly to 'demand' interventions like caesarean despite medical advice. This results in the self-portrayal by medical practitioners of themselves as servants, rather than manipulators, of the caesarean market. Such a heart-rending depiction is only enhanced by claims of pressure of medical litigation.

The midwifery response to such medical politicking is underpinned by accusations of medical paternalism (Lee and Kirkman 2008: 456), materialising as charges of bullying. Such allegations are closely linked to the institutionalisation of birth, limitation of midwifery practice and diminution of women's choice through medicalisation.

The rationality of fear of childbearing has long been recognised (Hofberg and Ward 2007), but *tocophobia* (or tokophobia) has only relatively recently been identified and defined as 'an unreasoning dread of childbirth' which is 'so intense that childbirth is avoided whenever possible' (Hofberg and Brockington 2000: 83). Tocophobia as a rationale for caesarean in the absence of other indications has been raised as a matter of concern (Leeman 2005). It is possible that a morbid and incapacitating fear of childbirth is all too real for a few women, but that this diagnosis may be used by both women and their attendants to justify unnecessary caesareans is a genuine possibility. The question of where 'blame' lies for this sorry state has been raised by Gian Carlo Di Renzo, who has astutely identified an alliance between the pregnant woman seeking to avoid 'nature's obligations' and the

> condescending obstetrician [evading attending] a labour while gaining more income and at the same time giving his patient the illusion of happiness.
>
> (Di Renzo 2003: 217)

Clearly, the politics of tocophobia and whether this term is merely an excuse for further medicalisation of birth urgently needs attention.

Decision-making in the context of caesarean is dynamic, being affected by a range of personal, professional, social and political phenomena. Despite allegedly 'absolute' indications being widely regarded as non-negotiable, the threshold for caesarean, like those operations which are performed for relative indications, is being lowered (Mander 2007). The politics of technological and professional influences on caesarean decision-making also need to be taken into consideration. The culture of both the institution and the society in which the woman gives birth affect the caesarean decision, which is associated with medical power being greatest where midwives are most marginalised (Wagner 2000). Decision-making power in the maternity setting, through the imposition of medicalisation, may resort to the rhetoric of choice, but such choice is little more than illusory, with lip service featuring prominently (Beech 2003). The politics of maternal choice are most eloquently illustrated by the debate around caesarean on request or 'demand'.

The widespread perception of the indication for increasing numbers of caesareans being *maternal request* is difficult to substantiate, despite being pre-valent in both popular and professional media (Arthur and Payne 2005: 17). Diony Young has referred to the misuse of data to support this perception as 'unadulterated fraud' (Young 2006: 171). The complexity of caesarean decision-making (see above) prevents the precise and accurate location of the decision; the party seeking to improve their caesarean credentials locates the decision with the other negotiating party (Lee and Kirkman 2008). Thus, obstetricians report a high rate of such requests, in contrast to childbearing women (Anderson 2006), but authoritative sources conclude that 'there are no credible data on the extent' of caesareans for maternal request (Bourgeault et al 2008: 106).

The perception of increasing maternal requests or demands for caesarean has been used to demean women's decision-making, by attributing such requests to other 'problems' being exaggerated, such as urinary leakage or sexual dis-satisfaction. According to Ivy Bourgeault and her colleagues, maternal request has also been reinterpreted as exemplifying obstetricians' respect for the childbearing woman's right to choose her mode of birth (Bourgeault et al 2008: 108). This international team of sociologists found that 'pressuring', 'prompting', 'advising' or 'offering' leads to the conclusion that maternal request is all too often physician-controlled (Bourgeault et al 2008: 113). These observations are sup-ported by Jennifer Fenwick and her colleagues in Australia, who found that obstetricians encouraged and reinforced women's tentative enquiries about caesarean (Fenwick et al 2010: 399). It is not impossible that maternal request for caesarean is most likely in commercially-oriented healthcare systems, where vested interests undermine women's confidence in their ability to give birth physiologically and endorse the philosophy of medicalisation.

Thus, caesarean 'epitomises' the philosophy of medicalisation of childbirth (Murphy 2010: 4). But this philosophy has been taken to new heights, affecting not only the birth itself but also birth decision-making. This has resulted in caesareans having been reclassified as unsafe, unless deemed to be safe by a medical practitioner (Lee and Kirkman 2008: 255). Such categorisation resonates powerfully with the findings of Meredith McIntyre and her colleagues who use caesarean to exemplify the problems associated with risk and its management (McIntyre et al 2011).

Risk

Always regarded as fact of life, risk has been converted into an unacceptable aspect of modern living (Jordan and Murphy 2009) which is an 'avoidable commodity' (Skinner 2008: 53). Lindsay Reid considers that the philosophy of risk-avoidance has seriously influenced midwifery since the original legislation (Reid 2011b: 221), when law-makers sought to protect women and babies from risk of exposure to unqualified practitioners. As Jennifer Hall and Meg Taylor reflect, though, women have long recognised the risks of childbirth (Hall and Taylor 2004: 47). Realising that birth may threaten that which an individual values is fundamentally important, not only for the woman, but also for those attending her. This realisation leads that individual to develop a trust in an agency which reduces the threat, be it their innate resources, a higher power, a particular practitioner or place of birth, or interventive techniques. Thus, as well as spontaneously-occurring risk (and safety) being perceived differently by actors in the childbearing scenario, remedies also differ.

While the risk culture appears to dominate, risk and safety are sometimes helpfully regarded as binary opposites; as shown by Ulrich Beck, fatalism and compensation have been replaced with risk and prevention (Beck 1992). Such polarity also emerges in the risk orientation of the medical model, unlike the social or midwifery model which focuses on assumptions that all is well until if and when 'something goes wrong' (MacKenzie Bryers and van Teijlingen 2010: 491).

Since the original legislators acquiesced to the philosophy of risk, the mushrooming of information systems for monitoring has elevated perceptions of risk to previously unknown levels (MacKenzie Bryers and van Teijlingen 2010; Beck 1992). Such techno-rational information systems are capable of increasing awareness of absolute risk (Skinner 2005), which comprises data on life activities, such as childbearing. These data present simplistic depictions of the effects of complex phenomena, such as place of birth, time of birth or the woman's Body Mass Index (BMI) (Sandall et al 2010). The reluctance or inability of many practitioners to interrogate the data results in acceptance of experts' interpretation of the desirability of hospital birth, advantages of 9–5 obstetrics and dangers of maternal overweight, respectively. Thus, perceptions of birth as risky are confirmed and enhanced and medicalisation, in the alleged interests of reducing risk and increasing safety, is embraced.

While absolute risk has been shown to play a significant role in the planning of maternity services, the effects of socio-cultural influences are ignored (MacKenzie Bryers and van Teijlingen 2010: 490). This is because these influences are difficult or impossible to quantify, comprising shared beliefs and values, concerning socially acceptable or tolerable risk. The post-modern view of risk denies the inherent riskiness of specific phenomena, attributing perceptions of risk to historical artefacts determined by socio-political influences (Skinner 2005: 26). Thus, in view of these differing meanings of risk, it may be that medicalisation has hijacked the risk philosophy, by taking advantage of what may be popular innumeracy, to assume control of childbearing that would otherwise be physiological.

The post-modern view of risk has been advanced by Nadine Edwards in the context of planning homebirth (Edwards 2005a). She explores the political nature of the global infiltration of risk into all aspects of living and, through requiring self-management and self-control, its tendency to inculcate passivity and submissiveness. Edwards advances her political analysis of risk to consider the neoliberal implications of a decreasing proportion of the population controlling an increasing share of world resources (Edwards 2008a). The transformation of health care in general and maternity care in particular into marketable commodities has undermined the role of the midwife, due to her focus on care, skill and making time available, which are anathema to organisations managing health services. Edwards argues persuasively that the debates around birth will be better understood when the midwifery philosophy of safety replaces the currently pervasive philosophy of risk.

It has been suggested that medical professionals have appropriated the risk philosophy to ensure their continuing domination of maternity services (MacKenzie Bryers and van Teijlingen 2010: 492). It may be, though, that midwives are not completely blameless in this respect, having employed the same philosophy in clinical encounters to preserve the hierarchical relationship between themselves and childbearing women (DeVries 1996). Medical practitioners have also been shown to draw on the philosophy of risk in individual clinical contacts. Sheila Kitzinger has identified how this philosophy may be used, not only to magnify the dangers inherent in a situation, but to actually 'construct' and 'assemble' (Kitzinger 2005: 81) such dangers in situations when, in reality, there is no risk to the woman or baby. Kitzinger further suggests that such fabrication is not unknown in persuading a woman 'into agreeing to, or better still, choosing an elective caesarean' (Kitzinger 2005: 81; page 91).

The assumption that has been made so far in this discussion of risk, and generally in the literature, is that 'risk' refers only to the possibility of adverse clinical outcomes for the woman and baby. It is necessary to mention the possibility and the political implications of other forms of risk operating in the maternity area. Reflecting that power is the common denominator in any situation in which risk is used as the rationale for refusing choice to women, Mavis Kirkham suggests that a 'perceived risk to their service' (Kirkham 2004: 271) is operating. Risks to the practitioner are likely to be closely linked to risk to the mother and baby, as Joan Skinner has identified (Skinner 2005: 55), but this is not inevitably so. A perception of risk by certain practitioners may be transferred to another discipline, as is the case with general practitioners who are reluctant to attend a home birth, resulting in conflict with women and midwives (Edwards 2005a).

Example: Risk assessment

Although the link between risk and harm appears to be clearly that this philosophy is intended to prevent avoidable harm, the real picture may be neither clear nor benign. The concept of iatrogenesis has been shown to be related to the philosophy of risk (Skinner 2008) and, more precisely, to risk assessment. Surveillance processes reduce the woman's self-confidence in her ability to give birth physiologically, which in turn affects her bodily functioning and makes the risk assessment a self-fulfilling prophecy. Research by Katja Stahl and Vanora Hundley in Germany examined the implications of risk assessment and categorisation of the woman into an 'at risk' group (Stahl and Hundley 2003). While recognising the good intentions of risk assessment, these researchers found that the large proportion of women labelled as 'high risk', were so categorised for relatively benign conditions. Most of these conditions, such as being aged below 18 years, would not have attracted the high risk label in other countries. The obstetricians who completed these assessments had minimal contact with the women, which resulted in the assessments often being incomplete and/or incorrect. Studying the effects on the woman's psychosocial state, Stahl and Hundley found that the correlation between 'at risk' labelling and poor childbirth outcome was weak to the point of not existing. The intention to benefit the woman and her baby is clearly not being fulfilled and the effect of labelling the woman was perceived as blaming and disempowering. Thus, such risk assessment was shown to have iatrogenic effects, as endorsed by Jane Sandall and her colleagues in their insightful probing of the political nature of the risk agenda in childbirth (Sandall et al 2010).

Less widely-accepted philosophies

The reasons for certain philosophies of practice being less widely-welcomed and implemented relate partly to the factors mentioned on page 87. Other factors influencing their acceptance emerge out of the discussion.

Normality

The philosophy of 'normality', or 'normalcy' in North America (Davis 2010), has introduced a fresh way of thinking about childbearing in general and labour in particular (Reid 2011b: 204). As well as such benefits, it has also introduced consternation about what it does or does not include (Young 2009).

Background

Normality has an interesting relationship with its spiritual predecessor 'natural childbirth', a term coined by Grantly Dick-Read in his 1933 publication (Moscucci 2003). Natural childbirth employed eugenic ideals to encourage a childbearing approach which constituted a backlash against the excesses of the interventive obstetrics then fashionable and introduced by Joseph B De Lee. To begin with, natural childbirth was any form of childbirth falling short of the full panoply of obstetric and anaesthetic interventions. Although 'natural' currently carries highly positive connotations, Steen Wackerhausen, a Danish philosopher, recounts that was not always so (Wackerhausen 1999). 'Natural' has been regarded as regressive and, in the 1950s, 'artificial' was considered more positively, indicating a forward thinking and scientific approach. Wackerhausen further defines natural as lacking 'human interference' (Wackerhausen 1999: 1109), a definition which proves useful in determining what is normal.

The concepts of normal and abnormal were introduced to midwives by the Midwives Act of 1902; through this legislation, medical practitioners assumed control over midwifery practice by limiting it to cases in which they had no interest, envisaged no financial gain and, hence, labelled normal (page 10). Throughout the twentieth century, though, some practices were moved from being part of the midwifery role to be subsumed into the 'abnormal' category, including assisted breech birth and multiple birth. Other practices, however, formerly considered abnormal and hence medical, were redefined and off-loaded onto the midwife, such as episiotomy under local anaesthetic, perineal repair, epidural analgesia top-up, ultrasound examination, and assisted birth using Ventouse (vacuum extraction).

Defining normal

These movements demonstrate that the definition of normality is in no way static, responding as it does to changing medical agendas. Perhaps because of such dynamism, this definition has attracted considerable attention and discussion. In her concept, analysis of 'normal labour', Debby Gould (2000) sought to clarify this Alice in Wonderland word and identified six distinct ways in which the term could be used:

(1) In statistical terms normality indicates that occurring most frequently. This definition disregards the woman's experience and the midwife's role, reflecting an environment of routinisation of birth.
(2) 'Upright' is the second interpretation, which Gould links to the woman's posture in physiological labour.
(3) 'Healthy' is a synonym for normal. This term is unhelpful because every birth should be maintained within the bounds of good health; however the means of achieving this may be far from physiological.
(4) For some women 'normal' has become an ideal for which to strive. Clearly, without probing the subjectivity of this meaning renders it useless.
(5) Normal, meaning 'not pathological', carries an aura of objectivity; but this is spurious due to pathology depending on diagnosis and interpretation.
(6) 'Natural' is the least unsatisfactory meaning of normal in Gould's classification. But, as mentioned already, natural brings its own historical baggage.

In his philosophical analysis, Steen Wackerhausen (1999) adopts the statistical meaning of normal as in Gould's first category. He shows, though, that what is normal may eventually come to be regarded as natural; but for this to happen, the phenomenon must be considered beneficial. So it is the value of the phenomenon, ie its goodness or badness, which is the basic criterion. For it to apply, the assessment of good/badness needs to be stated, together with the basis on which the evaluation is made, such as personal preference, education/socialisation, health benefits or reduced mortality/morbidity.

As well as these academic attempts to define normal, major organisations have entered the definition minefield (Young 2009). The WHO's (World Health Organisation) attempt has the advantage of brevity:

> spontaneous in onset, low risk at the start of labour and remaining so throughout labour and delivery. The infant is born spontaneously in the vertex position between 37 and 42 weeks of pregnancy. After birth, mother and infant are in good condition.
>
> (WHO 1997)

This definition is weak in that it relies heavily on the medical concept of risk (see page 96). It also permits a wide range of potentially iatrogenic interventions, such as augmentation/acceleration with oxytocics, CEFM, regional analgesia, episiotomy and manual removal of placenta.

In the United Kingdom, concern was such that the strangest of bedfellows (the Royal College of Midwives, the Royal College of Obstetricians and Gynaecologists, and the National Childbirth Trust) cooperated to form the Maternity Care Working Party, in order to resolve the definition conundrum:

> women whose labour starts spontaneously, progresses spontaneously without drugs, and who give birth spontaneously.
>
> (MCWP 2007)

While this definition allows for CEFM and augmentation by artificial rupture of membranes, regional analgesia is excluded.

A more recent attempt to define normal, which demonstrates that the problem has neither been resolved nor gone away, was made by a large group of women's health providers (Society of Obstetricians and Gynaecologists of Canada (SOGC), Association of Women's Health, Obstetric and Neonatal Nurses of Canada, Canadian Association of Midwives, College of Family Physicians of Canada, and Society of Rural Physicians of Canada):

> spontaneous in onset, is low-risk at the start of labour and remains so throughout labour and birth. The infant is born spontaneously in vertex position between 37 and 42+0 completed weeks.
>
> (SOGC et al 2008)

This Canadian definition, like the WHO but unlike the UK offerings, excludes the possibility of the foetus being in what is considered a 'malpresentation', such as breech.

Discussing these varied definitions of one universal concept, Diony Young (2009) concludes that it is local circumstances and practices which determine definitions, demonstrating the potential for some women to be penalised by regional terminology.

Although Holly Powell Kennedy suggests that 'physiologic' (sic) is preferable to normal, this term is far from user-friendly (Kennedy 2010). I would, therefore, like to recommend Wackerhausen's offering of a different meaning of normal which, if not helpful, at least provides food for thought. In order to avoid confusion between 'what is common and what is normal', 'Intervention-free' appears to be hopeful (Beech 2002b: 1). It is obvious that technological, medicalised, operative and instrumental births are not included. By redefining 'normal' as 'intervention-free', though, the questions soon emerge. Thus, it becomes necessary to address an even more challenging question, which relates to what constitutes intervention. It may be argued that any external factor which carries the potential to influence the progress of the labour should be included in this category. I suggest, therefore, that even the presence of an attendant, such as a midwife, or the move into a different environment, such as a birthing centre or maternity unit, may constitute interventions.

Initiatives

National initiatives have been introduced to support the normality agenda (NHS Wales 2006; Scottish Government 2009), but evaluation of their effectiveness is incomplete at the time of writing. Thus, the jury appears to be still out on the benefits of the midwife making a virtue out of necessity.

Woman centredness

Although the requirement for the woman to be central to decision-making and care provision in the maternity services appears too obvious to mention, the reality may be different. Originating with 'The Vision', an inspirational publication by the Association of Radical Midwives (ARM 1986), woman-centred care was eventually espoused by government publications (HoC 1992; DoH 1993). These publications brought the potential for 'transformatory' change within the maternity services (Phillips 2009), although the extent to which this potential has been fulfilled remains questionable.

Changing Childbirth defined woman centredness in terms of the 'Three Cs' – choice, continuity and control (Baker et al 2005). Mari Phillips, however, argues that it is the relationship between the woman and the midwife which is crucial to this concept (Phillips 2009: 20), and suggests that the following definition better fits feminist approaches to midwifery:

> women are acknowledged as active, conscious, intentional authors of their own lives and can occupy a powerful authoritative and controlling position in their childbearing experience.
>
> (Phillips 2009: 282)

The environment in which woman centredness develops is of considerable significance, as this philosophy is in 'marked contrast' (Baker et al 2005) to the

longstanding and ongoing medicalisation of birth (page 103). The organisational changes in the maternity services have also jeopardised the possibility of
the formation of the woman-midwife relationship though increasing bureaucracy
and centralisation (Phillips 2009). The operationalisation of woman centredness
was demonstrated in a qualitative research project by Sarah Baker and her colleagues (Baker et al 2005). Having collected data in England, these researchers'
findings were summarised understatedly:

> women-centred [sic] care designed to promote choice, continuity, and
> control was not their overriding experience.
>
> (Baker et al 2005: 332)

Phillips' qualitative study of woman centredness involved interviews with
childbearing women and midwives (Phillips 2009) and highlighted the need for
the woman to take responsibility for negotiating many aspects of her midwifery
and other care. This resulted in fragmentation of care during labour and afterwards, despite being 'known' to the midwife before and during her pregnancy.
These findings were not regarded as solely due to the midwife, but to the
system within which a large majority of midwives are employed and practise.
Thus, far from the woman being at the centre of all that happens in the
maternity services, Phillips concludes that the NHS is an anathema to woman
centredness and recommends the exploration of less orthodox or traditional
systems of maternity care.

CenteringPregnancy

One of these less orthodox or traditional systems is the North American philosophy
of care known as 'CenteringPregnancy' (Gaudion and Menka 2010). The brainchild of Sharon Schindler Rising, this 'copyrighted program design' (Schindler
Rising and Jolivet 2009: 365) comprises a form of group self-care based on the
philosophy:

> a dynamic union of health care provider and consumer holds the greatest
> potential for the personal growth of both. The consumer is viewed as an
> equal partner in care and works actively with the care provider to develop
> goals and appropriate means to reach those goals.
>
> (Rising and Lindell 1982: 11)

Since its inception, CenteringPregnancy has specifically sought to offer antenatal
care which effectively and efficiently answers the needs of women who are
disadvantaged socially, ethnically and/or financially (Schindler Rising and
Kennedy 2004). This specific orientation is welcome in a country with the
poorest maternal and perinatal outcomes of all advanced economies, due to
widespread poverty and the 'structural violence' of no national maternal health
care system (Wagner 2006; Lane 2008; Amnesty International 2010). In such

an overtly discriminatory system, that language of 'health care provider' and 'consumer' partnership may be politically necessary. Nonetheless, a more nuanced understanding and application of the philosophy and the model have been exported and evaluated in countries like Australia (Teate et al 2011), Sweden (Wedin et al 2010) and England (Gaudion and Menka 2010).

The ethos underpinning this philosophy encompasses dynamic shared learning within the group, with a midwife facilitator as leader. The learning activities are structured and time-limited for the group; the membership and leadership of which should be stable. The social aspects of the group's functioning are crucial, including sharing light meals. The antenatal checks happen within the group, with aspects being shared, such as blood pressure measurement (Schindler Rising and Kennedy 2004: 399). The place of male or other partners is not clear, as their presence obviously alters group dynamics, although some groups have identified unanticipated benefits from their participation (Schindler Rising and Jolivet 2009: 371).

Evaluations have shown benefits of this philosophy of practice to include improvements in preterm birth, readiness for labour, birth weight, breastfeeding, maternal satisfaction and perception of support (Ickovics et al 2007). Reports indicate the enthusiasm of stereotypical 'non-attenders' at childbirth education and antenatal clinics to join in centering groups. The childbearing women involved appear to relish the more balanced relationship with the care provider and the opportunity to share learning experiences in preparation for motherhood. It is my observation, though, that this system of care requires a high level of involvement, which some midwives may find demanding, although to others it will be satisfying. Additionally, personal experience suggests that its North American origins, including the requirement for formal training of facilitators in this philosophy, may not endear it to managers wary of innovation.

Other potentially relevant philosophies of practice

As midwifery becomes more firmly established in the twin spheres of academia and research, more philosophical and theoretical approaches emerge; these provide significant new insights into all aspects of the midwife's functioning and, particularly, her practice.

Maternal choice and control

Together with the much sought-after continuity, choice and control constituted the 'Three Cs' advanced by Changing Childbirth (DoH 1993). Maternal choice and control have contributed to other philosophies, such as woman centredness, and may be justified in underpinning the title in their own right. The authoritative series of research projects by Jo Green and her colleagues (Green and Baston 2003) demonstrate not only the significance of control to the child-bearing woman, but also its varied nature. These researchers have identified the location of control either internally or external to the childbearing woman; the former relating to the woman's body and behaviour and the latter to her input into decision-making or choices about what is done to, for or with her. Green and Baston reflect disappointingly that external control, over what staff are doing, is the form of control which women consider operates least frequently. This indicates that in the two decades since control was identified as a significant contributor to women's satisfaction with childbearing (Mander 1992), little progress has been made to return that control to them.

Choice and making choices are important aspects of control. The inter-dependence and complexity of choice and control are due to the belief and resource systems through which they are filtered (Snowden et al 2011). Thus, although choice is an aspect of control it also, if present, enhances feelings of control and satisfaction. According to Austyn Snowden and his colleagues, the woman's choice to seek to retain control of her labour and what is done to, for or with her is hugely significant to her. The researchers identify, though, that there may come a point at which the woman chooses to relinquish that control. The relinquishment choice, they argue, is not necessarily negative, especially if the woman confidently trusts those assuming control to follow her stated choices. In this way, it becomes obvious that choice and control as philosophies of practice are not held by the staff, but are determined by the woman with staff support and encouragement.

Partnership

The renaissance of midwifery in New Zealand has been founded on the political acuity of women, midwives and legislators. Throughout this political mael-strom the philosophy of partnership, with its alleged historical connotations, has been used to sustain midwifery's revival in the teeth of opposition from various quarters (Mander 2011a: 307). As refined in the first published version of the philosophy, partnership focused on normality, continuity and woman centredness (Guilliland and Pairman 1995: 34). Since then, this philosophy has formed a major plank of the New Zealand College of Midwives (NZCOM) mission, which states:

> Midwifery care takes place in partnership with women.
>
> (NZCOM 2012)

Recently partnership has become enshrined in the Competencies required by the statutory body, the Midwifery Council of New Zealand (MCNZ):

> Competency One 'The midwife works in partnership with the woman/wahine throughout the maternity experience'.
>
> (MCNZ 2012)

While obviously generally welcomed, the equitable relationship safeguarded by these illustrious organisations has been subjected to criticism due to its questionably universal relevance and its limited support for the midwife (Skinner 1999). These problems are aggravated by what has been shown to be some women's partial understanding of what partnership involves (Fleming 1998a). On this issue, the question of autonomy for the 'partners' appears to have been side-stepped, or even fudged (Pairman 1999). The imposition of one philosophy, no matter how well-meaning, across the board does not augur well for stable working relationships. Thus, the partnership philosophy is delivering less than it promised.

Salutogenesis

Although sharing a number of elements in common with the philosophy of normality (page 99), the origins of salutogenesis are immeasurably different. Aaron Antonovsky's work with holocaust survivors led to investigations of why some survivors demonstrated a much sunnier, even healthier, disposition than would be expected after such experiences (Antonovsky 1979). Antonovsky linked these positive orientations to the concept of 'Sense Of Coherence' (SOC) comprising making sense of life through comprehensibility, manageability and meaningfulness (Antonovsky 1996: 15). Salutogenesis and SOC are founded on an anti-pathogenic philosophy, which seeks to reject the West's preoccupation with disease and its prevention (Antonovsky 1987). Although 'health promotion' has become a cliché, Antonovsky originally used this term to motivate healthier lifestyles.

In midwifery, Soo Downe has applied salutogenesis to the woman's experience of birth, intending that this health orientation becomes a self-fulfilling prophecy (Downe 2010). The salutogenic philosophy is one of the factors leading midwifery to discard the medical approach of 'only normal in retrospect' (Percival 1970).

Matrescence

The ethnographic research on birth centres by Denis Walsh (2011) demonstrates the crucial importance of the woman's birthing environment. Such ideas, resonating with Michel Odent's (2003), emerge to show how the woman's 'nesting' instinct is all too often disregarded in favour of risk reduction or, so-called, safety. 'Nesting', however, involves the childbearing woman finding an environment in which she feels sufficiently attended and safe, without being scrutinised or interfered with, to allow her to labour optimally. If the woman's nesting is recognised and accepted by the midwife, her response involves supportive, permissive care which taps into 'a reservoir of protection and nurture' resembling a warm embrace (Walsh 2011: 192). For many women interviewed and observed in the birth centre study, this form of midwifery care reminded them of the loving security provided in childhood by their mother. Walsh envisages the reciprocal nature of nesting and matrescence which, when well-matched, enhance each other in a virtuous cycle, ensuring a birth experience satisfying both woman and midwife.

Independent midwifery practice

As mentioned above (section 5.3.2), it has been suggested that the philosophy of woman-centred care is difficult to apply in conventional healthcare settings, such as the UK NHS (Phillips 2009). For this, among other reasons, independent midwifery is a philosophy which has developed to meet the demand for an alternative form of care which satisfies the woman's needs as well as the midwife's:

> I wanted a job that would let me use my heart and mind rather than one where I had to sell my soul just to survive.
>
> (McHugh 2009: 165)

Unfortunately, but unsurprisingly, this alternative to standard midwifery care has not been greeted as enthusiastically as might have been hoped. Independent midwifery and its variably enthusiastic welcome are addressed in Chapter 7.

Control of midwives

Whether the control of midwives justifies being regarded as a practice philosophy is debatable. It may be that no philosophical movement exists to advance this aim, but external control over their practice has become accepted by many midwives as a fact of their working lives. I argue that this acceptance of having their practice controlled justifies its recognition as a philosophy held, certainly not by the controllers, but by those who practise under and endure this control. This philosophy of acceptance equates with occupational learned helplessness astutely identified by Mavis Kirkham (1999a).

In marked contrast to the reality of this external control, midwives prize their much-vaunted autonomy. Such external control is due in part to a nurse-dominated statutory body with little comprehension of the practice of midwifery outwith the straitjacket of medical domination (see Chapter 7). At the same time as genuine midwifery practice is constrained in a top-down manoeuvre, the midwife is held accountable by an alliance of convenience between litigation-obsessed managers and defensive medical practitioners. Until relatively recently the midwife supervisor constituted the third component of this unholy alliance, but supervision is being persuaded where its priorities lie (Stapleton et al 1998) and that these are no longer determined by management and medicine (Duerden 2009).

Two groups whose control remains problematical are gay and lesbian (LGBT) midwives and those midwives of black and ethnic minority (BME) background. LGBT midwives have long been ignored by and within the profession; this is despite, in every midwife's experience, their constituting a significant proportion of the midwifery workforce at all levels and their contributing similarly generously (Mander and Page 2012). The reluctance of LGBT midwives to self-identify results in an unspoken philosophy of homophobic discrimination, which curtails these midwives' effectiveness and deprives childbearing women and midwifery of a valuable resource.

The contribution of BME midwives has been recognised, alongside their experience of 'discrimination, harassment and restricted opportunities for professional development' (RCM 2000: 3). This RCM Position Paper correctly identified the situation, but concrete proposals for resolving it were not forthcoming, so the 'snow capped' organisation which is the NHS (Carvel 2003: 10), continues to be managed, even led, by a hideously white bureaucratic elite. Despite this observation, Paul Iganski and his colleagues found that some health authorities' recruitment strategies have been changed to feature more positive action (Iganski et al 2001). On the other hand, while some institutions monitored applications, these researchers found that these data were ignored in planning recruitment. Targeting strategies were found to vary hugely in their existence and effectiveness but, as with many interventions, they depended on individuals' enthusiasm rather than organisational policy. The need to satisfy the aspirations of both a multi-racial and multicultural clientele and staff has been shown not to be achieved by individual efforts or piecemeal interventions (Kalra et al 2009); this finding points up the requirement for drastic organisational interventions to change the philosophy of an otherwise intransigent institutional culture.

Conclusion

Based on the wide-ranging discussion in this chapter, I suggest that many philosophies of practice have been introduced in the maternity area. Featuring huge variation in their theoretical basis, I have shown that there are a range of factors which influence acceptance and implementation of these philosophies. I have endeavoured to demonstrate the extent to which these philosophies benefit, or even harm, those involved.

6 The state, governmentality and our maternity services

Introduction: making birth political

In the midst of their comprehensive introduction, Jo Garcia and her colleagues, editors of the original *Politics of Maternity Care*, cited a 'new political climate' which had begun to take hold in the early 1980s about the health services. This climate turned 'selfishness and the ability to pay into social virtues'. The editors implied that such thinking might yet affect commitment to the NHS as an important public institution (Garcia et al 1990: 2). Of course the immediate focus of their book was the intensifying medicalisation of childbirth within the NHS maternity services, done in the name of progress, with questionable consequences for women and their babies. In the decades since the book's publication, we have had ample scope to observe the escalating conflict and controversy about the adverse impact of the 'birth machine' (Wagner 1994) with its dual emphasis on risk and technology.

In this chapter, I want to examine the implications of what was an aside by Garcia and her colleagues about a changed political climate. I will explore the elements of that changed climate, how they have become central to the current politics of childbirth, and why it is important to get to grips with them in order to confront the birth machine. Along the way, I will draw on the work of several social theorists about contemporary efforts to achieve substantive agency over meaningful public issues. I will conclude with some suggestions as to where we can lay down challenges about good birthing and make the argument that this is an essential prerequisite for women, their families and communities.

We need to begin with the word 'politics'. The political philosopher, Sheldon Wolin, defines politics as a legitimised and very public contest by social groups, who are generally unequal in power, about the well-spring of available resources held by authorities for the good of the community (Wolin 1994: 11). Wolin deems actions political if, in spite of these contestations and inequalities, diverse interests do come together in 'moments of commonality' to 'promote and protect the wellbeing of the community'. He is quick to add that whereas the public struggles of politics are incessant, such moments of genuinely political action to secure wellbeing are rare.

The pressing need for good health services that would be free and open to all at the point of access was the rare commonality that became the cornerstone of the NHS. Richard Titmuss (2001: 56) described the 1946 NHS Act as one which gave personal freedom to the individual and professional freedom to the doctor, for the individual to go to a doctor without fear as to the cost, and, for the doctor to respond to patient need without fear that resources to treat the person would not be there. The premise of the NHS Act was equality: equal need, equal provision. Funded by income taxation, it was a great social feat. It was not without its critics and professional opposition at the outset, and yet fears that people would abuse the system were not realised. Over a long period, this was a largely workable, albeit complex system which, at its best, was seen as part of the fabric of communities. In a *British Medical Journal* review article on the fortieth anniversary of the NHS, a former Chief Medical Officer, George Godber, drew attention to the role of hospitals within the NHS system, and the need for the hospital to be 'part of the community it serves' so as to 'neither supplant nor control but supplement the work of their colleagues in the community' (Godber 1988: 40). Tellingly, Godber reversed this thinking in relation to the maternity services, seeing the hospital as having primacy, and not being just a backup resource for the community. Although opposed to a centralised bureaucracy running a health service, he admired Dugald Baird's post-World War II work in Aberdeen in centralising services for all pregnant women within a hospital obstetric department, arguing that this was a logical model, reflecting perceived improvements in maternal and infant safety. He admitted that the debate about the loss of home birth would have been 'less embittered' if hospital staff had been 'less rigid' in their responses to women with normal births (Godber 1988: 42).

Godber's comments only hint at the turmoil which was clear to so many by the end of the 1980s, and which influenced a number of the discussions in the Garcia book. For example, the incorporation of maternity units into general hospitals contributed in a major way to the damaging system of allocating work rotas by specialist area, antepartum, intrapartum and postpartum, rather than unbroken care for the individual woman by the same midwife. The result of this Fordism was that by 1979, almost two-thirds of NHS midwives were working in one area of care only (Robinson 1990: 77). The loss of continuity damaged women and damaged midwives. As women became more vocal about poor experiences of care, their traumatic birth accounts led to the work of birth activist groups such as AIMS. That work is rooted in enabling women and their families to overcome the deeply negative environment surrounding birth in our medically-dominated system. By contrast with that system, the strong sense of greater connectedness when birth has a more evident presence in the community has attracted new advocates. For example, it has recently been portrayed to an enthusiastic mainstream audience in the televised drama of Jennifer Worth's 1950s memoir, *Call the Midwife*, and has been discussed as something which midwifery needs to retrieve (Moorhead 2012).

Yet this is not a task of retrieving a lost past, even if that were possible or desirable. What we face is the political task to build an enduring space for women, birth and midwifery in the midst of contemporary realities that are reinforcing fragmentation and privatisation.

Governmentality and the NHS

The layer of complexity that is the NHS, the system within which the vast majority of women in the UK give birth, has created unique problems for midwives, not least because of the array of beliefs from the system's beginnings that have reinforced the move to medicalisation. Yet, as we know, in contemporary society the vast majority of women and the babies to whom they give birth are not actually ill. Moreover, the very notion that Godber admired, centralising their care for reasons of safety, has been steadily taken apart over the last 25 years, beginning with *Where to be Born? The Debate and the Evidence* and most recently, the Birthplace Cohort Study (Campbell and Macfarlane 1987; Brocklehurst et al 2011). Medicalisation and centralisation of maternity services are trends which have deepened, despite growing evidence about their associated damage to women and healthcare staff (Ball et al 2002; Healthcare Commission 2006, 2008; King's Fund 2008; Care Quality Commission 2011). We need to understand what has supported these adverse trends in the face of the substantial evidence about midwifery services that best sustain and safeguard good birth.

The state and its role in relation to midwifery services is the main focus in this chapter because it is the state that ultimately sanctions how these services continue to develop. The state is the caretaker of existing healthcare structures and of the taxation and funding streams which finance these and, in principle, within liberal democratic systems such as the United Kingdom, it is also accountable to all its citizenry for its actions.

Michel Foucault's work forms a necessary toolkit here. Foucault is the outstanding philosopher of our time about power and relations of power, and power is inseparable from the work of the state. Foucault uses the term 'governmentality' to describe what the state does. The myriad of apparatuses that are integral to governmentality – statutes, policies, programmes, monitoring and statistical mechanisms, and so on – carry effects and consequences of power which are part of their creation and use. State action very often contains simultaneously two modalities of power (Foucault 2002a). There is the power to impose – for example, to impose on the individual citizen participation in the national census, or attendance at school, or inclusion in compulsory MRSA screening programmes. There is also the power to dispose, making those same apparatuses freely available, for example, free state primary and secondary education and free health care, to be taken up as an accepted matter of course by its citizens. The power to impose and the power to dispose form 'technologies of normalisation' (Foucault 1980: 137), that is, technologies that contribute and give rise to our taken-for-granted participation in the social body as school-going children, pregnant mothers and so on. These are important subjective identifications for us in everyday life. In this sense, a pivotal element that Foucault has contributed to our understanding of power and governmentality is that the individual is also a body with 'a biopolitical reality' (Foucault 2002b: 137). It is the recognition of the importance of tending to biopolitics (by which Foucault means the work of responding to all the characteristics and problems of the people who constitute the population, for the good of the state), that national governments recognised when they first gave such prominence and backing to public medicine in the eighteenth and nineteenth centuries (Foucault 2004: 244).

Through its mechanisms of governmentality, the state focuses on the welfare of the population, which is a means to an end for both state and people. Individuals gain from government measures and the measures overall contribute to a more secure, economically sound, sovereign state. However, these apparatuses of government, as sources of power, also become ends in themselves, able to intensify and perfect their work according to their own lights (Foucault 2002a: 211). Above all, these apparatuses are enormously productive, linked to the vast number of bodies, professions, disciplines and institutions that are the accepted ways our society functions. Put together, the apparatuses and the linkages with all these other social bodies produce an astonishing range of knowledges about what we are and what we do.

The state can choose to legitimate some bodies rather than others to act in concert with it or on its behalf. This is what Foucault means when he argues that the points where the state intervenes in the lives of individuals are also points that create an extensive network of power relations which the state inevitably utilises for its own project (Foucault 1990: 77; Foucault 2002a: 219–20). These bodies have specific agendas to carry out, but in time develop their own interests and ways of doing things. An example of this is the National Institute for Health and Clinical Excellence, set up in 2002, to produce evidence-based clinical guidelines. NICE's initial function was cost-containment (Pollock 2004: 76) to make the NHS more efficient. To this extent, the interests of NICE converge with the interests of the state about the overall 'arithmetic' of care, but are not strictly the same. In relation to childbirth, NICE guidelines on intrapartum care and caesareans represent complex professional and commercial rationales about birth and, whenever lay representatives can make their voices heard, the needs, experiences and evidence from women (Chippington Derrick 2004). The state is concerned and interested in women's perspectives, however, only insofar as the final arithmetic matches its immediate needs and rationales.

The state can usually command greater power and will keep its own interests uppermost even when pressed to act differently by representative bodies, by bodies it appoints and by civil bodies. There is a strong sense in contemporary society, articulated by many citizens, that the state's actions, which should be for our wellbeing in our everyday life, are no longer 'ours' in any real sense that offer us safety and security. If we do not speak on the 'right' side of the direction in which the state wishes to go, we cannot affect the state's decisions in any clear democratic manner (Wolin 2006; May 2010).

This weight of complexity, lack of voice, and the sense of being unanchored are felt acutely in relation to the NHS. The layers of professional and ancillary workers that originally comprised the NHS and contributed to its standards of care have grown ever more intricate in the last several decades. It is fair to argue that the organisation of the NHS is now opaque to the point of unintelligibility on the part of citizens who require its services in their everyday lives. Few people will understand or be able to define the status of a Primary Care Group or Trust or an NHS Foundation Trust. Fewer still are able to follow the political rationales as to why these changes came about in 1999, 2000 and 2002 respectively, let alone the massive changes to the organisation and funding of the NHS in previous decades (Pollock 2004). We understand that there are private sector providers on whom healthcare is absolutely dependent: the manufacturers of instruments, supplies, new medical and diagnostic technologies, the pharmaceutical industry and so on, and that the NHS must pay for these services directly. We may be less aware of how and why it came to be argued that the financing of new hospital buildings needed to pass from direct funding by the state to the private sector. When the state still collects taxes from all its citizens to fund health services and can borrow money most cheaply on international money markets, how can it make sense to allow private healthcare businesses to build major public hospitals and then lease them back to the NHS? As it happens, these private consortia have duties to their shareholders, not to citizens at large, and in order to make a profit for the former, build at a far higher cost to the public purse than the state would incur (Pollock 2004: 52–7). The vast majority of the population continues to want the NHS as it was originally conceived: a healthcare service with treatments available to all which is free at point of use (Nuffield Trust 2011). There are problems with this position, not least a growing acceptance that as long as the NHS is 'free', the move towards still greater privatisation in the provision of individual services is not so important (Nuffield Trust 2011). The connection between the NHS being subjected to increasing staff cuts since 2009 and privatisation by the state (Leys and Player 2011: 143) has not yet been fully appreciated.

Perhaps the concern most germane to maternity services is what Foucault names as subjugation or dependency. We can argue that the NHS as part of the state's welfare system has 'imposed' a certain way of doing things on the individual who is dependent on these services. Anyone who rejects that position faces another power struggle: 'All persons or groups who, for one reason or another, do not want to accede to this ... find themselves marginalised by the very game of institutions' (Foucault 2002c: 369). Bearing in mind what Foucault says about governmentality and power, I want to sketch out how and why this has become so complicated and seemingly beyond our reach, before turning to what the implications are for midwifery and childbearing women.

State welfare and the background to the NHS

In one sense, the NHS was an extension of the state welfare system that the Liberal party constructed in the early decades of the twentieth century. State policy objectives from 1906 onwards reflected the acceptance of the need for unemployment assistance, social insurance and health care as a safety net for out of the ordinary life events, such as losing a job, having an accident which prevented one's working, or needing medical care for serious or chronic illness. This was not altruism on the part of the state nor was it altruistic on the part of the disparate groups, each with very different political motivations, which supported these policies. In the decades of rapid trade internationalisation and expansionist economic policies that preceded World War I (Hirst and Thompson 1996: 19–21), the welfare safety net came to be seen as a justifiable and necessary means to reconcile domestic conflicts and tensions about working-class poverty, ill-health and infant mortality, in order to regain and restore international military and competitive economic advantage (Searle 1971). There were concerns about the resulting burden on the national exchequer and about not alienating capitalists whose support the Liberal government required. The ideology of 'national efficiency' was used effectively to counter these concerns. Appealing to a number of disparate groups, arguments about 'national efficiency' emphasised that a state welfare system would contribute to worker productivity in a 'modernised' British society (Searle 1971: 54–68). Thus justified, the state took actions which included national insurance, pensions and maternity benefit, the latter paid to the insured worker only (Searle 1971, 2004). It also supported practical welfare interventions such as the medical inspection of children in schools and, at home, a more comprehensive surveillance of poor working-class mothers, a movement already inherent in the voluntary infant welfare movement (Searle 2004). It was argued that these measures would contribute to a more stable social order, albeit one that enforced strict class and gender divisions (Thane 1978; Brown 1978). Lloyd George asserted that it was not possible to 'maintain an A-1 empire with a C-3 population' (quoted in George and Wilding 1994: 80).

From our perspective, there are three notable points about this early twentieth-century programme of state welfare policies. First, it required a new practice of government (Searle 1971) for the state to shape these new policies in the direction it found most advantageous. This included an enlarged civil service that began to rely on co-opting relevant people into government. It also subtly changed how the work of the state was done, much of it no longer happening in open debate in Parliament, but nevertheless strongly influenced by competing interest groups who made their case in closed sessions without reference to the broader public (Searle 2004: 391).

Secondly, the welfare package as a whole and the specific 'medicalisation of social policy' (Searle 2004: 385) impacted on the boundaries between state and civil society. It ordered the lives of its citizens, especially the more economically and socially vulnerable, in ways that suited the state's interests and the professional groups steering this top-down programme. In Foucault's terms, this was a relationship of power that followed 'its own line of development', intent on becoming 'the winning strategy' (Foucault 1982: 794). This early programme of the welfare state laid down critical lines of engagement, the consequences of which have re-emerged to confront us in recent decades.

The final point relates to the social hierarchy within which midwives, health visitors and school nurses now found themselves. They gained in professional status, but at the same time were strictly subordinated and regulated and, in turn, were meant to regulate the women below them in social class and professional hierarchies (Searle 2004: 381; Kirkham 1999b).

The early layers of the welfare state were not sufficiently strong to withstand the impact of the 1930s' depression and savage international trade contraction. The economic crisis meant that unemployment benefit payments increased sharply in line with the massive numbers of people thrown out of work. This began to be viewed by orthodox Liberal economists as a burden on the Exchequer, which was too onerous (Kincaid 1975: 45–6). In response to such objections, and, pointing out the threat that the upheavals of collapsed trading systems and mass unemployment posed to capitalism as an economic order, John Maynard Keynes made the case for deepening state involvement. Keynesian theory held that stabilising business cycles and minimising the impact of recessionary trends could be done if the targets of full employment, economic growth and (to back these up) a welfare system for all citizens were set in place (Harvey 2005: 10–11). This had increasing salience in the wake of World War II. As Tony Fitzpatrick puts it, the justification for the post-World War II welfare state was the pressing need to 'save capitalism from itself' (Fitzpatrick 2001: 81–2). Keynes was not a socialist who sought to do away with the capitalist economy. In one sense, he agreed with classical liberal theory that the state must never intervene in the market. The latter would indeed balance itself in the long run, he believed. However, the social devastation that would ensue in the interim was not worth that price. Hence he argued that if the state supported the market with welfare measures and helped to encourage demand through various supports for the market, everyone benefited, albeit not equally (Harvey 2005: 11).

Overall, this was a form of 'class compromise' that became known as 'embedded liberalism'. The state could and did take a lead in economic and industrial initiatives and actively supported, and in some cases, owned and invested in industries to encourage market growth (Harvey 2005). State-sanctioned arrangements surrounded the market with a 'web of social and political constraints' (Harvey 2005: 11) and ameliorated the harsher impacts of the market for millions of low-paid workers. The Conservative MP, Quintin Hogg, summarised the value of the compromise this way in 1945: 'If you do not give the people social reform, they are going to give you revolution' (quoted in George and Wilding 1994: 49). At the other end of the political spectrum, social democratic theories about health and welfare systems argued in favour of the ethical obligation to respond to individuals' needs as the mark of a generous society. Thus Richard Titmuss wrote:

> the ways in which society organises and structures its social institutions – and particularly its health and welfare systems – can encourage or discourage the altruistic man; such systems can foster integration or alienation.
>
> (quoted in George and Wilding 1994: 82)

These remain crucial insights when we consider what we need midwifery to be within the NHS. However, positioned within the Keynesian model with the uneasy compromises that had been struck in that period, these theories about altruism could only work as long as there was economic growth.

The impact of neoliberalism and new public management on the NHS

One of the important tenets of classical nineteenth-century liberalism was that all economic, social and political choices on the part of actors, be it individuals or groups, needed to be formally free choices. What is meant by this is that the formal freedom to choose had to be guaranteed by the state even if, in practice, there were multiple social constraints on individuals about choices open to them. This notion was seen as a major plank in liberalism that extended the rights of full citizenship to all (Jessop 2002: 453). It was this emphasis on formal freedom that began to be used to dismantle the Keynesian post-war compromise about the state as an active agent working to support economic growth. Keynesian-influenced policies did help to bring stability and economic growth in the 1950s and 1960s. However, by then a strongly articulated series of beliefs, dating back to the 1940s work of Friedrich von Hayek, challenged the role of state intervention and regulation as destructive of personal freedoms. These arguments became known broadly as 'neoliberalism' because of their emphasis on removing any constraints on individual actors imposed by the state that might prevent the market from working freely.

As economic growth began to falter in western economies in the 1970s, the class compromise known as 'embedded liberalism' broke apart. The United Kingdom faced sharply rising rates of inflation and unemployment and there was widespread industrial unrest. One indication of this unrest was the struggle against technological innovation, in the form of automation and early computerisation of production which sought to radically reduce reliance on a skilled and unionised workforce (Hardt and Negri 2000: 267–8). At the same time, the argument that health and social welfare had become an intolerable burden on the economy, impeding marketplace freedoms, gained more adherents. The 1970s was a period of increasing disinvestment by the state in both current and capital expenditure for the NHS which, amongst other consequences, resulted in increasing workloads, poor staff morale and industrial action across the NHS (BMJ Editorial 1979: 288; Singer 2012). A significant point of tension was whether consultants would be allowed to treat private patients in NHS hospitals (Singer 2012), a break from what the NHS had represented up to that point.

In 1958, the prime minister of the day, Harold Macmillan, had resisted proposals from the then chancellor of the exchequer to cut overall welfare expenditure by £76 million, declaring that the government had an 'inescapable obligation to large sections of the community, the erosion of which would be both inequitable and unacceptable to public opinion' (quoted in George and Wilding 1994: 49). The argument that cuts in health and welfare were an erosion of a critical social good was vanishing. A long-running royal commission on the NHS reported in July 1979 that there was much to be proud of in the NHS, but 'the future state of the national economy will have an important influence on the NHS and its capacity to provide new or better services' (Royal Commission on the NHS 1979). In the event, it was the fundamental change to the political context that was to matter most. What David Harvey (2005: 36) terms 'a certain accordance of interests' was taking shape through overlapping sectors of corporate business, finance and technological development which sought the rollback of state regulation and welfare provision. This loose coalition came to the fore in the United Kingdom under Thatcherism in 1979 with a set of ideologies that had the potential to turn our social and caring relationships into commodities. It led to 'the financialisation of everything' (Harvey 2005: 33), beginning with the 1979 Conservative Party manifesto which announced the intention to open the NHS up to the private health care sector.

This constitutes the background to how from Thatcherism onward, and just as Garcia et al (1990: 2) feared, successive governments recast the NHS from a common good to being an inefficient behemoth that did not serve people well. It was spoken about as a growing drain on the exchequer, with hospital consultants and unionised hospital workers seen as having too much power (Pollock 2004: 36–7). The Thatcherite argument was that these trends could be halted and the NHS brought under control only through a series of what were termed 'reforms'. The language used to describe these reforms centred on the progress that would result with more productive and efficient services which could then expand to offer greater individual patient choice. Behind these superficially attractive arguments which stemmed directly from neoliberal ideology about market freedoms, lay the recognition that the administrative functions, operating plant, information technology and related data bases, along with specific diagnostic and treatment services of the NHS, could all be broken up into individual streams of profit-making for sale in a fast-emerging global market in healthcare (Pollock 2004; Sennett 2008; Leys and Player 2011). It was never made clear how to resolve the fundamental contradiction between the remit of private companies to make a profit for their shareholders and the duty to respond fully to the public good.

The fate of the NHS now hung on what was reconceptualised as a managerial problem. The term 'new public management' (NPM) developed in tandem with neoliberal notions, and borrowing from private sector managerial thinking, encompassed such objectives as slimming down public service bureaucracies and achieving better performance targets to gain lower direct taxation levels (Connell et al 2009). Drechsler (2005) refers to this as the 'quantification myth' whereby everything can be quantified while the need for qualitative judgement is discarded. Thatcher's government began the process by setting up general managements to oversee hospitals, cutting back the range of NHS services that were offered and outsourcing non-clinical services, including cleaning and laundry, to private companies (Pollock 2004). These reforms obscured the daily problematic realities of the NHS, which by the beginning of the 1980s included outdated buildings and operating theatres, worn equipment and a significant drop in numbers of doctors and nurses training to work in the NHS (Sennett 2008: 47). The drop in numbers affected midwifery as well which by that time was trying to re-articulate the grounds for its professional independence (Robinson 1990: 85).

Underinvestment in the frontline was considerable and cumulative in its impact. Healthcare experts argued that in real terms, by the 1980s, the NHS required a 2 per cent annual increase in spending to keep abreast of a growing population and growing complex needs. Instead, it was held to 1 per cent each year and told to make more efficiencies (Pollock 2004). In practice, the only way to do this was by cuts and restrictions in one area to fund services in another area. At the same time, management costs of total budgets more than doubled from 5 per cent to 12 per cent by 1995 (Pollock 2004). Under New Labour, these developments intensified still further. Between 1997 and 2007 alone, there were four major waves of reform and the NHS became 'a medical treatment system based on auto parts ... rather than patients in the round' (Sennett 2008: 47). Sennett notes that doctors had major problems fitting patients into this fragmentation of the body. Many knew that good care involved exploring the liminal space beyond the boundaries of a diagnostic checklist, and they 'create[d] paper fictions to buy themselves time from bureaucratic monitors' (Sennett 2008: 49). In 2006, the head of the British Medical Association stated openly to the government that its strategy of 'keeping prices down' while arguing that this would increase 'quality' was the strategy of supermarkets, not healthcare (Sennett 2008: 49).

Severing the NHS from what people had always identified as a social good did damage beyond the immediate challenge to the relationships between those who gave care and those who received it. The application of NPM entailed widespread institutional change with deleterious effects for democratic relations. The state had expanded and changed the relationship between itself and civil society at the beginning of the twentieth century to develop the welfare state. Now there was a 'declining publicness of public services' (John Baldock quoted in Clarke 2004: 27) as the state strove to accommodate a new 'arrangement between capital and the state' (Connell et al 2009: 333) which was taking primacy over the social good. For the NHS, for schools, for local departments, there was no longer an '"us" ... contained within a wider imagined community' but 'an isolated unit ... pitched into a partly real and partly phantasized life and death struggle against other units' (Hoggett 1996: 15). The emphasis on consumer choice and consumer rights obscured growing social inequalities (George and Wilding 1994: 42–3; Shaw et al 2005). More than the welfare state was being hollowed out: progressively, parliamentary democracy was also being vitiated. Valid political debate was being abandoned in favour of bringing together, 'dynamic markets' and strong communities so as to offer 'synergy and opportunity' (Tony Blair, quoted in Mair 2006). This was another way of describing increasing executive power working in tandem with non-elected groups of experts and vested interests which were beyond the reach of parliament (Mair 2006).

Accounts of expenditure by hospitals and health authorities, once routinely published annually and publically available, were now restricted because it was argued that they contained sensitive commercial data; they became exempt from freedom of information queries (Pollock 2012). In 2011, Hinching-brooke became the first NHS hospital to be handed over entirely to a private management consortium, Circle Healthcare (Leys and Player 2011: 75). A low-water mark in the wider public being able to hold the state to account about the NHS was reached in 2012. After an unprecedented suspension of the legislative process for two months because of public and professional disquiet, the Health and Social Care Act 2012 was passed. This Act repealed 'the duty of the Secretary of State to secure comprehensive health care throughout England' (Pollock et al 2012). This might be characterised as 'depoliticised democracy' (Mair 2006) where there is no longer a direct connection between what the citizen expresses as vital and the government she elects. Here we can see Foucault's logic about governmentality, that the 'game of institutions' (Foucault 2002c) has entered dangerous territory if the state legitimates certain interests over other interests to the exclusion of genuine political process.

Understanding midwifery's problems within the contemporary NHS

In his exploration of the current dilemmas within the NHS, Richard Sennett (2008) does not discuss midwifery specifically. However, he describes the frustrations for all clinicians as their scope to 'do good work' (Sennett 2008: 48) was radically reduced under the weight of all the reforms. Sennett speaks of low morale as nurses were forced to abandon older modes of relating to patients which had been central to good practice. The quantification project as it was applied to the NHS imposed targets which were meant to raise standards of care, but detracted from them, not least in the way care became more fragmented. Good clinical care required the space to listen in depth to individuals, to have a genuine dialogue and to reject 'quick fixes', undertakings which for all the emphasis on 'patient choice' had less value as the waves of reform rolled on: 'People have no experience to judge, just a set of abstract propositions about good-quality work' (Sennett 2008: 50).

Fragmentation of care severely affected midwives and their practice. They had already experienced an attack on 'good-quality work' during the 1970s as hospital birth was extended to include almost all women. Increasing numbers of women were subjected to routine interventions like induction of labour, with no clear evidence as to their value in reducing perinatal deaths (Chalmers et al 1976; Robinson 1990). There were new perspectives about birth and the value of skilled midwifery coming from midwives like Ina May Gaskin (1977), and the establishment of the Association of Radical Midwives in 1976 gave fresh energy to many midwives to confront medicalisation. The entire undertaking by Jo Garcia and her colleagues (Garcia et al 1990) was to document many of the negative changes as well as the potential for genuine change towards what women and midwives wanted.

Nonetheless, midwifery remained in a complex position during the 1990s and into the following decade. In that period, the work to strengthen understandings about what good birth comprises and how to support it effectively in clinical settings expanded enormously, while groups like AIMS and the National Childbirth Trust continued to raise public awareness about the consequences of indifferent or bad care. The parliamentary committee system was used successfully in this, and the notion of an established relationship with a midwife articulated by women was a centrepiece of the Winterton Committee Report in 1992 (HOC 1992). Continuity of care, however poorly understood (Murphy-Black 1992), occupied a core position in articulating what many perceived to be good midwifery practice.

The longstanding matter of midwifery's subordination to obstetric thinking remained an obstacle. Midwifery committed itself to a project of professionalisation in the hope that increased status and increased possibilities of developing vigorous research would help overcome older entrenched hierarchies that prevented autonomous practice (Robinson 1990). There was a growing sophistication in the analyses of what could go right fairly rapidly if there were a commitment to reorganising aspects of NHS maternity services (see eg Kirkham 2003, 2004; Shallow 2003; Downe 2004; Walsh and Downe 2004; Deery et al 2010). A series of policy documents at government level about the importance of midwifery-led care for women (DoH 1993, 2004, 2007) seemed to reflect evidence on this, at least in part. At local levels, women campaigned for birth centres (AIMS 2006) while from 1997, the work of the Albany Midwifery Practice in Peckham presented a viable community service with outstanding outcomes (Sandall et al 2001; Rosser 2003). Best practice midwifery was using rigorous evidence to separate itself from the flawed notion of consumer choice about birth and was focusing instead on the centrality of relationships in its care of women (Edwards 2005a, 2010; Kirkham 2010). By extension, this approach put midwifery in a different political position, in opposition to the NHS managerial model of targets and outcomes.

Yet the impetus to greater medicalisation and centralisation of care accelerated alongside the impact of NHS reforms, driven by managerial thinking (Sandall 1995: 202, 204), and the multiple applications of NPM. This convergence of interests and pressures led to standardised care resulting in what at least one midwife termed 'teflon-coated management' where 'neither blame nor responsibility could be attributed' (Deery et al 2010: 5). Strong pressures towards more medically-driven imperatives saw a sharp upward curve in interventions. For example, the caesarean rate rose again in the 1990s, 1 per cent in every year from 1995 onwards, raising alarm amongst midwives and birth activists. By 2001, it stood at 21.5 per cent for the United Kingdom as a whole, with London and Wales at 24.2 per cent (Boseley 2001).[1] Midwives were in danger of becoming a profession split by work practices within the NHS, with more having to manage on short-term contracts, even while they were arguing the case for greater autonomy and the need for community-based practices (Sandall 1995: 204). A cluster of problems amidst growing fragmentation contributed to an exodus from the profession with a number choosing to remain in health care, but significantly outwith hospital settings (Ball et al 2002).

This is similar to the experiences of Australian health workers struggling with the consequences of cutbacks to frontline services and the imposition of NPM (Newman and Lawler 2009; Sawyer et al 2009). Some left and went to work in the community where they could respond more fully to people's needs and were less constrained by hospital policies and protocols which were stifling skilled care (Sawyer et al 2009). Nurse managers who stayed found that their work was redirected away from the imperatives of individual patient-centred care towards targets and performance indicators as part of budget management. In practice, NPM left them with far less control over their clinical work while they saw scarce resources of time and staff absorbed by the data and other regulatory requirements with which to measure 'productivity'. NPM disempowered them as clinical leaders, leaving them angry and demoralised 'by the increased (and increasing) bureaucratization and politicization of health care' (Newman and Lawler 2009: 421). The term 'politicization' here refers to the politics of relocating health care to a business-oriented model. Although NPM is frequently couched in the language of 'facilitating', 'empowering' and 'enabling' clinical staff, its practice centres on doing the precise opposite by exacting conformity with that business model (Newman and Lawler 2009: 421).

To further complicate matters for midwifery, two other concepts came into extensive use in this recent period. The first one, 'governance', has often been used to indicate how well official bodies are responding to the second problematic concept of 'risk'. In the context of health care reforms, their use has been especially confusing. Deery et al (2010: 4–5) write about the negative effects that compliance with 'clinical governance' has had on midwifery in the NHS. The need to standardise care has been seen as an 'economic imperative' in line with state cutbacks to services, but also imperative to keep in step with the requirements of the CNST – Clinical Negligence Scheme for Trusts – in order to lower the costs of litigation (Deery et al 2010: 4–5).

Like NPM, the concept of 'governance' has its origins in neoliberal ideology and was first introduced by an expert on business management and entrepreneurial models (Cleveland 1972). Cleveland's argument, rapidly taken up in the United States, was that in a more complex world, the state, in order to continue to do the work of 'public administration' for its citizens, would need to make alliances with private organisations. This would entail a 'blurring' of the public and private, creating 'new style public-private systems that will be led by a new breed ... Public Executives, people who manage public responsibilities whether in public or private organisations' (quoted in Frederickson 2007: 283). This appears to be a benign notion, using all possible resources in an accountable manner. Governance actually does the reverse because it breaks the link between democratic mandates and elected governments who ordinarily instruct the state administration through legislative processes to do its work on behalf of all citizens. By contrast, with Cleveland's notion of 'governance' when the work of administering state duties and obligations is moved to private organisations, democratic accountability of the legislative and executive functions of government vanishes. As we have seen above, the private corporation has its first duty to its shareholders, not to citizens at large. Governance has been criticised as a mechanism which shifts us all from 'the bureaucratic state to the hollow state [of] third-party government', using 'market-based approaches' (Frederickson 2007: 285).

Transferred to the clinical area of the NHS, the term governance appears to say that if adherence to best possible evidence is employed in relation to pregnancy and birth, then individuals are fully protected; moreover, the CNST supports the individual should some unforeseen and catastrophic event occur. In practice, this results in the 'teflon-coated' management practices that Deery et al (2010) cite, so that a hospital trust justifies standardised maternity care, in line with its policies and protocols (which tend not to be evidence-based), as a way of protecting the hospitals and absolving responsibility in the case of an adverse outcome. What the CNST guidelines actually do is to put midwives into an impossible situation. Bound by the protocols and in fear of the consequences from within their hospitals if they deviate from these, they are unable to fulfil their duty of care to women as individuals (Kirkham 2011). They apply standardised care routines, actually creating risks to women and their babies because these standardised packages are not appropriate for each and every woman (Kirkham 2011).

Risk is as slippery a concept as governance when used in the contemporary NHS where, it is fair to say, the act of childbirth is saturated with discourses on risk (Murphy-Lawless 2012). As Mavis Kirkham (2011) points out, these are contributing to the 'general fear of birth' and to 'the fear of inaction which underpins the medical model of care'. However, risk discourses are strangely amorphous. Nikolas Rose comments that risk thinking is 'a motley array … of ways of thinking and acting' reformulated into an assumed authoritative discourse of 'vocabularies, techniques and responsibilities' (Rose 1998: 180). Like governance, this reformulation of risk benefits the status and approaches of some players within the complex topography of NHS maternity care, those who favour an intensification of medical interventions and those who supply the pharmaceuticals and technologies that support greater medicalisation.[2]

Like the term governance, risk is a term which obscures rather than clarifies. For example, we are told that a breech birth is high risk, making a caesarean preferable when what makes breech birth high-risk is a group of clinicians who are not trained adequately in dealing with breech birth (Cronk 1998). Another way of saying this is that it is cutbacks to skilled frontline midwifery staff that create genuine risks for women. The Healthcare Commission commented in 2007 that 26 per cent of respondents in their survey of women's experiences reported being left alone by midwives and doctors during or shortly after labour (Healthcare Commission 2007). More recently the Care Quality Commission has expressed concerns that, nationally, midwife staffing levels are not rising in response to the rising number of births and that there is severe understaffing in maternity units in southeast England (Care Quality Commission 2012; Campbell 2012). Lack of supportive one-to-one care does create genuine, not imagined risks (Murphy-Lawless 2012). The lack of a substantial commitment to securing space for midwifery has contributed to the quagmire in the NHS where, daily, midwives practice in fear rather than in response to women's needs (Scamell and Alaszewski 2012).

A parallel story about railways, maternity services and the NHS

Notions of change and progress are part of our commonplace expressions in daily life. We rely on phrases like 'things can only get better', 'moving on' and 'letting go' to show that we can overcome difficult events. 'Stuck in the past' is a rebuke to those who appear to refuse to change. The use of the disapproving phrase 'and to think of it [whatever "it" is] happening in this day and age' implies that we think we have already reached a point where things should automatically be better, as if it were a universal law that change is always a progressive good. That latter sense has been bound up with the very word 'progress' since the Enlightenment when scientific thinking secularised the future and argued that solutions to the world's dilemmas would be found through the sheer weight of science and civilisation (Williams 1983: 244–5). Yet we can see that 'progress' has mixed outcomes for many of us. We feel ambivalence and regret about patterns of change over which we exercise little or no control and we sigh in resignation 'That's progress for you'.

Governments in this neoliberal period have been generally keen to argue that they are making changes to major institutions in our society so as to achieve greater 'progress'. They like to use the words 'modernise' and 'reform' when they make their announcements implying that to resist change is to resist progress to a better world. The overriding problem is that the progress they desire is always cast in their terms of reference which may differ radically from people's clearly stated needs. In relation to the NHS, we have already seen that neoliberal reforms, carried out in the name of progress, have damaged our maternity services at fundamental levels. The NHS reforms have also damaged the confidence of local communities because their voices have most often been dismissed.

This is especially pressing in relation to growing health inequalities. The latest report on the triennial national confidential enquiry into maternal deaths (CMACE 2011) states that a number of issues may lie behind a stubbornly high maternal mortality rate. Maternal deaths are rare events in the United Kingdom. Even so, they should happen far less frequently than they do. Vulnerable women, women who are unemployed, women with multiple problems arising from poverty, women with problems of obesity, migrant women and women who are categorised as asylum seekers were the groups CMACE cited as being most exposed to a fatal outcome (CMACE 2011: 1–2). Maternal morbidity, stemming from the same complex backgrounds, is seen in increasing numbers throughout our maternity services (Mander 2011d). Women in such circumstances struggle with the embodied effects of inequalities that are the result of the many exclusionary actions of neoliberal regimes. These include the rollback of health services (Wilkinson and Pickett 2010; Global Health Watch 2011). In their commissioned report to the UK government, Michael Marmot and his independent review group argue definitively that health inequalities reflect deep social inequalities in British society (Strategic Review of Health Inequalities 2010). They also argue that the reduction in these inequalities benefits everyone in society (an argument that Wilkinson and Pickett 2010, also elucidate with their data). The Marmot Review recommendation in respect of children is to give every child the very best start in life, beginning with prioritising 'pre- and post-natal interventions that reduce adverse outcomes of pregnancy and infancy' (Strategic Review of Health Inequalities 2010: 22).

How is that to be done in concrete ways within the NHS? The CMACE report calls attention to some of the organisational failures that contributed to women's deaths, including poor or non-existent team working, poor personal skills on the part of staff, too little communication with women and too little consultation between health professionals (CMACE 2011: 2). These were issues raised in the investigation of ten maternal deaths in under three years in Northwick Park Hospital, London in the early 2000s (Healthcare Commission 2006) and which re-emerged more recently in relation to maternal deaths in two other large consultant units in the greater London area, Queen's in Romford and King George in Ilford (Boseley 2011; Care Quality Commission 2011). This information begs the question as to how we can ever hope to create a culture of safety within the NHS (Davies 2007a, 2007b) when conditions for midwives and other practitioners have worsened over the last number of years under the burden of more 'reforms' which have reduced resources while failing to increase numbers of frontline staff to necessary levels (Campbell 2012a).

With the economic crisis deepening in the wake of international banking failures in 2008, the government commissioned the McKinsey management consultants to look for 'unprecedented levels of efficiency savings' in the NHS while maintaining a 'world-class service' (Leys and Player 2011: 52–3). The McKinsey Report concentrated on two approaches, organisational change, including moving care services out of hospitals into 'cost-efficient settings', and immediate cuts to staff for immediate savings (Leys and Player 2011: 53). There were possibilities for the former approach which could also have marked a genuinely community-based and democratic dialogue with and between NHS frontline staff about services and access and keeping the NHS public. Other such dialogues were already in motion about local authority services (Wainwright and Little 2009). This might have had tremendous potential for relocating midwifery in to the community in group practices with clear routes and excellent communication with hospital-based staff. This was not the progress favoured, however, because the government wanted 'money in the tin' immediately (Leys and Player 2011: 53) and so the cutbacks ate into frontline staff.

Another response that has gathered advocates amongst more powerful groups of medical professionals is to rationalise resources and services through a programme of hospital centralisation, including closing as many as one in three of existing maternity units. These closures, it is argued, will contribute to the most effective clinical mass (Campbell 2012b, 2012c), part of the concept of 'centres of excellence'. The general secretary of the Royal College of Midwives, Cathy Warwick, has given voice to the fears of midwives about such moves, pointing out the dangers of 'baby factories' where women do not receive individualised care, midwives continue to leave because working conditions are poor and poorer quality of care is the outcome (Campbell 2010a). Data gathered from the greater London area on a rise in maternal mortality between 2009 and 2010 has raised concerns about the quality of health care for vulnerable women, raising concerns also about the strain on services (Bewley and Helleur 2012). In 2009, NHS figures indicated that women in labour were turned away or unattended because of hospital closures due to lack of staff and too few beds (Drazek 2009; Campbell 2010b).[3] Nelson-Piercy et al (2011) have noted that increases in indirect causes of maternal mortality are associated with sub-standard care, and in one-third of cases, classified as major failures of care where 'different care might have prevented the death of the mother' (Nelson-Piercy et al 2011). This data implies pressing questions about the deterioration of maternity care in large consultant-led hospitals and the wider community which the advocates of centralisation side-step.

Overall, there is a disturbing lack of clarity in the calls for centralisation. Obstetricians argue that there are two main reasons for increasing complexity in maternity care cases, which in their view require specialist consultant care: the numbers of women diagnosed with obesity and the numbers of women who are over 40 and are giving birth to their first babies (RCOG 2009; Campbell 2012b). The Royal College of Obstetricians and Gynaecologists also stated in 2007 that greater centralisation was required to give sufficient scope for consultant training and 24-hour cover (RCOG 2007). The evidence they used is disputed as being of poor quality and poorly understood, if not invalid in UK circumstances (MacFarlane 2008). Nowhere in their arguments, at least those in the public domain, is there any mention of the need for far more midwives working to provide one-to-one care with women, providing also the first-rate communication with the woman and with the clinical team. These are matters that the Care Quality Commission has repeatedly argued are vital if women are to be protected (Care Quality Commission 2011; Campbell 2012a). There is apparently no understanding that the skilled midwifery relationship, with the midwife as primary provider, in settings with either caseloading or group practices, supports vulnerable women to better outcomes (Reed 2008; Leap et al 2011). There is no indication that they fully understand how obesity is strongly correlated with rising rates of social inequality (Wilkinson and Pickett 2010; Buck and Frosini 2012).

Obstetricians also seem to be confusing maternity care with the critical care required for, say, acute coronary events (Campbell 2012b) and with an eye to the demands for 24-hour cover and reduced medical working hours laid down by the European Working Time Directive. Do these experts hear only their own voices? Is this any different to where the NHS was at the time of its institution, with the voices of consultants louder by far than those of midwives, and centralisation of women's care into hospitals the preferred political choice? Have consultant obstetricians understood why it is crucial to act on repeated calls for greater numbers of midwives in appropriate settings within and outwith the hospital over the last decade in order to ensure safer birth for all? We now know from the Birthplace Cohort Study that for women with no complicating factors, consultant care is least appropriate and most costly (Brocklehurst et al 2011). Of course there is a need for critical care for a minority of women. However, given data on growing health inequalities, would it not be infinitely more sensible to search out how we are going to get better care in the community, with midwives as lead carers for vulnerable pregnant women, and far better linkages to hospital care as and when it is needed? We have the data to prove the efficacy of such approaches (Reed and Walton 2009; Leap et al 2011; McCourt et al 2011; Mclachan et al 2012) whereas the data may be beginning to run against centralised hospitals for this very population (Bewley and Helleur 2012).

The call for centralisation is far from straightforward in other respects. Decisions about mergers for some London hospitals are now being made by the so-called Cooperation and Competition Panel – CCP (Levy 2012). This may not strike the ordinary citizen as the appropriate venue for such an important decision that affects many different communities. Yet we know that the Health and Social Care Act will ratchet up the pressure to keep costs as low as possible and that this will include hospital closures in order to open up services for competition. One of the promised clinical advantages resulting from centralisation is the establishment of 'high-tech and comprehensive centres', yet these centres are unlikely to come together unless there is a significant number of private patients to fund them (Leys and Player 2011: 138–9). The CCP is one of many new bodies now involved in decisions about the structure of NHS services and reports directly to MONITOR. The latter is the UK regulator which has the task of regulating 'NHS foundation trusts based on the risks they face and how well they manage these', stepping in if problems are not being identified and addressed (MONITOR, http://www.monitor-nhsft.gov.uk/). We are told that MONITOR 'maintain[s] a risk-based approach to regulation ensuring our actions are timely, focused and proportionate' (MONITOR http://www.monitor-nhsft.gov.uk/). What can this actually mean as the very system MONITOR is meant to oversee is imposing cuts to yet more staff, while MONITOR itself is meant to promote competition? This latter remit falls under the EU regulatory body, the Competition Commission. Does MONITOR's risk-based approach reflect the consequences of the imperative to cut staff or does it reflect corporate business risk modelling in line with EU competition strictures? If the latter task takes precedence, does this mean that MONITOR seeks to protect profits by diminishing what they perceive as the least profitable forms of care? For ordinary citizens, this language and these perspectives are unlikely to excite confidence in their endeavours, any more than the newly-installed 'health and wellbeing boards', which are meant to act as forums about the NHS locally, will restore any genuine sense of control.

Once more, we are squarely in the territory of neoliberal governmentality. At the very same time citizens are told they will benefit from the reforms of NPM as applied to the NHS, they face emphases on service delivery that reflect the interests, anxieties and preoccupations of corporate capital. It is estimated that the current value of health services provision to the private sector is approximately £24.2 bn (Boffey 2012). The interests of the most powerful medical groups, intent on retaining their own spheres of influence, including NHS consultants, are being renegotiated in line with these preoccupations. Perhaps this is why we hear so little of the critical work that falls to midwives to secure safety in birth for women.

From a quite different location on the national map, the reconfiguration of the railways provides a sobering case study about safety and profit. In his stunning essay on the Hatfield rail disaster of 2000, Ian Jack (2009) lays out in punctilious detail how the headlong rush to extract as much profit as possible from the privatised railways had deadly consequences for ordinary citizens. Four people were killed that day in Hatfield and over 100 were injured. This crash followed the Southall crash in 1997 which took the lives of seven people and the Ladbroke Grove crash of 1999, where 31 people were killed. After many decades of under-investment in the railways, these crashes followed the Railways Act of 1993 which sold off the railways, rolling stock and management to a series of companies. The immediate cause of the Hatfield crash was a 100-foot length of rail which had buckled and cracked. The story of the cracked length of rail is also the story of how a skilled engineering inspectorate that maintained British railways was abandoned because the workforce was seen as too costly. A 'hotchpotch of private companies linked together by a gigantic paperchase of contracts overseen by a bunch of quangos' (Jack 2009: 62) lost no time in dismantling the inspectorate that oversaw the work of 39,000 people who had ensured that every foot of rail across the UK was 'walked', examined and reported on at least twice a week. The number of workers inspecting the rails declined to approximately 15,000 while skilled engineers found their experience and voice being subordinated to business managers with backgrounds, for example, in the hotel industry.

Jack explains what former chief railway engineers explained to him, that rails are 'living things' in that they move and change constantly under the weight of the trains they carry and thus need constant care. Once the system of railroads, trains and timetabling was fragmented amongst so many companies, it was not in the interests of any single company to run trains in conjunction with proper rail maintenance or to take full responsibility to inspect and replace rails more frequently. Five years after the Hatfield crash, two companies were convicted of violating the Health and Safety Act and fined a total of £13.5 million.

Hatfield should stand as a cautionary tale in respect of NHS reforms and the calls for centralisation. Measuring the impact of centralisation on maternity services differs according to one's position. Like the rail engineers, frontline workers, the midwives, have a multifaceted understanding of what safety is. Those in positions of power, who are under pressure to change the ways that services are delivered and financed, will be reluctant to use that multifaceted approach. They are far more likely to rely on a delimited set of indicators about what comprises the 'obstetric safety' that centralisation is meant to ensure.

The Manchester reconfiguration is currently the most quoted example by enthusiastic advocates of centralisation in the NHS (Campbell 2012b, 2012c; Dowler et al 2012). The controversial reconfiguration, given the title Making It Better (MIB), began in 2004 with the work of the Greater Manchester Children, Young People and Families Network, a group, we are informed, of expert clinicians and managers who bore the subtitle: Network Approach to Achieving EWTD Compliance (European Working Time Directive). Objections from the general public to the centralisation process itself proved futile from the outset, so the issue was how would it be done? With the intention of creating eight 'centres of excellence', a principle argument on the part of consultant obstetricians and neonatologists who were part of that Network, was that very low birth weight babies, representing less that 1 per cent of all babies born, would be better helped by centralised maternity services: this was about 'moving forward' and would 'save the lives of up to 30 babies every year' in the greater Manchester area (MIB press release 2007, quoted in Davies and Rawlinson 2010: 5).[4] This projection was never followed up with hard evidence, nor did it take into account the broader range of care needed by women with vulnerable pregnancies (Davies and Rawlinson 2010: 5). Other arguments in favour of centralisation included a projected reduction in the number of babies being born and therefore a need for fewer maternity units with a proposed closure of four units altogether. This reduction in birth numbers failed to materialise (Davies and Rawlinson forthcoming).

A number of 'options' for the process were drawn up by a healthcare management company. It would appear that the first report did not find favour with this Greater Manchester Network and another company was commissioned to propose different options (Davies and Rawlinson 2010: 4–5). A 'public consultation process' was then begun in the Greater Manchester area with the distribution of information leaflets outlining the second schedule of options. This consultation and the volume of responses it generated was subsequently lauded by the Network as the 'largest ever received in the NHS' (Greater Manchester Children, Young People and Families Network 2010: 3). However, like the old fairground conjuring game of thimblerig, the preferred alternatives expressed by the wider community kept disappearing off the table. In the case of Salford, for example, the original proposal to retain the neonatal unit in Salford's Hope Hospital vanished. It was one of only two units in the Greater Manchester area accredited by the Royal College of Paediatrics and Child Health (Davies and Rawlinson 2010: 4). With it went the proposal to retain Hope Maternity Unit which, under the CNST, had a ranking of Level 3, the best rating that can be obtained, and which was listed as the eighth safest maternity unit in the United

Kingdom by the Healthcare Commission (Davies and Rawlinson 2010: 3). With 3,100 births in 2009, Hope Maternity Unit had a caesarean rate of only 18 per cent, well below the national average (Drazek 2009).

The reconfiguration was completed in 2012 despite bitter community opposition (Dowler et al 2012). In Salford alone, community and locally-based clinicians were meticulously organised in their rejection of the proposals and the process of consultation. Their work included the local Salford Maternity Forum. Indeed, the community used every public forum available to them to express their profound concerns. They saw their objections rendered meaningless, with evidence ignored and accountability denied (Davies and Rawlinson 2010; *Salford Star* 2010; Davies 2011b). A member of the Manchester NHS primary care trust board has since argued about the closure of the four units that 'Maternity units which aren't providing the best possible care, perhaps because they don't have enough staff, should not be championed; instead they should be shut if necessary' (quoted in Campbell 2012b). However, it was one of the eight hospitals chosen to be a 'centre of excellence' that had a poor performance record: it closed its doors to women in labour 26 times alone during 2009 because of too few staff and beds (Campbell 2010b).

The consequences of the closures have yet to be fully absorbed, but thus far, one of the planks of the original MIB plan, optimising healthcare services for women and their children, has fallen afoul of problems with staff and units which are so busy that women are transferred home as soon as possible after birth (Davies and Rawlinson 2012). Early discharge would be a good plan for many women if there were adequate backup in the community, but follow-up is poor with only three postnatal visits permissible in most Trusts (Davies and Rawlinson forthcoming). During exceptionally busy periods and when staffing levels are lower than the optimum, hospital managers rather than midwifery managers are taking decisions to keep units open despite pressures on staff, leading to concerns about overall safety. These are circumstances in which we can predict a steady rise in operative interventions because of the lack of sufficient midwifery cover. In Salford itself, an excellent community midwifery team has been disbanded and services have now been divided amongst four separate NHS Trusts.

Salford endures high indices of multiple deprivation: higher numbers of lone parents, high unemployment, lower life expectancy, poor social housing, poor public transport links and low levels of car ownership (Davies and Rawlinson 2010: 8; Office for National Statistics 2010). At 27.9 per cent of its population, Salford has a rate of obesity above the national average and the second highest in the North West, and this is directly linked to the depth of social inequality within its boundaries (Fisher 2008: 2). The recent King's Fund report shows the increasing class divide in health, with the poorest five times more likely to have a poor quality diet (Buck and Frosini 2012). In 2008, the Salford Strategic Partnership drew attention to the importance of healthy eating for pregnant women and encouraging breastfeeding (Fisher 2008: 4), and Salford City Council set the specific goal of ensuring that breastfeeding and healthy weaning would be established as norms in Salford by 2010 and that by 2020, the rates of obesity would be cut significantly (Salford City Council 2008). The Salford programme is the type of action meant to form the core of public health policy, in response to the Marmot Review, so as to improve the health of the poorest very speedily (DoH 2010b). Yet, the changes resulting from the reconfiguration make such goals unreachable. It will be far harder for women to have the scrupulous ongoing maternity care, pre- and post-birth that the Marmot Review has so strongly recommended if health inequalities are to be reduced for very young children (Strategic Review of Health Inequalities 2010: 22). The reconfiguration makes explicit the emptiness of official rhetoric about the health of vulnerable citizens. Finally, a recent review of the data on mergers in the NHS and their outcomes, concludes: 'Post merger, financial performance declines, labour productivity does not change, waiting times for patients rise and there is no indication of an increase in clinical quality' (Gaynor et al 2012: 2).

In a period of sharp economic contraction, cuts to vital public services are already disproportionately affecting disadvantaged communities (Hastings et al 2012). This is why it is all the more crucial that maternity services are protected. The progress that Greater Manchester communities needed in any reconfiguration was a secure infrastructure for an extended midwifery service in the community: individual care for women and babies and caseloading midwives able to achieve all-risk cover because they were also provided with swift access in and out of specialist hospital services, and birth in hospital as required. This approach, supported by abundant data as we have seen above, would have ensured the relationship between midwife and mother which is at the heart of safety (Edwards 2005a; Hunter et al 2008; McCourt and Stevens 2008; Reed and Walton 2009; Kirkham 2010), not the industrial approach to care which does material and emotional damage to women and to midwives who burn out (Dykes 2009; Edwards 2008b).

The changes that were made to maternity service organisation in Greater Manchester benefited the interests of a number of elite medical service providers and managerial groups sliding across the porous border of public and private with often confused agendas.[5] The plethora of consultative and decision-making groups was exclusive nonetheless. The notion of 'stakeholders' proved to be entirely insufficient for any inclusive decision-making about maternity care and other forms of community representation in this neoliberal period (Edwards 2005b, 2005c; Murphy-Lawless 2006). Accountability was here reduced to a business model focused on inputs and outputs and transferred illegitimately to the public sector (Walker 2002: 65, 66) in the sense that we, the demos, ordinary citizens, never agreed to this version of accountability. For all the vaunted praise about a consultation process and not a little dismay that communities, Salford especially, resisted so vigorously (Dowler et al 2012), at no point were individuals and community groups who put forward responses considered seriously. There was no mechanism of power whereby their opposition could become concrete. There was no overturning of votes because in third party government, that is, where the governing is done through a network of non-elected organisations such as the Greater Manchester Network above, there is no voting. Instead, in this 'diminished politics' (Rancière 2007: 11), where decisions are distributed to us, the demos, rather than created by us (Rancière 2007: 20), there could only be an appearance of democratic engagement called 'consultation'. In fact there was no structure whereby any of the elite decision-making groups could be held to account for their actions. The Manchester reconfiguration exposes the inherent conflict between the business contracts with those to whom aspects of the health services are contracted out (managers, service providers, commercial medical research institutes and so on) and the communities who used to have a social contract with the institutions of representative democracy (Walker 2002: 65–6). Foucault (2002c: 374) has argued that what we must articulate is our right to have access to a 'means of health' which he defines as 'everything that is at society's disposal' to help create health. This right, the right to safe, reflexive midwifery care, was overturned in the closure of Salford maternity unit. The midwives, now scattered, must think just the same as the railway workers who were interviewed before the Hatfield crash and who comprised the rump end of what was once a dedicated, skilled workforce: 'If the public knew the full picture, it would be horrified. There are accidents waiting to happen' (Jack 2009: 63).

Using train metaphors to dismantle midwifery's fears

The shape of neoliberal governmentality in relation to the NHS and the searing consequences for women, midwives and our maternity services are becoming clearer. This is why documenting precisely how midwifery is being undone is so important. We need that firm basis of analysis to make midwifery once more political in Wolin's sense, that is, identifying how, against the grain of contemporary state engagement, we can establish a commonality about an undertaking that genuinely promotes and protects wellbeing (Wolin 1994: 11).

Rosemary Mander has written extensively in Chapter 7 about the attacks on the Albany midwifery practice. The sudden closure of the Albany in 2009 was a shocking event for an internationally validated practice which had contributed so much to our understanding of how to sustain good birth (Leap et al 2010). Its closure has brought us more sharply still to the realisation that midwifery is acceptable within the NHS (indeed within Britain) only so long as it does not disrupt the dominant story about childbirth. That story is based on the presupposition, unchallenged in official and professional regulatory discourses, that birth is becoming ever more risky and therefore requires still greater medicalisation, still greater 'insurance' against 'something' going wrong.[6] In a blind refusal to see the 'something' that has already gone wrong, those same discourses sustain increasingly fragmented services in our unequal society which, as we have seen, is the source of genuine risk for women in birth. Beneath the language of 'making it better', this is the story of the Manchester closures and it is why the Albany was seen as such a political threat to an interconnected set of professional and corporate interests which have absorbed the NHS (Pollock 2004; Whitfield 2006). The rhetoric about changing the NHS to a series of more decentralised, smaller organisations that were not-for-profit, and were open, flexible and responsive to local need was found to be empty when challenged by just such a practice.

The Albany, supported for 12 years by singular midwifery leadership from within King's Hospital, was a mainstay in the Peckham community. At the time of the Albany's closure, Peckham was ranked as the fourteenth most deprived district of 354 districts in England; the Jarman Index of deprivation listed one of the highest scores for the areas served by Albany midwives (Jarman 1989; Sandall et al 2001). The Albany stood at the apex of community midwifery practice in the NHS precisely because it fulfilled all the requisites of the most rigorous international evidence we have to hand: caseloading, inclusive one-to-one midwifery care for all women, place of birth determined by the woman, access and transfer to first-rate obstetric facilities as women required, accompanied and cared for by their named Albany midwife throughout, and excellent postnatal support for 30 days after the birth. The support ran beyond the postnatal period and included the voluntary involvement of many mothers in ongoing birth education classes in the Albany. These were often vulnerable women, as the example of one mother who had six births with the Albany shows (Reed 2007). Many of them were poor, marginalised women, single mothers, women of colour, non-national women without legal status as refugees and so on: the very women cited by the final CMACE report (CMACE 2011: 1–2) as most likely to have very difficult, if not tragic, outcomes to birth.

The Albany midwives were fully accountable to the women for whom they cared, in the sense of being 'deeply ingrained in everyday life' so that 'inter-dependencies ... have precedence over individual interests' (Walker 2002: 71). It was the polar opposite of the input/output version of accountability used within neoliberal governmentality. The Albany's was the accountability that builds family and community lives, making a formidable basis for a democratic politics. It is little wonder that feelings ran high amongst the over 100 women who had their care abruptly terminated and the wider community which had lost its practice. The Albany Mums and the Albany Action Group campaigned very hard and, as with groups in Salford, turned to every possible public representative forum to have their case heard. In one forum, a hearing of the Southwark Health and Adult Social Care scrutiny subcommittee in June 2010, a number of people from King's College Hospital were questioned by committee members, after the Albany Mums had outlined their case for the Albany to be restored (Beech 2010). King's representatives were confronted with a number of crucial discrepancies about the CMACE 'London' report on the Albany and the Southwark Council committee subsequently wrote formally to King's about these points (AIMS 2010a: 16). Sadly, just as with the efforts made by Salford community groups, the Albany Mums found that the Southwark Council subcommittee had no real power.

During the period of the Albany's work, King's College Hospital became a foundation trust which entailed its becoming an independent financial entity, free to enter into contracts with the private sector and to create corporate partnerships. It was also released from compliance with DoH guidance and regulation about its operations (Pollock 2004: 71–3). Given this loosening of accountability and with the lines between public and corporate business increasingly indistinct, it is no surprise that the Peckham community was not successful in getting the Albany restored. It was not possible through any official mechanisms of government to have removed from the King's website, the statement that the Albany had 'poor outcomes' and that its 'safety record' was open to question. According to that statement, King's Trust had reached this conclusion on the basis of an internal review of its own records, having already contracted CMACE to carry out an 'independent investigation' that was not a 'statistical report' (King's College Hospital NHS Foundation 2009). It will require detailed freedom of information searches, document retrieval and interviews to determine all the conflicted background circumstances to the Albany's closure, a future doctoral research project that will pursue the failure of NPM and its language of governance. For now, we can only observe this semantic confusion about records, numbers and non-statistics as yet another example of an unaccountable regime that ordinary citizens are unable to challenge.

The aftermath of the Albany closure is worth examining in light of Wolin's explanation of how contemporary states work. They combine an intricate blend of formal political power, power de jure and power de facto which includes 'the complex of modern science-technology and corporate capital' (Wolin 2004: xvi). Within this melange, formally constituted government departments are 'encouraged to become "leaner", to delegate more authority to sub-units, to "privatise" their services and functions, and to govern as much as possible by executive orders' rather than by more time-consuming legislative processes (Wolin 2004: xvii). This is the background to the rise of what are known within UK government structures as 'arms-length bodies' (ALBs) that go back to reforms imposed first by the Thatcher government in 1988 as part of NPM. Also known as quangos or non-departmental public bodies, ALBs were meant to increase the efficiency of service delivery; they have come to be viewed as inefficient in their work, poorly-defined and inconsistently organised (Gash and Rutter 2011: 95–6). Dominant in the DoH, they are peculiar groupings, some with executive functions, some with regulatory functions, some with statutory status, while some are independent, but receiving some government funding. Their titles, names, duties, membership, and even their existence change frequently.[7] Amidst their business management language about 'efficiency 'and 'accountability', the widespread existence of ALBs, which themselves are frequently commercialised entities (Whitfield 2006: 16), brings to the fore troubling issues about what kind of power devolves to them, and how and by whom their internal decisions are made (Greer and Hoggett 1999: 236). ALBs appear to be a decentralising of power and a move away from a tradi-tional bureaucratic and hierarchical organisation. For the NHS, however, the imposition of a market and compulsory competition in the NHS has entailed 'far more coercive forms of control' by central government over budget and policy, resulting in far greater standardisation of practices (Hoggett 1996: 11;

Greer and Hoggett 1999: 250). In fact, the decisions of ALBs appear to be limited in range, focused on 'strategy' rather than policy. This is an important distinction. Policy should be about determining in a coherent manner courses of action which are consonant with public values (Greer and Hoggett 1999: 237–8). 'Strategy' is far more concerned with 'organisational postioning' and with creating a case for a body's ongoing work (Greer and Hoggett 1999: 237). Any given ALB will be alert to the need for strategy over policy in environments that are very sensitive to unstable political conditions (Greer and Hoggett 1999: 237), the result of overlapping state, corporate and professional interests.

Three ALBs were involved in the closure and aftermath of the Albany debacle: CMACE, the Nursing and Midwifery Council (NMC) and the Council for Healthcare Regulatory Excellence (CHRE). The first, CMACE, the national confidential enquiry on maternal deaths, started its life in modern times as a triennial process in 1952, funded by and reporting directly to the Minister for Health. This also meant that a Minister had to stand over its work in reporting to Parliament. By 1999, it had been subsumed under the umbrella of NICE, another ALB, and the direct line of accountability to the minister of the day and hence to Parliament had gone. The Enquiry moved twice more, by 2009 becoming an independent charity, with less government funding for its work. As such, it developed research facilities to carry out local audits on a fee-paying basis and it was in this capacity that it undertook the contested report about the Albany (Davies and Edwards 2010; Yentis 2011).[8] In 2010, CMACE failed to win a competitive tender for the continuing confidential enquiry process and has since ceased to exist.

In Chapter 7, Rosemary Mander has commented on the role of the CHRE and the NMC in relation to the fitness to practise proceedings that are being sought against one of the former Albany midwives, Becky Reed. The CHRE, also due to change its title in 2012, has now completed its extensive investigation of the NMC and has concluded that the NMC has 'problems at every level and is at risk of losing public confidence' (CHRE 2012). On the basis of the CHRE review, we can conclude that the NMC is not in a sound position to carry out fitness to practise proceedings against Becky Reed, given its problems and its reliance on the contested CMACE report. The internal processes of the NMC may be seen as bearing the hallmarks of ALBs: being unaware or even uninterested in what the connection should be between its work and collective values held by the broader society about the common good, involved instead in the 'strategic behaviours' ALBs feel forced to adopt. These latter 'are either means towards the organization's survival and/or growth or towards the private advantage of organizational actors' (Greer and Hoggett 1999: 239–40). In the wake of the CHRE report, the NMC website continues to list documents about its 'strategic vision' and its 'corporate plan'. How can this corporate language speak to midwives struggling in untenable circumstances (to which the NMC itself has often contributed) and to the women for whom they care?

We can also conclude that there are acute problems at other levels of the so-called regulatory process, including the supervisory structures for midwifery that can make fitness to practise proceedings less than safe. There are three further points to be made. This regulatory soup of ALBs is too complex to be reachable, understood and used with confidence by citizens. Secondly, although it gives the appearance of protecting our individual rights, it cannot do so because it is in no way democratically accountable. It is what Wendy Brown (2001: 12) describes as a society 'increasingly administered' by 'bureaucratic agencies' that make us less safe and more unequal. The final point is that this regulation is not neutral. Hospitals such as Northwick Park and Queen's Hospital, Romford, where women actually died, received warnings, but were not closed down.

This lack of regulatory accountability is bound up with the fundamental issue of the lack of democratic equality, a messy impasse that is particularly acute in relation to the Albany's closure. On all sides, that decision has entailed deep hurt and injury. That is precisely why attention to equality is vital because the capacity and power to injure have also been deeply unequal. In order to have genuine democratic voice and accountability about these contested issues, to see what can be learned, and to see how matters can be different in the future, there is a need to assume an equality of purpose amongst all the women and midwives involved and all the organisations involved in the Albany crisis. That is a political task, given the mammoth embedded inequalities of neoliberal governmentality that we have already observed. Suddenly, without warning, the Albany's closure brought about what Jacques Rancière (1999: 32) terms a meeting between two logics, the logic of that neoliberal governing which he terms a 'police logic', and an 'egalitarian logic'. Egalitarian logic was built into the Albany and the way it functioned in developing the mother-midwifery relationship. It was based on the competence of the former and the skill of the latter. That logic spilled out into families and the Peckham community. The community recognised at once that losing Albany was losing a lifeline. The police logic, on the other hand, has seen the state, along with the interests and instruments it favours, acting literally at arm's length from democratic accountability, co-opting midwives who are willing to act as regulators to carry out and give an appearance of order to practices which are illegitimate.

In the meeting between these two logics, the police and the egalitarian, there was a depth of injury. Injury and hurt in some form or other were sustained by the mothers and families whose babies were born with unexpectedly poor outcomes, including one perinatal and one neonatal death (the core of the CMACE 'London' report). The babies would have had these outcomes regardless of place of birth, mode of care and degree or type of intervention (AIMS 2010b; Davies and Edwards 2010) as Rosemary Mander has written. There was the shock to the midwives when babies in their care had poor outcomes. Women, parents and future mothers and fathers who might have relied on the Albany lost its care. The Albany midwives lost their work. Becky Reed, reported to the NMC about her fitness to practise, lost her livelihood, damaging her vocation as a midwife. Peckham was deprived of the enormous social good that the Albany had contributed through its outstanding work.

There is also the perception of injury which has an entirely different structure (Scarry 1985: 51–7). Midwives in King's College Hospital felt the force of this upheaval as did other clinical staff in King's who were involved in proceedings against the Albany.[9] They, along with King's managerial bodies, must have felt the institution's reputation to be adversely affected by the ensuing national and international furore over the closure, hence the statement on the King's web-site. One can presume that the individuals in the various regulatory layers also perceived an injury to their reputations because of their roles. At a glance, however, comparing perceptions of injury with the actual consequences of the Albany's closure, we can see that there cannot possibly be an equivalence of hurt and injury between that sustained by the community and that which the institutions have experienced.

The lack of equivalence is what the community recognised at once, spurring them to make this political for the common good. They did not doubt either their capacity to act or the necessity to act about what they had lost. They did not need to be sanctioned to act. In Rancière's terms (Rancière 1999; May 2010), the recognition of the community's equality to speak created a new political space. The Albany closure 'rearrange[d] what and how we perceive, mak [ing] us see something new or different' (May 2010: 40). It remade 'the field of our experience' (May 2010: 40). As traumatic as this experience has been, we have the Albany as the model about what good birth should comprise at community level. Crucially, we also now understand the necessity of political action, of holding to account the presumed authority of discourses and structures which are intent on eliminating the spaces for good birth and the care that secures safety for women. In 1940, the cultural theorist Walter Benjamin mused about the famous saying from Karl Marx that revolutions are the loco-motive for progress in world history. Benjamin deftly recast that image of trains and progress: 'Perhaps revolutions are an attempt by the passengers on this train – namely, the human race – to activate the emergency brake' (Benjamin 2006: 402). The ongoing protests and actions about the closure of the Albany have let us see how vital it is to activate that emergency brake on behalf of midwifery to halt the 'progress' towards which we are otherwise hurtling.

Democratic politics and midwifery

Foucault writes about the necessity to 'open up' a concrete problem in such a way that it 'cuts across' how we ordinarily see that problem, and thus makes it political (Foucault 1991: 376). If we can do this, enable the political task to emerge, we gain 'a different ... understanding of ourselves and our possibilities' (Brown 2001: 112).

That has been the objective of this chapter: to explore the politics of the British maternity services as currently structured and to ask whether they can provide the settings where midwives can consistently support good birth. We have seen how the state expanded its work in the twentieth century, albeit reluctantly, to take up its responsibilities for the health of its citizens as a clear social good. We have seen the state side-step that undertaking in recent decades and discard crucial commitments about health services and about democratic accountability to its citizens. And, despite the thesis of a common good that underpinned the founding of the NHS, we have also seen that the overarching structure of the NHS and the tendency to centralisation under the control of obstetric medicine always posed problems for midwifery because of the latter's subordinate status to obstetrics. Those problems have deepened even while the direction the state has taken, dramatically increasing its dependence on the market, has added overwhelmingly to the burden of problems midwifery faces. In too many instances, midwives in their daily clinical work, in academic settings, in their professional organisations and in regulatory roles, find that they can be on the right side of the 'game of institutions' (Foucault 2002c: 369), only if they too side-step their obligations as midwives and go quiet on their personal commitment to good birth.

To cope with these realities, midwives commonly resort to what Susan Watkins (2012) terms 'presentism', and speak of taking small steps. This statement is made almost in desperation. It is unanchored with no clear long-term intent or a clear focus on how these small changes might be sustained. It is a remedy wrapped up in 'the illusion of an endless present, oblivious to historical developments taking place outside' (Watkins 2012: 87). In that endless present of small steps, midwives stumble and their efforts are overtaken and quickly dissolved before they realise what has happened. Untutored in a democratic politics, accustomed to hierarchies, midwives remain unfree to discern fully that these institutions where they are embedded are 'institutions that embody and systematise ... disorder' while appearing 'settled and innocent' (Watkins 2012: 99). There is nothing settled and innocent about institutions which are doing damage every day to pregnant and birthing women and their babies, and to the project of midwifery.

Yet outside these damaging institutional confines that are determined by groups and agendas representing the very opposite of the intentions and obligations of midwifery, midwives in the United Kingdom have created outstanding examples of care and carried out outstanding research. They have laid down the basis for a midwifery that is political. Invariably, where this has occurred, midwives have found themselves working in tandem with and supported by women as mothers and as birth activists and, sometimes, with and by a handful of courageous doctors. This suggests that a democratic politics, grounded in equality of being and purpose presents the only secure future for midwifery.

The push to get to this democratic politics arises from the urgent need to understand how matters can be different on the part of 'those who have no part' (Rancière 1999: 15), no voice, no contract. It thus entails a 'thinking and reasoning' which is 'ethico-political' in nature (Kishik 2012: 38). Each time this democratic politics takes shape for midwives: in standing out against the decision to close down a badly-needed local midwifery unit; in refusing to cease their clinical work with vulnerable women despite the imposition of new 'protocols';

in transforming their practice guided by local women's maternity committees; they accomplish what Jacques Rancière terms a '*partage du sensible*', forming the shared meanings and subjectivities of 'those who participate by acting together', wherever that need arises. This is a democratic politics that always comes from below, that is premised on equality, and that is a dissensus: it dissents from and challenges a policing logic that otherwise thrives on hierarchy and exclusion (May 2010: 21–2). It is careful, deliberate, self-determining, linguistically alert. 'People decide to act' (May 2010: 144). Of its very nature, the dissensus they create cannot be co-opted by a hierarchy 'that denies so much to so many' (May 2010: 42). Such movements do that work of remaking, creating a new field in our understanding of childbirth. This remaking is there in the story of Montrose Midwifery Unit in Scotland which owes its journey to midwifery to local women (Winters 2007; section 8.3.2); in the significance of the Albany's work for Peckham; in the story of the Albany's closure and the bizarre disciplinary actions taken against Becky Reed; in fitness to practise hearings which have had to be taken away from the incompetent regulatory bodies for nursing and midwifery and put before a formal court system (Edwards et al 2011). Thus we have learned to think radically differently about the relationship between a woman and her midwife where both are fully engaged in an experiential learning to support that woman to birth her baby in best possible circumstances.

Midwives and women will build extensive support when they ask questions collectively: in whose name are these new policies and protocols being sought, in whose interests? In whose interests is this research being carried out and whose agenda does it really serve? Who really benefits from this form of regulation? Is it not really about control and conformity in order to protect indefensible practices of institutions while the midwife who practises ethically is cast off? From where within the body of midwives has support arisen for this welter of inauthentic actions and deceitful positions? As Todd May argues, 'the mere ability to refuse to cooperate with a police order constitutes a significant resource' (May 2010: 41). Midwives will gain by becoming political in the ways that thinkers like Wolin, Foucault and Rancière show us. They will be tested in learning to build a dissensus, but they can learn to become fearless in their truth-telling (Foucault 2001: 112–13), discovering also the truths about themselves.

Notes

1 Upon publication of these rates as part of the first National Sentinel Caesarean Section Audit for the UK in 2001, the then president of the Royal College of Obstetricians and Gynaecologists, Bill Dunlop, stated 'It is important we don't overreact and say this is a worrying rate and therefore it must go down'.
2 See Barbara Perkins (2003) *The Delivery Business: Health Reform, Childbirth, and the Economic Order* for an account of the profit-making potential of new technologies in birth.
3 In the 2009 annual report to the Nursing and Midwifery Council, the local supervisory authority for the north west reported that in Liverpool Women's Maternity Unit, over 500 women were unattended during birth for that year (Drazek 2009).

4 Although these reform programmes rely heavily on the disconcerting use of words such as 'transparency' (disconcerting because it should be taken for granted that democratic processes of decision-making are open to all), in fact Sarah Davies and Heather Rawlinson had to resort to freedom of information requests about many aspects of the proposed configuration in Greater Manchester (Sarah Davies 2012, personal communication). Similar to the status of current NHS accounts (mentioned above, Pollock 2012), not being released because of what are deemed sensitive commercial interests, Davies and Rawlinson will not have had that complete data about the range of decisions being made because it will have been withheld from freedom of information for the same reasons.

5 The confusion of agendas for obstetricians who are unable to see wider social contexts emerges in a report for the Health Protection Agency (Wloch et al 2012), on rates of infection after caesarean (the Health Protection Agency is an ALB which raises funding for its work from the EU, amongst other sources, and which also runs commercial services). The research on data from 14 hospitals across England on 4,107 caesareans in 2009, concluded that of the 394 women, most of whom had minor infections after surgery, with 25 suffering more serious infections, overweight and obesity were cited as major factors in women who developed infections. Rather than centres of excellence focused on the end point of consultant care, what women who are overweight or obese require is ongoing one-to-one care by a midwife to support improved health during pregnancy obviating the potential for infections, obviating also the too easy resort to caesarean (Reed 2008; Schmied et al 2011; McNaughton 2011; Abenhaim and Benjamin 2011).

6 The intensifying connections between ill-defined notions of risk and requirements for insurance cover poses growing complications for intervention-free childbirth. The private healthcare and health insurance industries are huge markets across Europe, aided by the binding nature of the World Trade Organisation GATS (General Agreement on Trade in Services) which opens up all services which were once designated as public services to competition. In the UK, the NHS CNST is now being questioned by a number of trusts who are seeking alternative commercial insurance providers (Clover 2012). The debate about whether issues of clinical negligence should even be handled by insurance and whether there is not a more just and non-profit-taking series of mechanisms to ensure protection is not being held. While decisions about national healthcare policies are not determined at EU Commission level, competition policies about healthcare as a marketable service fall under the EU Competition Authority (to which MONITOR in the United Kingdom is subject) because of GATS. The application of GATS as an international treaty to which the EU is subject has opened the way to intensive trade lobbying at EU level about the marketing of healthcare provision and health-related services which include insurance (Rich 1999–2000; Arnold 2005; Blomgren and Sundén 2008). Given the focus of the health insurance industry on financial incentives (Rich 1999–2000), we can see a perverse connection between expanding schedules of obstetric risks that open up further the scope for medicalisation, while midwifery is further restricted (Murphy-Lawless 2012). The EU Directive 2011/24/EU requires professional indemnity insurance under terms of reference that will bring an end to independent midwifery in the United Kingdom by 2013 (Heckel 2012). Andy Morton (2011: 12) argues that the directive reframes 'social rights to healthcare around the economic principles of the market will only serve to further undermine social healthcare provision'.

7 A recent review by the Treasury states that the numbers of ALBs, now thought to be over 900, are to be reduced and their functions reformed, to increase 'efficiency' and 'accountability' to the public under new freedom of information legislation and an expanded role for the Parliamentary Ombudsman only (HM Treasury 2010), but does not mean direct accountability of these bodies to Parliament. This constitutes extraordinarily circular reasoning even by the standards of contemporary government.

8 For its 2009 report on perinatal mortality, CMACE accepted full-page commercial advertising from Philips about its electronic foetal monitoring equipment (http://www.hqip.org.

uk/assets/NCAPOP-Library/CMACE-Reports/37.-June-2009-Perinatal-Mortality-2007. pdf). In the 2010 and 2011 reports (the latter its final report on perinatal mortality), CMACE carried advertisements from the Chiesi pharmaceutical corporation (http:// www.hqip.org.uk/assets/NCAPOP-Library/CMACE-Reports/35.-March-2011-Perinatal-Mortality-2009.pdf; http://www.hqip.org.uk/assets/NCAPOP-Library/CMACE-Reports/ 36.-July-2010-Perinatal-Mortality-2008.pdf). The understanding by ALBs that theirs is a commercial undertaking is underscored by the Care Quality Commission which has entitled its new quarterly series of reports on its inspections, 'Market Reports' (see Care Quality Commission, http://www.cqc.org.uk/public/our-market-report).

9 In the wake of the Albany's closure, a report in the national press drew attention to an internal report on King's maternity services which stated that maternity services were so overstretched, there were insufficient beds to cope with the increasing numbers of birthing women (AIMS 2010c).

7 Musts to avoid: how not to do statutory regulation

Having addressed, in previous chapters, themes and issues underpinning and arising out of political manoeuvring in childbearing, I move on now to examine examples of issues using specific situations. In the light of the themes and issues outlined previously, these examples illustrate the implications and effects of political manoeuvring. In this chapter, I examine how politicking may produce, possibly unexpectedly, untoward outcomes, before moving on to potentially beneficial results in Chapter 8. Largely UK-oriented, this chapter's examples demonstrate how inter- and intra-disciplinary power issues have unfolded and serve to show that political manoeuvring is far from invariably successful. These examples also illustrate the complexity of the system of which the childbearing woman is a part, the existence of recurrent patterns of power, and the effects of forms of resistance and social action which are oriented to change.

The Nursing and Midwifery Council

In the United Kingdom, the Nursing and Midwifery Council (NMC), whose origins and activities have already been mentioned briefly (see Chapters 1, 2, 3 and 5), came into being in 2002 following the demise of the UK Central Council for Nursing Midwifery and Health Visiting (UKCC; NMC 2010a). These statutory regulatory bodies are descended from those established in the opening years of the twentieth century with the stated aim of protecting the public from incompetent, unqualified or otherwise unsafe practitioners. That there was a 'me too' element, following the introduction of medical registration, is apparent from the NMC's English nursing-oriented history of 'how we got to where we are today' (NMC 2010a).

To appease midwifery concerns about nursing's domination of the statutory regulatory bodies which it ushered in, the Nurses, Midwives and Health Visitors Act (HMSO 1979) legislated for the establishment of a Midwifery Committee. This body has a majority of midwife members and, supposedly reassuringly, the NMC is obliged to consult it on all midwifery-related matters (Reid 2011b: 132). That the Midwifery Committee is merely a sop to midwives becomes clear with the realisation that *requiring consultation* is all too different from implementing the counsels of that consultation.

It comes as no surprise that some of the criticisms which led to the demise of the UKCC are appropriately being levelled at its successor organisation. These include exceeding its role, a misdemeanour for which the UKCC was justifiably criticised during the Jilly Rosser debacle of 1988 (Jowitt 2008). This criticism has more recently been targeted at the NMC (Beech 2002a), as this body was reminded of its threefold role of protecting the public, ensuring the competence of practitioners and safeguarding ethical practice. On the more recent occasion the NMC was overstepping the mark by seeking to compel all practitioners to hold Professional Indemnity Insurance (PII). But, as Beverley Beech typically perceptively reminded the NMC, PII may indemnify families, but there is no way that it will 'prevent a practitioner from acting negligently in the first place' (Beech 2002a).

A further criticism points up the similarities between the memorable disciplinary cases of Jilly Rosser and of Jan Jennings in the 1980s under the UKCC regime and current ongoing NMC-adjudicated cases (Edwards et al 2011). What all of these cases share in common is their reliance on 'obstetric safety' (Edwards et al 2011: 5), which is quite different from the health and well-being of the mother and her baby. Even the Department of Health has found it necessary to admit that safety is a subjective, rather than an absolute, concept (DoH 1993). So the NMC's rigid enforcement of pointless medical protocols, in the name of 'safety', may be just that.

Another, characteristically insightful, comparison between the UKCC and the NMC is found in the writing of Tricia Anderson (2004), who drew attention to the damage which both of these bodies have inflicted uniformly on women and midwives. The damage to midwives, originating with medical practitioners, is to condemn them to acting as agents of both control and oppression of child-bearing women. These two forms of damage, Anderson maintained, resonate with Jane Salvage's observation of nurses' experiences under the UKCC (Salvage 1985). Thus, as nurses were scarred almost three decades ago, midwives are now vulnerable to similar wounds inflicted by the successor regulatory body.

As I have mentioned already, the NMC's *raison d'être* is protecting clients and patients from unsatisfactory standards of care; as the NMC website proclaims:

> Our job is to protect the public.
>
> (NMC 2010b)

While this claim appears simplistically straightforward, Nadine Edwards deconstructs this rhetoric from the viewpoint of a birth activist (Edwards 2004). She emphasises that the term 'protection' is too value-laden to be a stable concept; as both women and midwives are uncertain about who or what is being protected and who is doing the protecting. The idea of the NMC protecting the woman and, particularly, her baby implies that the woman is unable and/or unwilling to protect herself and her own child; this suggests that she is something less than responsible and knowledgeable and calls into question her ability to mother her baby.

Edwards argues that 'protection' constitutes idealistic rhetoric, but its reality relates more closely to control, by ensuring compliance with policies and practices. Such control is operated indirectly by obstetricians, through the more-or-less willing medium of the midwife. Edwards recognises the NMC's recommendation of holistic and supportive midwifery care, but such care is not always feasible in a medically-dominated bureaucracy, like the UK health service. She argues that, if the NMC rhetoric of protection is to be translated into reality, it is women's autonomous decision-making that needs to be safeguarded. It is this safeguarding role which the NMC should endorse and facilitate for the midwife. Such endorsement would require amendments to the NMC documentation to remove inconsistencies between regulations and standards and to focus explicitly on woman-centred values, such as engagement and enhancing the mother-baby relationship. Edwards goes on to advocate that the NMC should recognise and encourage unique midwifery knowledge and practice, such as support for the woman and for midwife colleagues. The 'restrictive climate' (Edwards 2004: 163) in which midwifery operates, she argues, should be converted into a 'can do' culture with the maternity system being under the constructive influence of the NMC. This, it is hoped, will result in women becoming more autonomous and, not only the public, but also midwives being better protected by the NMC.

The problems of the NMC have not passed unnoticed and have, at the time of writing, recently been investigated by the Council for Healthcare Regulatory Excellence (CHRE). The CHRE, formerly the Council for the Regulation of Health Care Professionals, is a super-regulator brought in to resolve public distrust following a series of medical scandals. As a result, this quango is tasked, not with finding professionals treated too harshly, 'but for instances where they appear to have been treated too leniently' (Lewis 2010: 151). The CHRE report (2012) recommended 15 changes in leadership, culture, finance and operational management. Disappointingly, the report resorts to the time-honoured panacea of 'leadership' which it, probably naïvely, anticipates will bring culture change in the NMC to restore the confidence of all involved and affected. A career civil servant with what is probably fitting experience with the Health and Safety Executive, Mark Addison has been appointed to oversee these changes.

In summary, the situation of any statutory regulatory body is not an easy one (Thynne 2006). Such bodies, though, are a crucial aspect of ensuring the confidence of the public in services on which they have a right to rely. Statutory regulators are also fundamental to the achievement and maintenance of professional status by an occupational group. In spite of these strengths, any regulatory body is obliged to learn from the misdemeanours of its predecessors and to identify its constituency and respond appropriately to it. I venture to suggest that the NMC has disregarded the former and, through its politicking to maintain control and to curry favour with medicine and management, neither has it yet fulfilled the latter obligation. These shortcomings on the part of the NMC have had particularly dire consequences for two, not unrelated, groups of midwives. Because of the grave implications of these consequences for childbearing women, midwives and midwifery, I make no apology for now addressing these two examples separately.

Independent midwives

The first of the two examples of midwives who have suffered at the hands of the statutory regulatory body, the NMC, are the Independent Midwives (IMs). It is necessary to recognise the political nature of the service which IMs offer, largely because of the various threats which beset them. Their practice is, theoretically, no different from that of any other midwife. But their freedom from the checks and balances of working within the NHS maternity system serves to elevate their practice on to a higher plane. Their marginal status, largely due to only a small number of midwives being able to practise independently, may simultaneously both strengthen and weaken their position, as will become apparent.

Strengths

While some may choose to differ, I would certainly regard IMs' independence from the maternity system as their major strength. The statutory regulatory framework within which the IM practises is the same as for any UK midwife (Reid 2011b), but personalised, woman-centred care is facilitated by the midwife not being restricted by unit or trust policies and protocols (Edwards 2005a: 30). While some NHS midwives are able to provide a high standard of care, practising outwith systematic constraints means that the IM is able to offer care of a standard beyond the wildest dreams of many NHS midwives. IM care almost invariably happens in the woman's home, although the midwife may accompany the labouring woman into hospital, should transfer be necessary; according to Carrie McIntosh, this would probably only be as a birth support partner or advocate (McIntosh undated: website). My personal observation is that the IM's care may not unreasonably be regarded as the gold standard, in that it reflects evidence-based, holistic continuity of carer. This high standard may *per se* cause discomfort among those midwives prevented, by the system, from offering it.

The woman's previous experience, possibly of institutional birth (Milan 2003; Symon et al 2010), is often a major factor in her decision to access and possibly employ an IM. The qualitative study by Melanie Milan (2003) demonstrates that, not only does the IM assist the woman to achieve a satisfying birth experience, but the IM goes an extra mile by helping the woman to reach some degree of resolution of her previous trauma. Such a doubly positive outcome is clearly a further strength of the IM.

Weaknesses

The small number of IMs may be regarded as a weakness. Allison Ewing states that IM-UK currently incorporates 90 members (Ewing 2012) and, for reasons which will become apparent, that number is unlikely to increase. That they form such a small minority of the midwifery workforce is only able to aggravate IMs' marginal status and, thus, to increase their vulnerability to criticism and censure. IMs, though, may have made a virtue out of a necessity by transforming this potential weakness into a strength, which has happened partly as a result of their shared ideology and partly because of the common challenges faced by all IMs (Hunter 1998).

Clare Winter reports that in 1985 this group was founded and named itself the Independent Midwives Association (IMA; Winter 2002: 15); it later became IM-UK (Independent Midwives UK), an Industrial and Provident Society which is able to access government support (IM-UK 2009a: 608). The close links between IM-UK and the Association of Radical Midwives (ARM) reflect IMs' 'philosophy of birth being a normal physiological event and [the need for] practice as a real midwife' (McIntosh website). This philosophy contrasts markedly with the maternity services' norm of an increasingly interventive and technological approach to childbirth; for which reason this strategy is likely to need to be defended against criticism. Thus, the IM is required to ensure that practice is as evidence-based as existing research permits. Such an approach to practice, which clearly verges on the defensive, has become an accepted fact of independent midwifery life.

The costs incurred by the childbearing woman of employing an IM may render this form of care unattractive and vulnerable to accusations of being private care (Hunter 1998; Mander 2011b). Such hostile accusations could not be further from the truth. Although the 'complete package of care will cost you between £2000 and £4500 (approx)' (IM-UK 2009b: 750), IMs believe fervently in the NHS (Winter 2002: 15) which, they consider, has been moved away from providing woman-centred care and its original altruistic principles. This sense of regret is obvious in the words of IM Allison Ewing:

> However, at present, the only way I can provide that level of service to other women is to practice (sic) outside the NHS.

A further apology for or justification of the costs of independent midwifery is found in the writing of Mary Cronk. Adopting an emblematically provocative stance, Cronk compares the historical relationship between the woman as employer and the midwife as employee (Cronk 2000). This relative balance of power favours the woman, unlike when the midwife is employed by a trust or health board. The employed midwife is required to adhere to the protocols, policies and procedures dictated by the employer. Such adherence inevitably means that similar obedience is required of the woman. If the woman needs to be certain of freeing herself of such constraints, an IM may be the solution because the only alternative, private obstetric care, carries an increased risk of caesarean (Kirkham 2004: 270; Mander 2011b: 395).

The significance of independent midwifery

Independent midwifery matters to the childbearing woman who opts for this form of care. Although this is clearly important, I venture to argue that the existence and continuation of IMs is of even greater significance to midwives and the midwifery profession. I have referred to the high standard of care which IMs are able to offer as the 'gold standard' (page 144), meaning the best possible available. This is no exaggeration, as IMs are unconstrained by the policies, demands and resource limitations of health service provision. This lack of restriction means that the IM is able to provide individualised care, due to not being required to care for two or three women simultaneously undergoing highly interventive and medicalised labours. Thus, the IM is able to focus on the woman and her baby.

The further significance of independent midwifery arises, at least partly, out of the requirement mentioned already of some degree of defensive practice. In the knowledge that the IM does not have a huge bureaucratic organisation to come to her aid should it be necessary, the IM must practise using up-to-date research evidence and within the guidelines published by the statutory body. It is my personal observation that, although IMs are few in number, I have seen them using the NMC Code (2008) far more frequently than other midwives. Thus, it is my contention that IMs serve as exemplars to other midwives, by demonstrating what being 'with woman' really means. As Billie Hunter succinctly observes, rather than an anachronism, IMs have become 'role models for ideal practice' (Hunter 1998: 85).

On what may be a less positive note, though, I suggest that as midwifery in other settings becomes institutionalised, routinised and reduced to the minimum permitted by bureaucrats, the torch of real midwifery is being kept alight by this small band of midwife pioneers. The benefits to midwifery are widely unrecognised as are the costs to the individual midwives who practise independently, which I address now.

Threats to independent midwifery

The place of independent midwifery as an inspirational beacon of how midwifery could and should be practised is vulnerable to a number of threats from a variety of sources.

RESEARCH

Following a previously good press (Weig 1993), independent midwifery has suffered from adverse publicity resulting from a large quantitative research project (Symon et al 2009). Claiming an interest in the choices available to the childbearing woman, Andrew Symon and his colleagues investigated any differences in outcomes between childbearing women accessing IMs and comparable women using NHS maternity services. Unsurprisingly, the findings attracted considerable attention in the popular media. This was because, while many clinical outcomes were significantly better for IMs' clients, perinatal mortality rates for this group were presented as disconcertingly high. The authors concluded that the solution lies in planning 'to expedite transfer to a suitable facility' (Symon et al 2009: 8) should serious problems present.

A damage limitation exercise in the form of a qualitative follow-up study (Symon et al 2010) managed put flesh on to the bones of the initial study. This follow-up study relied on the notes maintained by the IMs attending women with poor outcomes; and it clearly demonstrates the frame of mind in which the women involved embarked on their pregnancies and, eventually, their labours. Many of these women were determined, on the basis of their previous experiences, to avoid NHS and hospital care at all costs. Their determination was such that, had the IM not agreed to attend her, the woman would have chosen to give birth unattended. Each of the women was clearly aware of any risks inherent in the planned birth and was prepared to accept those risks. The IMs involved were able to achieve that most basic, yet often challenging, characteristic of the midwife of being truly 'with woman'. In view of the recommendation of the initial study relating to transfer mentioned above (Symon et al 2009: 8), the reports of the women's admission to hospital in labour are highly paradoxical. The transfer of these women, when they had agreed, was marred by miscommunication and scepticism of the IM's account of the seriousness of the woman's condition. The logic of the medical staff attempting an assisted vaginal birth, when a surgical birth was clearly indicated, suggests some form of perverse point-scoring exercise. The tragic outcomes, however, were compounded by such arrogance.

As so often happens on these occasions, the threat to IMs' public image, exerted by the initial report (Symon et al 2009), may not have been invalidated by the findings of the follow-up study (Symon et al 2010).

PROFESSIONAL INDEMNITY INSURANCE

Until 1994 Professional Indemnity Insurance (PII) was available to all UK midwives, including IMs, through their membership of the Royal College of Midwives (RCM); although NHS employed midwives are also covered by the Clinical Negligence Scheme for Trusts (CNST) organised by the NHS Litigation Authority (NHSLA; Barnes 2012; IM-UK 2009a; Anderson 2007). Because IMs' risk status has been, erroneously, regarded as comparable with obstetric practitioners, the RCM's insurers were faced with increasing the premiums paid by midwives as well as medical practitioners, their main source of business (Warren 1994; Dimond 1994). In 1993 the RCM chose to ballot its members to ascertain whether NHS midwives were prepared to subsidise the higher premiums allegedly being incurred due to IMs' practice. The membership ballot decided against supporting IMs, so the RCM withdrew the availability of PII to them. This resulted in the paradoxical situation that:

> the only professional body catering solely for midwives chooses not to include those who may actually wish to make use of such cover!
>
> (Hobbs 1997: 13)

Other commercial cover continued to be available until 2005 (Hopkins 2009), but annual premiums have escalated to more than an IM earns in a year

(IM-UK 2009a). The result is that IMs have been forced to either cease practice or 'go bare' as far as insurance is concerned. Although this arrangement is not ideal, it has worked for IMs to inform their clients of this situation. The last commercial insurer had withdrawn from IM insurance because it was no longer lucrative, and they were unprepared to insure IMs because of the persisting comparison between obstetric risk and that of IMs. The level of risk envisaged is clarified by the Flaxman report, which shows that the level of claims to the CNST for obstetric cases is far higher, ie double, those for surgery which is the next most claim-prone specialty (FPL 2011: 67). This purportedly high level of risk also underpins lawyer Catherine Hopkins's unbalanced and uninformed diatribe against independent midwifery (Hopkins 2009), which draws on health service and supervisorial examples of harm unrelated to independent midwifery practice. Such deplorable ignorance only endorses Tricia Anderson's astute observation that the PII issue is 'a game only lawyers can win' (Anderson 2007: 4).

Following their recommendation that a midwife:

> in advising, treating and caring for patients or clients, has professional indemnity insurance. This is in the interests of clients, patients and registrants in the event of claims of professional negligence.
>
> (NMC 2010c: 8)

The NMC has continued to grapple with the problem of PII; Pontius Pilate-like in their decision-making alacrity, the NMC has stated:

> indemnity insurance could nevertheless be obtained were independent midwives to form a limited company and were then subsequently contracted by the NHS. However, outside the NHS clinical environment PII could not be obtained.
>
> (NMC 2012: section 12.4)

This recommendation resonates sadly ironically with an ongoing tragedy which is discussed below (page 152). The PII issue, however, has been seized from the hands of the NMC by the European Union which requires Member States to ensure that by the end of 2013:

> systems of professional liability insurance, or a guarantee or similar arrangement that is equivalent or essentially comparable as regards its purpose and which is appropriate to the nature and the extent of the risk, are in place for treatment provided on its territory.
>
> (EU 2011: 4.2(d))

This requirement reflects the prevalent view of PII as a benefit to the client, rather than a commercial enterprise which advantages the insurance industry and constrains the organisation and provision of care.

INDEPENDENT MIDWIVES' HARASSMENT BY THE NMC

As I have mentioned already (page 142), the statutory regulatory body makes great play of being tasked with protecting the public from any midwife whose standards have fallen below those expected of a competent practitioner. Such a banality is self-evident and such action is occasionally necessary, even for mid-wives practising independently (Rodgers 1999). With such observations in mind, the functioning of the NMC relating to IMs deserves closer scrutiny. While it is all too easy for IMs to find themselves before disciplinary panels, such as the NMC Conduct and Competence Committee (CCC), facing allegations of professional misconduct, it is considerably more difficult for other occupational groups. Medical practitioners, for example, are only able to be reprimanded for *serious* professional misconduct, making them relatively immune from censure (Beech and Thomas 1999). Marsden Wagner recounts the usual practice of orthodox medical practitioners, even following a tragedy such as a perinatal death, being:

> a hospital review committee meeting behind closed doors but it will not come to the attention of the public or legal authorities.
>
> (Wagner 1995: 1020)

Panels of the CCC comprise three people, one of whom must be a 'peer' and have expertise in the area under consideration (Griffith et al 2010: 46); while this latter requirement may sound unproblematical, for IMs this has often proved difficult. The term 'midwives' may imply a homogeneous occupational group, but exer-cises such as the RCM ballot in 1993 (page 147) clearly show that this is far from the case. The RCM ballot demonstrated NHS-employed midwives' limited understanding of the significance of independent midwifery (page 152). While the peer or 'due regard' member of the CCC panel is required to be on the same part of the register as the 'registrant' (defendant), that is a midwife, it is uncertain whether that midwife will have any experience of the area of practice under investigation. Not only will their experience be inadequate and/or inappropriate, they may not admit this and may be assumed by fellow panellists to be an 'undeclared expert witness' (Jowitt and Kargar 2009). This possibility becomes disconcertingly likely with the lack of any requirement for genuine expert witnesses to be called (Beech 2009: 4). In a particularly unfortunate case against an IM (DP) in England with an 'unblemished record' for 25 years (LSAMO 2006 in Davies 2009: 10), the 'due regard' panel member:

> was a midwife, with [only] nine years experience; a labour ward manager in a consultant obstetric unit. Because he was the only panel member with midwifery experience, his opinions went unchallenged.
>
> (Davies 2009: 11)

This case hinged on the IM's auscultation of the foetal heart, her forbearance regarding vaginal examination and her agreement to a woman in apparently normal labour moving into a birthing pool. The IM's adherence to evidence-based practice (EBP) was, effectively, being condemned by a midwife whose only experience was of the administration of medicalised maternity care in a consultant-led institution.

The role allocated by other, particularly lay, panel members to the 'due regard' has also been highlighted in other contexts. The others' reliance on the 'due regard' to interpret research evidence, on matters such as foetal heart monitoring, called into question the value of the lay input in the case of an IM in Scotland (Beatrice Carla; Beech 2009: 4). In this case the lay and nurse members had incorrectly assumed that if some observation is good, then more is better.

The investigatory process administered by the NMC has been widely criticised for its lack of humanity on the grounds of its duration. Beverley Beech argues that the time taken for supervising authorities and statutory bodies to complete their investigations according to their rules and regulations constitutes a breach of the human rights of the accused person (Beech 2009: 5). Margaret Jowitt and Ishbel Kargar maintain that these cases 'often take years to come to resolution' (Jowitt and Kargar 2009). In the case of the midwife in England mentioned already (DP), she was practising conscientiously for four years while awaiting the NMC panel hearing; after which time she found herself being judged unsafe to practise and to be removed from the register. Such an unconscionable and inhumane lapse of time may be linked to failings in the administrative processes by the NMC (Jowitt and Kargar 2009). Cancellations and adjournments at short or no notice and the mishandling or loss of vital documents only endorse the impression of malign inefficiency.

In a broader context, Marsden Wagner draws attention to what might be called the 'camaraderie' among those in a position of judgement over the person accused (Wagner 1995: 1021). In his example the influence is exerted by locals who share a common background, which is often male and medically-oriented. Such commonalities tend to disadvantage someone like a midwife, who is unlikely to be either, especially if her practice is other than mainstream, medicalised maternity care.

Reminiscent of Wagner's 'behind closed doors' (see above Wagner 1995: 1020), Beech focuses attention on the double standards operating (Beech 2009: 4). Hospital incidents tend to be reviewed internally; on the other hand, those in the community, being more distant from the medical power base, are likely to be referred to the NMC for full investigation. This means that the 'out-of-hospital' practitioner is at greater risk of being disciplined than her hospital-based colleagues (Jowitt and Kargar 2009), and any shortcomings in hospital practices persist.

In his insightful analysis of the global situation, Wagner discusses the implications for the practitioner whose practice is regarded as deviant from the local standard (Wagner 1995: 1020). He defines such deviance in terms of attending home births, practising in a birthing centre or practising independently. Such 'unorthodox' practice is, effectively, being punished for exerting a threat to those values held dear by orthodox practitioners, by which he means 'income, practice style, prestige, and power' (Wagner 1995: 1022). Heterodox practice, in the form of questioning routines and supporting women's decisions, is more likely to engender the application of sanctions through referral to the NMC (Beech 2009: 4).

The tendency or need for IMs to adhere to EBP, mentioned previously (page 145) may *per se* represent a reason for IMs to be penalised Wagner (1995: 1022). While medical rhetoric explicitly espouses EBP, this medical *enfant terrible* argues cogently that much obstetric intervention is based, not on research evidence, but on locally held opinions forming a clandestine consensus. In this way, local orthodox practitioners come to fear for the 'legitimacy or supremacy of the standard of practice' (Wagner 1995: 1022).

Up to this point in considering the NMC handling of IMs, I have been looking mainly at the experience of the individual. The existence of a community of IMs, though, means that individuals' adverse experiences inevitably carry implications for other practitioners who espouse similar ideologies. This scenario is suspiciously sinister in view of the disproportionately large number of referrals of independent midwives (Jowitt and Kargar 2009) who, these authors maintain, must expect to be referred for investigation at least once during their working lives. They go on to argue that many referrals are an all too easy way for NHS managers to resolve difficulties which come down to little more than human resources problems. The effects of such perverse referrals represent an unspoken order to other IMs to fall into line with medical orthodoxy and, as such, exert a strong deterrent effect on midwives contemplating practising independently (Wagner 1995: 1022).

On the basis of these examples and arguments serious questions arise concerning the extent to which the NMC claims of protecting the public are justified. What appears to be emerging from this discussion is that the statutory regulatory body is more concerned with maintaining the status quo by punishing behaviour which it and medical practitioners consider to be deviant or heterodox. Unsurprisingly, the term 'witch hunt' has come to encapsulate the attitude and behaviour of the regulatory bodies towards those practitioners, particularly IMs, who practise outwith the state system.

INDEPENDENT MIDWIVES AND OTHER PERSONNEL

The sensitivity of the relationship between the IM and NHS-employed midwives sometimes proves challenging (McHugh 2009); it has been explained by Ishbel Kargar as a form of jealousy at the freedom experienced by IMs (1987). Similarly, Lesley Hobbs ironically warns IMs that they should 'not expect to be welcomed with open arms' by hospital colleagues (Hobbs 1997: 65). Such antipathy also emerges out of Sarah Roch's sorrowful expression of shame 'that midwives are so ungrateful and disloyal' to this group of colleagues (Roch 1994: 247).

The relationship between IMs and other midwives has been clearly illustrated by these comments, the outcome of the 1993 RCM Ballot and the behaviour of the NMC; transfer of the childbearing woman to hospital, though, appears to engender particular friction. As Jowitt and Kargar observe, if there is a poor outcome after a woman has been transferred, it is certainly not the hospital input which is the subject of investigation (Jowitt and Kargar 2009). These authors reflect on the tendency, also highlighted by Symon and his colleagues (Symon et al 2010), of the admitting staff to disregard, not only the accompanying midwife, but also the records which that midwife conscientiously brings with her. The staff may decide that the woman will not have been in labour prior to admission and they certainly ignore the care which she has been given up to that point. Jowitt and Kargar perceptively observe that:

> It is ironic how often poor record keeping crops up in such cases while these 'poor' records are not even read.
>
> (Jowitt and Kargar 2009)

As well as the non-use of existing records, staff more generally may behave to an agenda. This behaviour appears to be an attempt to establish the fault of the accompanying midwife. Symon and his colleagues, in a series of IMs' cases with poor outcomes, identified three cases in which the staff failed to act on the midwife's account of the urgency of the situation. These authors consider that such disbelief, and the ensuing delay, was a factor contributing to the perinatal deaths, citing an example:

> In one case the independent midwife believed the obstetric registrar into whose care the woman was transferred 'was out of her depth'. She would not communicate with the independent midwife, and after four attempts at ventouse extraction a fresh stillbirth was delivered by cesarean [sic] section.
>
> (Symon et al 2010: 284)

This poor relationship between the admitting staff and the accompanying midwife is epitomised in the case of a midwife in England (DP) who diagnosed a previously unknown breech presentation when the woman was in established labour. On admission the baby was known to be in a good condition but, following breech extraction and prolonged resuscitation attempts, the baby died (Beech 2009; Davies 2009). That the woman and the baby were both well when they arrived at the hospital, suggests that the subsequent investigation focusing solely on the IM's care was, to say the least, perverse.

These examples show that it is not only the woman and baby who suffer when a woman is transferred into obstetric care.

The Albany Midwifery Practice debacle

In the previous section I sought to address the issues relating to independent midwives generally. I now move on to examine one notorious example of the behaviour of the UK statutory regulatory body towards a certain group of midwives and one midwife in particular.

Background

Some of us recall the heady days of the early 1990s, when Nicholas Winterton chaired the path-breaking House of Commons Select Committee on Maternity Services (HOC 1992); this was the precursor to the more familiar Report of the Expert Maternity Group, often known as 'Changing Childbirth' (DoH 1993). It was in that buoyant milieu that a group of forward-thinking independent midwives in South East London sought a route by which they could offer midwifery care, of the standard provided by IMs, free of charge to NHS clients (Reed and Walton 2009: 142). In this way they could overcome a potential criticism of independent midwifery (page 145), while offering women all the advantages of the '3Cs' promoted by Changing Childbirth. Thus, in 1994, the South East London Midwifery Group Practice (SLMGP) was established as a group of self-employed, self-managed midwives with a practice manager. In 1997, following changes in personnel, financial support and contractual arrangements, the group became the Albany Midwifery Practice, which was based in a leisure centre in Peckham and contracted with King's Healthcare NHS Trust to provide care for 216 women per year (Sandall et al 2001). The Practice's location in this part of London meant that the women clients would be living with high levels of deprivation.

Since 1994, the Practice has become a beacon of exemplary practice in a darkening maternity scene, through offering continuity of care and carer, a vision of childbearing as a normal part of the woman's life and relationships built around respectful partnership. The woman's risk status has constituted no barrier to midwifery care and women have been encouraged to birth their babies in their setting of choice, with their known midwife. Evidence-based information has been provided for women with the aim of facilitating sound decision-making (Reed and Walton 2009: 146).

Because the Albany midwives recognised the prototypical nature of the Practice, statistical data were collected assiduously and an authoritative evaluative Report was prepared and published (Sandall et al 2001).

Albany outcomes

The evaluation involved mailing the King's Maternity Services Questionnaire to 447 women, of whom 299 gave birth in hospital, 42 gave birth with Trust midwives at home and 106 were cared for by the Albany Practice (Sandall et al 2001: 7). The response rate overall was 52 per cent, with highest response rates from women attending the Albany Practice (58 per cent), followed by those giving birth at home.

Women attended by Albany midwives felt more involved in decision-making, perceived the midwives as being more available and reported being given more information (Reed and Walton 2009: 152). Of the women accessing Albany midwives, 69 per cent did not use pharmacological pain control, significantly more of whom stated 'no pain relief was required' (Reed and Walton 2009: 152);

this indicates that the Albany women were better prepared for labour, better supported in labour, or both.

The evaluation was positive, stating:

> Throughout the women's responses, there is a clear pattern of woman centred care being offered and of partnership with women, which may contribute to the positive evaluations of antenatal care and good clinical outcomes.
>
> (Sandall et al 2001: 56)

And:

> The overall conclusion is that the Albany practice have [sic] been successful in achieving the objectives they set for themselves in agreement with the Trust.
>
> (Sandall et al 2001: 81)

There were a few cautious provisos related particularly to research methods, but the existence of 'considerable misconceptions' among trust midwives were also noted (Sandall et al 2001: 81).

The case

Into this midwifery Garden of Eden, though, slithered the serpent of acrimonious censure. The Albany Practice concurred with the advice of the statutory regulatory body, mentioned above (page 148), that independent midwives organise themselves to contract their services to the NHS (NMC 2012: section 12.4). Similarly, the Albany Practice resolved the problem of payment, necessitated by IM practice, as suggested by a system of contracts with NHS institutions (Hunter 1998: 87). The limitations of these, probably well-meant, counsels have been laid bare by the Albany case. The inherent risk involves damaging most those most reliant on and those with most invested in such innovative developments.

THE SEQUENCE OF EVENTS

The various parties involved in this unsavoury shambles are in agreement that, although previously relationships may been less than ideal, the Albany case originated in late 2008 after a baby died following care by an Albany midwife (Jowitt 2009; Yiannouzis 2010). The death of a baby is a tragedy for the family, and the midwife sorrowfully scrutinises her care and seeks the help of her Supervisor of Midwives. But the loss of a baby is a distant yet constant risk, particularly for women from more deprived backgrounds. It was after this baby's death that the effects of hypoxic ischaemic encephalopathy (HIE; page 157) began to emerge as an issue (Edwards 2012). At this point the Trust managers suspended the Albany home birth service.

Just over 12 months later, in December 2009 following a neonatal death, the Albany Midwives were subjected to accusations from the Trust of responsibility for a disproportionately high number of cases of HIE (Phipps 2010; Reed 2010). Becky Reed, one of the original Albany midwives, argued with good reason that the figures presented to support the accusations were at least partly incorrect, and the subsequent corrections favoured the Albany Practice (Reed 2010: 4). On the basis of the initial and seriously questionable data after a few weeks, despite 12 years of commendable provision, the Trust terminated the Contract (Edwards et al 2011). It was at this point that the findings of a number of different, yet interrelated, investigations began to kick in.

THE INVESTIGATIONS

First was the series of cases which comprised the erroneous data which prompted the suspension and termination mentioned already.

Unbeknown outwith the local management circles, a supposedly independent review was commissioned from CMACE (Centre for Maternal and Child Enquiries, undated). This Report, bizarrely entitled 'The London Project', would have been kept under wraps, had not a freedom of information order been raised by the AIMS Committee (Edwards 2012). The credibility of the CMACE document has been called into question by variably authoritative sources (Phipps 2010; Davies and Edwards 2010; AIMS 2010b) resulting in its findings being widely ridiculed. The criticisms focus on the sample, time frame, research method, diagnosis, poor understanding of the woman's prerogative, anonymity of the panel and assumptions of medical authority and advantages of hospital birth.

Following the commissioning of the CMACE report in January 2009, the Albany midwives continued to challenge the original data, given to CMACE by the Trust and upon which the report was based. Following their persistent demands for corroboration of the data, the Trust finally commissioned an Internal Audit in June 2009, which was prepared by a renal nurse at the hospital (Casley-Ready undated). Based on the findings of this audit a statement appeared on the Trust website, stating that: 'We have become concerned about the safety record of the practice in comparison with the Trust's overall maternity safety record. Our records show that whilst Albany delivered babies for 4% of all King's births, those births accounted for 42% of our full term babies born with Hypoxic Ischaemic Encephalopathy … '. This Internal Audit has subsequently been critiqued by two professional statisticians, both of whom question the findings' reliability. The damning statement, however, remains on the website at the time of writing. Most authoritative were the criticisms by Alison Macfarlane, formerly statistical advisor to CMACE's predecessors:

> In the absence of information about sources of the case series, the defini-
> tions and inclusion criteria used, the longer term outcomes of the babies
> who survived, the extent to which the babies included and all babies
> delivered at Kings had factors which were associated with neonatal

encephalopathy and the lack of denominators and statistical power, it is impossible to draw any inferences.

(Macfarlane 2009 in Reed 2010: 4)

Although Katie Yiannouzis maintains that the CMACE report 'highlighted serious concerns involving the Albany Midwifery Practice' (2010: 193), the authors of the Report itself forbore to make any recommendations that the Albany Contract should be terminated (Davies and Edwards 2010).

The Coroner's Inquest which was held to investigate the 2009 case, mentioned above, came to the conclusion that there was no evidence of any neglect in the care provided by the midwives (Edwards et al 2011: 4).

The midwife who has featured most prominently and has suffered most in the course of this sorry saga, Becky Reed, was required to submit her midwifery records for scrutiny in the course of two Supervisory Investigations (Edwards et al 2011: 4; NMC 2010d). On the basis of these investigations this Midwife was referred to the Nursing and Midwifery Council (NMC); as this referral has involved only one of the Albany team of midwives (Edwards et al 2011: 4), the experience of Becky Reed is addressed next.

ONE PARTICULAR MIDWIFE

The enthusiastic support which Becky Reed has received from midwives, among others, during the Albany case is evidenced by her short-listing for the 2012 BJM Midwife of the Year award (Davies 2012). Meanwhile, she is appropriately scathing in her analysis of her treatment at the hands of the Trust and the statutory regulator. She attributes her experience of being made a scapegoat partly to the Albany Practice being beyond the day-to-day control of the health care system (Reed 2010). Thus, the independent Contract, negotiated to ensure that the Albany Practice was able to function as a self-managed and self-employed group, has proved a rather mixed blessing. To illustrate the narrow-mindedness of the context in which the Contract operated, Becky Reed quotes a trust spokesperson as praising the advantages of keeping all 'services in line with the same national clinical and safety guidance and standards' (Reed 2010: 5). Such railroading of maternity services, though, clearly contradicts governmental pretensions to the provision of individualised or woman-centred care.

THE ROLE OF THE STATUTORY REGULATORY BODY

In January 2010 Becky Reed was referred to the statutory regulatory body, the NMC, by her Supervisor and Head of Midwifery, Katie Yiannouzis. An Interim Conditions of Practice Order for 18 months, the maximum permitted, was made at an NMC hearing in September 2010. This Order required a programme of supervised practice which 'should have clear learning objectives that address the shortfalls identified in the Supervisory Investigation Report' (NMC 2010d). An NMC review in April 2011 revoked this Order, on the basis of reports on Becky Reed's supervised practice and multitude of testimonials, liberating her to practise as a midwife. The statutory regulatory body, though, has continued to pursue its investigation.

The NMC documentation relating to the investigation, comprising 543 pages with five A4 sides of allegations, was received in March 2012 (Reed 2012). Although the documentation was found to be incomplete, Becky Reed was given less than one month to respond. The documentation comprised, in the main, a report by an expert witness who is a midwife educationist which bears a disconcerting resemblance to the seriously discredited CEMACE report (undated; page 155). The expert witness focused on five cases with alleged poor outcomes, for three of which Katie Yiannouzis was the Supervisor, but had not commented at the time. For three of the cases Becky Reed was not the lead, but the second midwife, although no other Albany midwives have been either investigated or disciplined. One of the cases was referred to the NMC by the parents, but the finding reached was 'no case to answer' and a supported practice order made (Davies et al 2012). For one of the cases, which was the main subject in the original referral, the inquest in 2011 found that the hypoxic episode occurred during pregnancy, with no indication of neglect by the midwives.

This brief summary clearly indicates that the expert witness was doing little more than recycling the disreputable document produced by CEMACE and the internal report provided by the Trust. She is obviously far from achieving the NMC's remit to 'comment on the care given by the registrant and the conduct of the other midwives' (Davies et al 2012).

Thus, writing more than three years after the original incident, there is no sign of the statutory regulatory body realising, even less rectifying, the dreadful implications of its dysfunctional handling of this case. This means that due to the NMC's malign inefficiency and at a time when she is most needed, another far-sighted, inspirational and fundamentally human midwife is languishing, employing her inestimably valuable skills outwith UK midwifery practice.

HYPOXIC ISCHAEMIC ENCEPHALOPATHY (HIE)

Largely unknown among midwives before the Albany case because of its specificity to paediatrics (Page 2012), this term was only introduced in the late twentieth century (Mysak 1968). Its significance in the Albany case, though, demands that it be scrutinised. Its spurious precision has led to this term being largely abandoned (Kurinczuk et al 2005). While it clearly carries connotations of brain damage, associated with lack of oxygen and poor circulation, leading to cerebral palsy, it fails to indicate when and how such damage may have occurred. This matters because in the CEMACE report 11 cases were considered in which the babies had 'apparently suffered an intrapartum event leading to hypoxic ischaemic encephalopathy' (CEMACE undated: 5). That a large majority of these babies (nine out of 11) were born in the maternity unit with medical involvement in the care tends to pass unreported (Davies and Edwards 2010). As with many neonatal conditions the signs, symptoms being unavailable in such pre-verbal human beings, tend to be poorly-defined. So suspicions of differences in muscle tone or feeding ability may be labelled as HIE or, the now preferred term, neonatal encephalopathy.

The term HIE is generally considered, as indicated by the CEMACE report, to imply that the hypoxic episode occurred during labour. In her authoritative analysis, Margaret Jowett establishes, though, that such incidents are six times less frequent than hypoxic episodes occurring during pregnancy (Jowett 2010). These incidents may be attributable to any of a range of maternal or foeto-placental conditions. Thus, the implication of blame with which this term is loaded (Phipps 2010) was used to incriminate the Albany midwives when there was no certainty about the timing of any untoward events.

Margaret Jowitt and Sarah Montagu further scrutinise the term HIE and identify a more sinister picture. This is due to the likelihood of litigation following a diagnosis of HIE with the ensuing massive financial costs to, for example, the trust. These authors suggest that the Albany Practice's remarkably low perinatal mortality rate may be associated with their low-intervention philosophy. Jowitt and Montagu go on to consider whether these midwives were in fact protecting the largely deprived childbearing women in their care from obstetric interventions which would have brought about even more, and even more serious, morbidity in their newborns (Jowitt and Montagu 2009). This contention is supported by the Albany perinatal mortality rate of 4.9 per 1,000, compared with the average rate for the area of 11.4 per 1,000 (Reed and Walton 2009: 156). This like-lihood of the protective effect of the Albany practice leads into consideration of the significance of HIE.

Hypoxic ischaemic encephalopathy is thought to derive its significance from the possibility that it was caused by neglect or substandard practice on the part of the Albany midwives. The reality of its significance, though, may be surprisingly dif-ferent, as implied by Becky Reed when she writes 'we look after [the women] until their babies are a month old, we know their stories and how their babies are doing' (Reed 2010: 4). This 'knowing' is crucial to this case because there has been no long-term follow up of the babies diagnosed with HIE, so knowing that a baby is growing into a healthy toddler calls into question the accuracy of the diagnosis and implied prognosis (Davies and Edwards 2010).

The supposedly higher incidence of HIE admissions among 'Albany babies' needs to be considered in the context of the Albany's low admission rate to the neonatal unit (Jowitt and Montagu 2009). The Albany babies tended to remain *in utero* longer, so preterm births and ensuing admissions were correspondingly low. Thus, admissions of Albany babies would have attracted considerable attention by virtue of their rarity, and exposed the babies to a battery of investigations suggesting the possibility of a condition such as HIE.

INTERPRETATION

How may the observer interpret these events? What is the reality of this as yet unfinished saga? Becky Reed argues that the Albany practice has been penalised for its temerity in threatening the risk management orientation of the health system. She argues the powerful influence of risk management over all decision-making in the NHS, which serves to medicalise maternity services and deprive women of choices about their childbearing experience (Reed 2010: 5).

Writing on behalf of the NCT, however, Belinda Phipps suggests that a more sinister agenda may have been operating to bring about the demise of the Albany Practice (Phipps 2010: 35). Phipps agues that 'difficult management issues' (Phipps 2010: 35) existed, with which the trust management were not competent to cope. This sorry scenario resonates with the picture which I have presented of a lack of understanding verging on hostility between hospital-employed midwives and Albany midwives (page 154). Such acrimony may not be surprising in view of the diametrically opposed philosophies espoused by the two different groups of practitioners. Phipps charitably suggests that, in referring the Albany case, the managers may have been seeking 'guidance as to how to move forward' (Phipps 2010: 35). Employing CEMACE and the NMC to obtain such guidance, though, is heart-breakingly disappointing. Such recourse to the statutory regulatory body, though, is far from novel. This was the discouraging conclusion reached by Margaret Jowitt and Ishbel Kargar in their analysis of the shortcomings of the NMC on midwifery matters:

> When an NHS midwife is referred to the NMC it often appears to relate to a failure of management to resolve workplace issues such as a breakdown in working relationships rather than clinical concerns per se.
>
> (Jowitt and Kargar 2009: 22–3)

Thus, the NMC appears to be permitting itself to be exploited by NHS managers to do their dirty or 'arm's length' work for them; thus no costs accrue to the service, but monumentally immeasurable costs are visited on the midwives on the receiving end of NMC judgements. In this way, the statutory regulatory activities of the NMC appear to have been jettisoned in favour of protecting, not the public, but the management functionaries.

THE SIGNIFICANCE OF THE ALBANY CASE

The significance of this case is found to affect differently the various groups involved. Some of the paradoxes of the Albany case engender serious concerns about the competence and rationality of the management and its decision-making. As mentioned already, the NMC has been inefficient and lackadaisical in its assigned aim of protecting the public from unsafe practitioners. The Trust managers demonstrate similarly paradoxical behaviour; on the one hand they praise the Albany Practice describing it as 'an excellent example of midwifery practice for others to emulate' (Yiannouzis 2010: 193). On the other hand, this manager terminated the Contract on grounds of the safety of 'our women and their babies' (2010: 193). A further example of paradoxical thinking is found in reports that, while accusations of unsafe practice are being levelled at Albany midwives, the very same, allegedly unsafe, staff are being offered alternative posts as midwives within the Trust (Davies and Edwards 2010: 261).

In terms of the impact of the management deficiencies on childbearing women, the NCT argues that contracts with groups like the Albany need to be drawn up at a higher strategic level (Phipps 2010: 35). In this way women are likely to be able to exercise genuine choice in their childbearing, as has been facilitated by the Albany midwives (Reed 2010: 5).

The meaning of the demise of the Albany Practice for women has been outlined by Margaret Jowitt drawing on a feminist argument:

> midwifery respects and honours the power of the female body to do what it was designed to do, to give birth. Nowhere is women's power more evident than in the act of giving birth; it can feel like climbing Everest, and we get it handed to us on a plate – but without support it can feel like being thrown to the lions. I believe that our patriarchal society is afraid of women's power. ... Giving birth can be one of the most empowering things in a woman's life – or it can be profoundly disempowering.
>
> (Jowitt 2009)

The significance of this case for midwives is not very different, with the empowerment of midwives carrying potential to enhance the choices for the women they attend. The 'incredible' support of women for the discontinued Albany Practice midwives indicates a collaborative relationship developing into a virtuous cycle (Reed 2010: 5). Less optimistically, the reverse scenario may also materialise through disempowerment, with midwifery being:

> in danger of losing its very identity through NHS control of the ways midwives are allowed to work and NMC rulings on midwives who work in different ways.
>
> (Jowitt 2009)

For midwives the meaning of this case is that it exposes a climate of fear (Kirkham 2010). Such fear results from anxieties about differences in modes of practice and about midwives liberating themselves from management constraints to achieve excellence in care. Rather than the ideal of midwives working together to instil confidence in each other and in childbearing women, conformity to systematic and hospital norms have become priorities. The disheartening result is a 'lowering of everyone's expectations of maternity services' (NMC 2010: 13).

The significance for maternity care lies in the Albany midwives' gold standard practice being unilaterally terminated. As an exemplary innovation, the Albany succeeded in achieving enviable breastfeeding rates and home birth rates among women in an area of profound and multiple deprivation. Thus, the Albany

Practice was able to operationalise government policies relating to public participation and the reduction of institutionalisation. The irony of the demise of this beacon of policy implementation was not wasted on Jenny Hall (2010: 3), who referred to it as 'the way to be practising'. The breadth and impact of the ripples which are spreading out from this unsavoury case are not to be underestimated, in the form of national and international recognition of the Albany midwives' ability to 'inspire the rest of the NHS, managers and midwives alike' (Jowitt 2009).

Midwifery supervision

The supervision of midwives by their midwifery colleagues creates the impression of being an ideal arrangement for ensuring high standards and supporting practitioners. But, having mentioned the history of supervision (page 58) and its potential for control (page 107) already, it is now appropriate to consider the political realities of Midwifery Supervision.

A large majority of UK midwives are employed in the NHS, as are their Supervisors (SoMs), an arrangement which means that those involved appear to make Supervision function reasonably smoothly. Because of fear of errors and ensuing vilification, though, such apparent smooth functioning is largely due to 'NHS midwives [being] obedient creatures' (Kirkham 2011: 13). While relationships as toxic as these ensure that the maternity care system operates efficiently, the potential for innovative and individualised care tends to be stifled. The Supervisor-manager whose supervisee is a forward-thinking midwife finds herself in a cleft stick facing a conflict of interest. Where do the Supervisor's priorities lie? Should excellence be promoted or is a smoothly-running service a greater good? These questions are explored by Margaret Jowitt and Ishbel Kargar in their insightful analysis of the role of Supervision in protecting the childbearing woman and the midwife from 'NHS management bullying' (Jowitt and Kargar 2009: 23). These authors conclude that SoMs' ability to offer protection is limited.

The Supervisor of an Independent Midwife (IM) is particularly likely to face such quandaries. This is because the IM's client will have opted out of the NHS system of care (page 144) and is likely to be seeking care which is something other than the standard NHS package. In such situations, if there is a less than ideal outcome, the Supervisor needs to be very clear about whether the midwife may have practised outwith the Midwives Rules and Standards or merely overstepped local practice guidelines.

Sarah Davies probes the case of an admirable Independent Midwife whose Supervisor was unable or unprepared to differentiate between these two standards (Davies 2009). The midwife found herself being referred to the Nursing and Midwifery Council, which was sufficiently seriously ill-advised to find her guilty on three counts, none of which were evidence-based or NMC requirements. Heartbreakingly for the midwife and midwifery, she was struck off.

Supervisors have traditionally been drawn from the ranks of midwifery managers. It is fortunate that that arrangement has been discontinued. Less fortunately, though, the narrow organisational mindset which managers brought to Supervision has, for all too many supervisors, survived.

Medical politics

A case which bears comparison with the Albany midwives' sorry saga is that of obstetrician Wendy Savage (Wagner 1995; Jowitt 2009). Beginning in 1985, this particular *cause célèbre* has become known as the 'Savage Enquiry' due to the books it engendered (Savage 1986; Savage 2007). The precise issues involved in this case may never be entirely clear, but the picture portrayed by popular and professional media represented a cabal of male obstetricians confronting the woman-centred practice of their female colleague.

A 'ploy', used in both the Savage and the Albany cases to disgrace the prey, has been highlighted by Wagner (1995: 1020); this manoeuvre involved trawling through all of the subjects' midwifery or medical records in the hope of finding a flaw on which to build a case to discredit the practitioner. The incidents thus identified instigated Savage's suspension on the grounds of her reluctance to perform (unnecessary) caesareans. The conflict with her male colleagues, however, was due to her unwillingness to follow the policies and practices to which they fervently adhered. Her penalty for not towing the 'party' line was suspension from practice. This case eventually ended with her exoneration in 1986 (Pratten 1990).

One interpretation of this case is that the usual laddish behaviour among the obstetricians was expected to apply pressure to Savage, to coerce her to bring her practice into line. Unfortunately, her medical brethren underestimated her political abilities in manipulating the media, public and professions on her own behalf. The political ramifications of this case extended, though, beyond the obstetric fraternity at the London Hospital. Savage was successful in harnessing support from childbearing women and their representatives, with visions of a shared ethos of maternity care (Zander 2007). Midwives also allied themselves with Savage to offer what Luke Zander terms 'woman-centred care' (Zander 2007: xiii), although the phrase had not been applied to maternity by 1985. The third 'very significant' supporters took the form of the local general practitioners (GPs; Zander 2007: xiii); herein lay the other foundation of the medico-political conflict. The GPs' interest in maternity care included personal and professional, as well as financial, components. They sought to continue their maternity practice, which Savage encouraged in the interests, allegedly, of low-tech domiciliary maternity care. In reality a large majority of this care was provided by midwives, who derived no benefit from the generous payments to GPs. Savage's opponents, though, were becoming increasingly wise to the irrelevance of GP maternity care.

It may be to the credit of Savage that she shepherded her supporters to overcome obstetric opposition, but we should be clear that this case related more to medico-political manoeuvring than to women's health.

Maternity in the Republic of Ireland

I have already addressed some of the political issues relating to maternity care in the Irish Republic on pages 27 and 55, focusing on interpersonal issues, maternal death and active management, respectively. Although my earlier discussion has implications for strategic planning, the primary concern has been on the clinical level. I now seek to address the implications of certain national issues for maternity and midwifery.

Ireland constitutes an excellent example because the overpowering medicalisation of Irish maternity services, combined with a predominance of private health care, creates an unwieldy imbalance of power between medical practitioners on the one hand and childbearing women and midwives on the other (Matthews and Kelly 2008). It was hoped that the KPMG Report on maternity provision in the greater Dublin area (Matthews and Kelly 2008) would resolve this impasse by encouraging the Health Services Executive (HSE), the organisational arm of the Irish Department of Health and Children, to act on its recommendations. This would have increased the provision of out-of-hospital and non-medical care; but the demise of the Celtic Tiger has been blamed for even the KPMG Report's modest aspirations being unlikely to materialise. At 16.8 per 1,000 population (ESRI 2012), the country has the highest birth rate in the European Union and the recommended changes in the infrastructure are crucial for hospitals strained to breaking point (Siggins 2011).

The KPMG aspirations related to increasing the provision of midwifery services in Midwifery-Led Units (MLUs; KPMG 2008: 11; AIMSI 2008). But not only have the new MLUs not come to fruition, one of the two existing MLUs is under pressure; additionally, small community-based services have been forced to contract or close (Murphy-Lawless 2011a). Economic factors have been credited with being the reason for these closures, but other agendas are also operating. This is evidenced by, first, the high caesarean rate of 'over 26%' (ESRI 2012), which squander finite resources but are not subjected to financial stringencies. The second significant pointer is the serious under-utilisation of one of the MLUs, in Cavan, thought to be associated with obstetricians' reluctance to jeopardise their fee income (Murphy-Lawless 2011a: 7).

The statutory regulation of midwifery in Ireland has been transformed by the passage of the Nurses and Midwives Act which was signed into legislation on 21 December 2011 (ISB 2011). The transformation is beginning to be operationalised by a Commencement Order taking effect from midnight on 31 December 2011. The reception of this legislation has been mixed, with little to celebrate, but I endeavour to identify the good news first.

The good news

The Nurses and Midwives Act (NMA) repealed the previous legislation, the Nurses Acts, which had not deigned to recognise midwifery's existence. Thus, 'It restored the standing of Irish midwifery as a separate profession for the first time since 1950' (Murphy-Lawless 2012: 68).

The indeterminate news

At the time of writing, there is some uncertainty about the effect of the new statutory regulatory framework on midwifery. Under the new legislation, the extant body, *An Bord Altranais* (ABA, the Nursing Board), will be replaced with *Bord Altranais agus Cnáinhseachais na hÉireann* (the Nursing and Midwifery Board of Ireland). Although the Irish government claims to recognise 'midwifery as a separate and distinct profession' (Harney 2010), this recognition is both less than convincing and familiar to UK midwives. The NMA provides for the establishment of a Midwives Committee to advise the Board on all matters pertaining to midwifery practice. This arrangement is reminiscent of the UK situation in which a Midwifery Committee (page 141) was created to offer advice to the NMC on midwifery matters. As Jo Murphy-Lawless observes, the Irish Midwives Committee will have no binding effect (Murphy-Lawless 2011b: 24), making it precisely comparable with its UK equivalent.

The not so good news

It may be that such comparisons with the NMC should have been included with the even less good news, but I have chosen to err towards optimism, as the outcomes remain to be seen.

The new Irish legislation failed to grasp the opportunity presented to provide midwives with self-governing professional status. Andrew Symon observes that other occupational groups in Ireland have been granted such status (Symon 2011) and AIMSI catalogues countries in which midwives have been awarded independent status (AIMSI 2010). That midwives in Ireland have been denied such status and remain under the nursing yoke disheartens women's representatives:

> The dominance of nursing has restricted midwives' professional development for over half a century.
>
> (AIMSI 2010)

A development, which may replicate the problems encountered in the United Kingdom, is the new concept of clinical supervision (Healy 2010). It is unclear how the clinical form of supervision will differ from the midwifery supervision with which UK midwives are all too familiar. There is a possibility that clinical supervision for midwives in Ireland may approximate to the healthier, more therapeutic, form employed by occupational groups such as counsellors, but this is not yet clear. That such optimism may be unjustified is plain from the legislation's emphasis on disciplinary procedures (ISB 2011: Parts 7–9) and other publications (Mills et al 2011).

The most disconcerting aspect of this new legislation is that part (section 40) which discriminates against the 'self-employed community midwives' (SECMs or IMs) (ISB 2011: 39). Although superficially complying with the EU Directive (EU 2011: 4.2(d)), this legislative discrimination takes the form of requiring midwives to maintain indemnity insurance (PII). SECMs must sign a 'Memorandum of Understanding' (MOU), which is a service level agreement with the HSE to obtain PII. The criteria forming the basis of this MOU are stringent; they exclude the SECM from attending at home certain groups of women in childbirth, including older women and those with prolonged rupture of membranes, a BMI ≥30 or a history of surgery, such as previous caesarean (Murphy-Lawless 2012: 69). The penalties for a midwife attending such a woman for homebirth are clearly stated:

> a fine not exceeding €160,000 or ... imprisonment for a term not exceeding 10 years or both.
>
> (ISB 2011: 39)

By no means overstating its catastrophic nature, this legislation has appropriately been summarised as 'criminalisation of midwifery' (Murphy-Lawless 2011b: 24i) and in breach of the European Convention on Human Rights (Symon 2011: 193iii).

On balance

Ireland has a long and painful history of obstetric intervention (Murphy-Lawless 1988). Against the backdrop of the highest birth rate in Europe (ESRI 2012; UN 2011) being addressed by 'An embedded and deeply conservative obstetric profession' (Murphy-Lawless 2011b: 23i), such a litany of tragedy surprises no one. The prevailing dogma and domination, it is hoped, will not be permitted to persist.

Conclusion

In this chapter I have shown that there is a wealth of examples which show disconcertingly clearly the pitfalls of statutory regulation. These examples should serve as a dire warning for those states currently developing regulatory systems to support and facilitate midwifery practice. Midwives and others in these newly regulating states should and must learn from these salutary, but unfortunately not unique, examples.

The twin concepts of risk and risk management have emerged repeatedly, carrying the implication that these concepts exist to protect the childbearing woman and her baby. The reality of risk management strategies, though, is somewhat different. All too often these techniques are applied to protect practitioners, together with the 'interests of hospitals, health authorities, and ultimately, the state through its regulatory bodies' (Murphy-Lawless 2012: 70). Thus it appears that the statutory regulatory agencies are undertaking the control activities which constitute others' dirty work. As I suggested above (page 158), this is the dirty work of, for example, indolent or otherwise reluctant employers. A further insight into these agencies' less than scrupulous activities is that they comprise the government's dirty work, as the electorate witnessing such behaviour would jeopardise politicians' careers.

8 Promising practices: how it can be done

I scrutinised, in Chapter 7, the extent to which benefits of midwifery care can be threatened and invalidated by the political intervention of agencies such as the statutory regulatory bodies. Far from optimistic, Chapter 7 presented a 'warts and all' analysis of certain challenges facing midwifery practice. In this chapter I examine the reverse side of the coin to assess whether the midwife is able to, despite challenges, practise real midwifery and what the outcomes are likely to be. Thus, I scrutinise whether and how the midwife is able to be sufficiently political to manipulate the environment within which she practises to benefit all concerned. To do this I plan to draw on illustrations of local and international examples of hegemony being applied beneficially in maternity care.

The political implications of these promising practices arise from not only the manoeuvring by which they are achieved, but also out of their effects. This focus is necessary as alterations in practice inevitably affect the balance of power between providers and users of midwifery services; thus the political implications of these developments need to be recognised and addressed. First, though, a little consideration must be given to the 'benefits of midwifery care', which I have mentioned already.

Benefits of midwifery care

While it is not easy for me as a midwife to be objective on such matters (Walsh and Devane 2012), midwifery's association with more positive outcomes than other models of care is becoming increasingly apparent. The other model with which midwifery is often compared is the medicalised 'obstetric-interventive' (Wagner 2001: S27) approach to birth. So, rather than putting the woman into a submissive 'patient' role during the birth, the midwife seeks to facilitate the woman's own ability to give birth as she wishes. In this way, the woman undergoes a transformational experience through which she comes to recognise her own ability, even strength, to mother her child and her family. Such empowerment provides the solid base on which self-esteem, family relationships and new individuals may be nurtured.

The evidence on which assertions of such benefits are based is becoming more authoritative, having begun over three decades ago (Mander 2001). Roberto Sosa and his colleagues serendipitously happened on the beneficial effects on birth outcomes of a friendly person being present (Sosa 1980). This chance finding spawned an epidemic of randomised controlled trials (RCTs) in the hope of identifying the vital ingredient (Hodnett et al 2011). That support in child-bearing, by a person such as a midwife, brings beneficial outcomes for the woman and baby has been established beyond dispute; the precise mechanism by which it operates, though, is not yet entirely clear.

What form does this care take?

Midwifery is firmly bound to the culture in which the woman gives birth, so the form of midwifery care varies correspondingly. While in some settings the midwife has traditionally practised relatively autonomously (van Teijlingen 1990), in others such autonomy is more novel (Mein-Smith 1986). The picture is yet more complex as within one country, or even locality, differently authentic or woman-centred forms of midwifery practice may be identified (Page 2010). As I mentioned previously (page 144), in the United Kingdom Independent Midwifery most closely approximates to genuine midwifery prac-tice but, for reasons which I discussed, that practice is threatened. As in many states, the majority of births in the United Kindom happen in medicalised set-tings (Wagner 2001). That situation is beginning to show the green shoots of change, which started as a reaction to the routinisation of interventive practice in the 1970s (Flint 1986). The rate at which this change occurs is affected by a number of factors.

Place of birth

While it is generally assumed that out-of-hospital birth empowers the childbearing woman and facilitates authentic midwifery practice, at least until recently, research has focused largely on institutional birth. An example is a meta-analysis by Sharon Brown and Deanna Grimes which reviewed studies involving nurse-midwife practice in a range of institutional and community settings (Brown and Grimes 1995). Although randomisation was notable by its absence, these studies sought to compare nurse-midwifery with obstetric practice. These researchers found midwifery to be associated with significant differences in terms of less analgesia, anaesthesia and foetal monitoring and fewer episiotomies, forceps-assisted births, artificial rupture of membranes and intravenous infusions. Apart from the nurse-midwife's practice being more woman-friendly, there were no major differences in outcomes.

Like Brown and Grimes' meta-analysis, Vanora Hundley and her colleagues in Scotland studied the care of 'low-risk' women, but in a midwife-managed birthing unit situated just 20 yards from the consultant-led labour ward (Hundley et al 1994). While significant differences were identified between the midwife-managed unit and labour ward in foetal monitoring, analgesia, mobi-lity, and use of episiotomy, there was no change in type of birth or neonatal outcomes. Unsurprisingly, in view of this unit's novelty and its proximity to the labour ward, this RCT demonstrated disconcertingly high transfer rates.

These studies show that, even in relatively medicalised environments of maternity units, midwifery care brings advantages. Few disadvantages have been demonstrated, apart from those inflicted by research protocols, such as eligibility and transfer criteria.

Increasing interest in out-of-hospital birth has progressed simultaneously with the development of a stronger evidence-base (McCourt et al 2011). Midwife-led units (MLUs) and birth centres (or alternative birth centres in the United States) are differentiated mainly by their staffing arrangements, but there remain huge variations in their location and organisation (Hodnett et al 2010). While UK birth centres tend to incorporate a midwife-led ethos, in more medicalised health care systems different personnel are involved. Midwife-led care may take the form of a team of midwives sharing responsibility or may be more indivi-dualised through a caseloading approach. The systematic review by Marie Hatem and her colleagues showed the many established benefits of midwife-led care as compared with other approaches (Hatem et al 2008); these include less use of regional analgesia and fewer episiotomies or instrument-assisted births. Midwife-led care has also been shown to be associated with the woman being more likely to be cared for in labour by a 'known' midwife and a greater likelihood of feeling in control in labour. There is also a greater chance of the woman experiencing a 'normal' birth and, at least, starting to breastfeed.

A birth centre located in a medical facility is known as an alongside or integrated birth centre (IBC; Hodnett et al 2010) to differentiate it from a standalone, iso-lated or freestanding birth centre (FSBC), which is discrete from any health care provision (Nicoll 2006; Walsh and Downe 2004). For those who value medical supervision of uncomplicated childbearing, FSBCs may be a step too far, making the 'home-like' environment of the IBC preferred. Clearly, though, the proximity of medical resources to an IBC will affect the woman's confidence and the midwife's practice. A number of authoritative RCTs focusing on IBCs, though, have established the benefits to the woman, in terms of her health and satisfaction, and have identified no disadvantages for her or her baby (Hodnett et al 2010). Despite methodological weaknesses in the studies located, a structured review of FSBC outcomes reached broadly similar conclusions, summarised in the less-than-enthusiastic maxim 'safe unless proved harmful' (Walsh and Downe 2004: 228). These authors do, however, advance the place of birth debate by implying, without using the term, the iatrogenic potential of institutional birth for low-risk women.

For those who regard hospital birth as a potential cause of maternal and perinatal iatrogenesis (Olsen and Jewell 1998), planned home birth presents a solution. The Cochrane review by Ole Olsen and David Jewell, though, deplores the dearth of suitably-sized studies to support such a conclusion. The research in this area has tended to either vilify home birth and/or to demonstrate less than scientific methods. The former includes a US study by Joseph Wax and his colleagues using an epidemiological approach (Wax 2010), which led to the conclusion of a tripling of the neonatal mortality rate. This study, and the journal which published it, has been rightly and authoritatively pilloried on methodological grounds, such as sampling and statistical errors (Gyte et al 2011). Concerns about the safety of home birth among some community midwives, however, may result in 'the hospital being brought into the home' (Edwards 2005: 90; Steen 2012). Attempting a global picture of planned home birth, Judith Fullerton and her colleagues identified the massive variability in the conditions under which women give birth at home (Fullerton 2007). Their wealth of data, while recommending public policy developments, permits them only to be able to draw 'generally favorable' (Fullerton 2007: 330) conclusions.

The lack of 'strong' research on home birth, Patricia Janssen and her colleagues argue, should lead to childbearing women's views compensating for statistical power (Janssen et al 2009). These researchers collected qualitative data from 559 women (response rate 82 per cent) as part of a large evaluation of an innovative midwifery programme. The overwhelmingly positive views may be dismissed as little more than characteristic of a volunteer sample; but the women's comments about 'Knowledge, Skill, Competence, and Professionalism', 'Empowerment', 'Birth at Home as Family-Centered' and 'Home Birth as a Way of Maintaining Control, Avoiding Intervention' resonate with more general findings.

The impact of midwife-led care was brought home to me through an innovative project undertaken in a major city in the People's Republic of China (Cheung et al 2011). In a country experiencing precipitously rapid development, the high status of medical intervention is a relatively unchanging aspect, so this midwife-led normal birth unit (MNBU) challenged longstanding and widely-held assumptions. In the MNBU, interventions to accelerate labour for the convenience of staff were reduced by more than 50 per cent. Particularly remarkable was the finding that, with China's caesarean rates occasionally reaching 100 per cent (Huang 2000), the rate in the MNBU was lowered to approximately one-quarter of the standard labour ward's rate. The difficulties facing midwifery in China, though, are reflected in the MNBU midwives' limited ability to bring down the astronomical episiotomy rate. In the standard labour ward the rate reached 94.2 per cent whereas, despite the best efforts of researchers and management, the MNBU episiotomy rate remained stubbornly fixed at 77.9 per cent. The persistently routine use of this intervention reflects the local cultural environment. In such a powerfully patriarchal society, the one child policy obviously circumscribes most women's childbearing aspirations (page 64) and the midwife has long been cornered into defensive practice.

How it happens

The beneficial effects of midwifery care being provided in these woman-friendly settings arise out of the relationship which develops between the childbearing woman and the midwife. While it may be possible for such a relationship to form within an institutional environment, the values of the institution tend to outweigh and confound the development of profound engagement (Kirkham 2000b: 236). The skills necessary for the formation of a meaningful relationship begin with the midwife's confidence in both her own abilities and that of the woman whom she is attending. Such confidence facilitates the woman's trust in both the midwife and her own ability to give birth as she wishes. Thus, this relationship becomes a virtuous cycle in which the woman, crucially, feels well-supported.

In such a mutually beneficial situation, the power and control ordinarily available to the midwife becomes shared and loses any negative features, leading to a positive birth experience. Denis Walsh and Declan Devane (2012) write about this relationship formation in terms of the development of 'agency', first, by the childbearing woman with an empathic midwife. The continuing contact during pregnancy and the presence of the midwife during labour were found to be crucial to the woman's perception of agency. These researchers compared this development of agency with the woman's autonomy through decision-making and action to achieve empowerment. Such agency involves the woman, not only retaining responsibility for her decisions and actions, but also deciding if and when the time had come for her to relinquish responsibility and allow the midwife to assume a more traditionally directive role. Of course, such a relationship means that the woman is able to resume her agency when she feels ready.

The second type of agency which Walsh and Devane identify applies to the midwife practising in an MLU (Walsh and Devane 2012), which may assume a form of autonomy. This agency pertains at various levels, such as in the organisation of the MLU, or at a clinical level in making decisions about a woman's care which might be regarded as risky in a more routinised institutional environment. These researchers advance their argument by suggesting that the midwife practising in a more traditional setting might be prevented from exercising agency by the pressure of time required to complete allotted tasks. While the woman's agency may be permitted to operate in such a setting, the sheer scale of the institution acts as a deterrent. These researchers argue that it is the 'smallness' of the birthing environment, and the associated availability of time, which is crucial to relationship formation and more favourable birthing outcomes in an MLU. Thus, cultural and organisational aspects of midwifery constitute fundamentally important features which may either impede or enhance the woman's 'good birth'.

Promise fulfilled?

The possibility that midwifery is able to deliver benefits is considerably more than that. A number of better- or lesser-known examples serve to illustrate the reality of what midwifery provides. These examples are variably well-established and from various countries and continents. As well as being good news stories, these examples demonstrate the crucially important role of political manoeuvring if the midwife is to achieve the sought-after outcomes for herself and the woman for whom she provides care.

The Dutch midwife

The midwife in Holland is widely-held, and holds herself, to be the epitome of idealised midwifery practice (De Vries et al 2009: 31). Such status is based on the Dutch midwife's long and honourable history (Marland 1996), her championing of home birth with admirable outcomes (CBS 2012) and her recent and current portrayal (De Vries 2004).

The practice environment

Although presently undergoing the changes and challenges faced by most developed countries, the socio-cultural milieu in which the Dutch midwife practises is essentially prosperous, enlightened and healthy. These factors, which are unlikely to be unrelated, are evidenced by infant mortality statistics which are consistently lower than, for example, US figures (WHO 2012). Healthy lifestyles feature prominently and home birth is a standard aspect of life, rather than the problem into which it has been relegated elsewhere (De Vries et al 2009). In this idyll the midwife, practising independently, attends birthing women who are 'low risk', although terms like 'physiological' and 'simple' are preferred. Women considered at higher risk of complications, referred to as expecting a 'pathological birth', are attended by obstetricians in secondary or tertiary institutions (Pieters et al 2010). Despite being reassured that this distinction is unproblematical, it appears artificial to the point of inaccuracy, as health problems may both manifest and resolve themselves during a woman's childbearing experience. This somewhat questionable distinction, though, is ratified in the Obstetric Indications List (*Verloskundige Indicatielijst* VIL 1999).

Status

The social and professional standing of the Dutch midwife is enhanced by her history and her independent position, which verges on entrepreneurial. The small number of midwifery schools in the Netherlands, four in total, and the few places available result in serious competition for those places (De Vries 2004). The stated rationale is to ensure that employment is available for those who qualify, but elitist agendas may be operating.

Another aspect of the high status claimed by the Dutch midwife is found in her professional allegiance. Midwives in many countries are endeavouring to distance themselves from other occupational groups in order to clarify the true nature of the midwife's role (Mander 2008). In the Netherlands, however, the reverse process is occurring, involving the midwife allying herself with and actually presenting herself as a medical practitioner (Cairoli 2010). While De Vries contends that this is merely a legal nicety (De Vries 2001: 284), in support of Ester Cairoli's view I have certainly encountered the full, proud explanation of the Dutch midwife's superiority to those elsewhere due to her enhanced status through her medical orientation.

Politics

In many countries in the early twentieth century, the midwife found herself in conflict with other occupational groups as she has sought control over her own professional activities (Jackson and Mander 1995). Hilary Marland claims that the Dutch midwife avoided such acrimonious conflicts, preferring to refer to the negotiations in the Netherlands as the 'midwife debate' (Marland 1995: 317). As in other settings, midwives and their practice were supported by a range of powerful agencies. Unsurprisingly, for financial reasons, opposition came from their competitor provider of basic (*eerstelijn*) maternity care, the general practitioners (*huisarts*). Obstetricians declined to support their medical brothers in this debate, having no wish for competition from that direction. Playing a crucial but not over-committed role in negotiations, the government committee (*Raad*) eventually ruled in favour of the midwife, confirming the *status quo* for this practitioner whose regulation had long predated her medical competitors.

Primaat

The Dutch midwife's longstanding contribution to the health of local communities had been recognised by regulation since the eighteenth century (Marland 1993: 192), whereas her medical brothers were required to wait for another century for such recognition. The enhancement of her status by such early acknowledgement of her role can only have been assisted by the primacy or protection given to her practice by other legislation. The *primaat* (priority), which may have been introduced to save money for the insurers or to ensure attendance of the professional more experienced in physiological birth, penalised women for *not* employing a midwife. This operated by the midwife being paid preferentially if she practised in an area where a *huisarts* also offered maternity services. Thus, the Dutch state has effectively provided the midwife with a 'monopoly over normal obstetrics' (Abraham-Van der Mark 1993: 4). So the *huisarts* could only be employed for a physiological birth where no midwives practise. Such preferential treatment of the midwife by the state has been, to say the least, unusual (Cairoli 2010). For the ordinarily less powerful occupational group to be favoured by such generous fiscal arrangements defies the conventional logic of professions; in such 'turf wars' the power holder is invariably the victor.

*Obstetric Indications List (*Verloskundige Indicatielijst *VIL 1999)*

Closely linked to *primaat*, and having a similar effect in protecting the midwife's practice from competitors, is the Obstetric Indications List (VIL 1999). First drawn up in the early decades of the twentieth century, the List comprises a protocol of conditions in which the *eerstelijn* care provider must transfer the woman to obstetric care (DeVries 2001). It was around this list that *primaat* eventually foundered. Ironically, the original rationale for re-examining the List was concern about the increasing number of hospital admissions of childbearing women; that such concern continues to be justified is evidenced by the persisting fall in the home birth rate to 20 per cent (Davis-Floyd and Bonaro 2012: 62). This persistent fall is widely perceived as being due to medical manipulation, ie expansion, of the Obstetric Indications List, so that fewer women are able to give birth at home and the power base of the Dutch midwife is jeopardised.

Politics, privilege and practice

While not belittling the exemplary practice of the Dutch midwife, close examination of her background shows clearly the favourable environment in which she has long practised. On the one hand, it is tempting to conclude that it would be difficult *not* to be successful in such a privileged *milieu*. On the other hand, though, the Dutch midwife deserves credit for recognising that effective midwifery requires the convergence and manipulation of societal, occupational and political influences.

Montrose Birth Centre

Despite the ever-present threats posed by being part of cash-strapped health care systems, some birthing facilities have emerged as beacons of good practice (Murphy-Lawless 2011a; Davies 2007c; Winters 2007). In Scotland the Montrose Maternity Unit, a standalone unit (FSBC) 30–45 miles from consultant provision, exemplifies such innovation. The threat of closure was overcome by the type of campaign, largely organised by users, with which we have become all too familiar. Midwife Phyllis Winters, reflecting on the relationship developing with users following the unit's reprieve, recalls the 'defensive attitude or negative response' (Winters 2007: 12) among midwives, and she gives credit to the perseverance of the users in encouraging woman-centred change. The midwives were persuaded by figures showing the benefits of the newly forward-thinking unit, with rising birth rates and falling transfer rates. One of the attractions of the Montrose unit, waterbirth, developed into its unique selling point (USP), with the majority of women giving birth in water (Winters 2007: 13).

User representative Avril Nicoll and her colleagues trace the story of how waterbirth became the norm in this small east coast town (Nicoll 2005). With the help of the charity AIMS (page 19), educational activities were organised for women, user reps, midwives and health visitors; evidence was produced of the enthusiasm for waterbirth and the reduction in perineal damage. Identifying the threat posed to midwives, particularly in the 'itch … to be hands on and doing' (Nicoll 2005: 12) and concerns about the baby's colour, the workshops began to address such anxieties. That these concerns have been overcome is demonstrated by one-third of births featuring a physiological third stage, an episiotomy rate of 2 per cent (Nicoll 2005: 13) and an intrapartum transfer rate of only 8 per cent (Nicoll 2006: 3). These enviable figures represent a high standard of care, even when compared with similar facilities (Hogg et al 2007).

The users' input into the Montrose unit is not unique, as in FSBCs the management team may include service users (Nicoll 2006: 3). Thus, the role of the woman, working with the midwife, in retaining and maintaining this exemplary facility is clearly apparent.

The Albany Midwifery Practice

Although the Albany Practice featured prominently in Chapter 7 on how *not* to do maternity politics, this warning related to the regulatory environment and most definitely not to the Albany *per se*. The wealth of research evidence demonstrates all too clearly the successful outcomes achieved by the Albany midwives (Sandall et al 2001; Reed and Walton 2009). These successes have been attained through a focus on woman-centred care as advanced by the 'Changing Childbirth' Report (DoH 1993). This focus has been operationalised through meticulous attention to communication, information-sharing and facilitating women's decision-making, particularly relating to home birth. Details of the successes of the Albany Practice are provided in Chapter 7 (page 152), so are not duplicated here.

The New Zealand Experience

In many ways midwifery in New Zealand has faced, and continues to face, challenges similar to those encountered in other developed countries. The New Zealand remedy, though, has been uniquely different from, and potentially more successful than, others.

Developments

The scarcely believable developments in New Zealand midwifery in the closing years of the twentieth century are often recounted with reference to the country's history. This reference for some reason proudly and not infrequently goes back as far as the Treaty of Waitangi (1840), which is regarded by some as the point at which the wrongs of the colonial power began to be rectified (Guilliland and Pairman 1995; Orange 1984). More relevant midwifery history, which includes familiarly global and peculiarly parochial features, is traced by Valerie Fleming in her characteristically questioning manner (Fleming 2000).

As the second half of the twentieth century became established, like many developed states, New Zealand faced a surge of counter-cultures seeking to overturn the old order; especially vulnerable were the technological, professional and patriarchal aspects which had established themselves to control childbearing (Mein-Smith 1986). One example was the Auckland Homebirth Association, founded in 1978 following the Parents' Association, and comprising feminists who described themselves as consumers (as was common then), with a few midwives who actively sought to redress medicalisation of childbearing. This group endeavoured to encourage the home birth option, undermined by the medically-dominated but midwife-staffed maternity units, to regain birthing power. The momentum of the Homebirth Association was fuelled by the widespread acceptance of the Nurses Act (NZLII 1971) which, in removing midwifery autonomy, merely confirmed the *status quo*.

Midwives reacted more strongly to the Nurses Amendment Act (1983), which required homebirth midwives to be registered as nurses and provoked the formation of 'Save the Midwife'. Although this association comprised mainly service-users, the issues succeeded in uniting homebirth midwives with their hospital-based colleagues. In response to the Obstetric Regulations of 1986 the Homebirth Association and Save the Midwife came together in overtly political activity to oppose the total annihilation of New Zealand midwifery.

At this time the Midwives Section of the New Zealand Nurses Association (NZNA) established the Direct Entry Taskforce, which transformed itself into the New Zealand College of Midwives (NZCOM) in 1989. As well as pursuing the goal of independent midwifery practice, NZCOM founded itself on the principle of 'partnership', as illustrated by its equality between midwife and non-midwife women members. Crucially important to the explicitly political activity of NZCOM was the involvement of Helen Clarke, the then Minister of Health and later Prime Minister (1999–2008). It was this 'dream team' of politicians, politically-astute consumers and midwives which ensured the swift and, to some, surprising passage of the Nurses Amendment Act (1990). Through this legislation women choose their birthing attendants and midwives practise independent of medical and nursing constraints.

Partnership

The development of New Zealand midwifery shows the fundamentally crucial relationship between midwives and childbearing women, which underpinned the New Zealand midwifery model of partnership (Guilliland and Pairman 1995). This model is now built into the country's midwifery legislation:

> The Midwifery Scope of Practice: The midwife works in partnership with women.
>
> (MCNZ 2005)

Despite this legal authority, partnership is not without its detractors (Mander 2011a). Part of the problem of partnership relates to the term's lack of any precise meaning. It may be little more than a professional friendship (Pairman 2000), although it carries an aura of egalitarianism (Skinner 1999; Freeman et al 2004). The relationship is more likely to be one of interdependence (Fleming 1998b), but anxieties have arisen that the term fuels insatiable aspirations (Ozturk 2004).

The remarkable passage of the Nurses Amendment Act (1990) left a vacuum which had been occupied by negativity about nurse and medical control of childbearing. This void needed to be filled by a professional project representing the newly autonomous midwife. The partnership model fitted the bill admirably, being defined originally as comprising four philosophical foundations:

(1)   pregnancy and childbirth are normal life events;
(2)   midwifery's primary professional role is with women experiencing a normal pregnancy, labour, birth and postnatal period;
(3)   midwifery provides women with continuity of caregiver throughout her (sic) childbearing experience;
(4)   midwifery is women-centred (Guilliland and Pairman 1995: 34).

After its original publication (NZCOM 1990), the partnership model underwent its first major trial later that year. This trial was not at the hands of the usual sources of threat, but from midwives in the form of the International Confederation of Midwives (ICM; Fleming 2000: 197). While clinical partnership could be condoned by this august body, organisational partnership by including women and their representatives on the College's board of management was an innovation too far. Once more NZCOM's political leaders swung into action, guaranteeing the acceptance of this revolutionary concept and New Zealand's continuing membership of ICM.

Outcomes

Although the recent development of New Zealand midwifery reads like a fairy tale, the new organisation and freedoms are not the complete story. It remains to be seen what difference this midwifery revolution makes to childbearing women and to midwives. That women and midwives have made changes in the provision of care during childbearing is indisputable (Davis and Walker 2010; Mander 2005), whether changes are being made to measurable outcomes, such as caesarean rates, remains to be seen (Douche 2008; Ozturk 2010: 16; Gibbons et al 2010).

North American midwifery politics

In considering the politics of midwifery in North America the urge to address separately issues relating to the two major states in the land mass is almost irresistible. Because of these countries' crucially different positions on the same issues, however, I seek to make comparisons by analysing their development and current situation thematically. Variations exist, not only between the two countries, though; inter-state and inter-provincial differences further complicate this convoluted picture.

History

Disconcertingly little attention is given to first peoples' midwives (Kennedy 2009: 416), so North American midwifery history is widely regarded as having started with European immigration. At that time care in childbirth was provided by neighbours and midwives who served their own migrant community (MacDonald and Bourgeault 2009: 89; Bourgeault and Fynes 1997: 1052; Jackson and Mander 1995). It was when the migrants sought to free themselves from the baggage of their old countries' culture, that the scientific orientation espoused by medical practitioners was preferred to the traditional services of home-grown midwives. Thus, medicine's power base became established and medical practitioners prepared to eliminate the potential threat exerted by local midwives by annihilating midwifery *per se*. Childbearing came to be redefined as a problem and, as women were considered unsuited to attend births, male medical attendance became perceived as a prerequisite for survival. In the United States the 'midwife problem' was identified by Joseph B De Lee, together with strategies to resolve it (De Lee 1915); while in Canada physicians implemented a policy of 'denigration and erasure' of midwifery from the mid-nineteenth century (MacDonald and Bourgeault 2009: 90).

The success of these medical manoeuvres extending into the twentieth century is well known. Midwives became alegal in Canada, practising only in reservations, and non-nurse midwives survived only as 'granny midwives' in the United States (Fraser 1995; Rooks 2007).

Resurgence

The renaissance of midwifery happened somewhat differently in the two countries. In the United States Mary Breckinridge founded the Kentucky Frontier Nursing Service based on Episcopalian principles in the late 1920s to provide *inter alia* midwifery care. At about the same time, philanthropic ideals underpinned the development of the New York Maternity Center Association (Rooks 2007: 13). In both countries the emergence of counter-cultures in the 1960s favoured midwifery, although in Canada this process began from a uniquely low base, as the majority of the country had been without midwives for over a century (page 60). Margaret MacDonald and Ivy Bourgeault argue that this long-term 'midwifelessness' served to kick-start a woman-centred form of midwifery in Canada more effectively than the gradual redevelopment found in their southern neighbours.

Occupational relationships

Perhaps because of its more recent development, the relationships between the different types of midwives, and with other professions, are more straightforward in Canada than in the United States. Although it tended to be known as 'obstetric nursing', nurse-midwifery has long been consigned to the remote North of Canada to attend 'native women' who, as patients, hold little attraction for medical practitioners (Bourgeault and Fynes 1997: 1057). In the United States it was nurse-midwifery on which the Kentucky Frontier Nursing Service and the New York Maternity Centre Association were founded. Thus,

US midwifery has long endured strong links to nursing, with which Canadian midwifery has been relatively unencumbered. Providentially, nurse-midwives and lay midwives in Canada envisaged, in the early 1980s, the advantages to both of joining forces to present a united front in the face of common threats. The nurse-midwives anticipated achieving greater autonomy and the possibility of a desirable homebirth practice. At the same time, lay midwives considered that an alliance with nurse-midwives would enhance their general acceptability. These developments were threatened by a coroner's inquest into the death of a baby boy born at home in 1985. The 'verdict' was the establishment of an unashamedly pro-midwife Task Force, including a lawyer, physician and nurse-midwife, to investigate legislating to legalise midwifery. The Task Force recommended that midwifery should become a self-regulating profession, free of either medical or nursing domination (Eberts 1987). The legislation was enacted in Ontario in 1991, with other provinces following suit.

The relationships between those who practise midwifery in the United States are infinitely more complex and decidedly less harmonious. Differences arise out of nurse-midwives' nursing orientation and from the resistance among many practitioners to submit themselves to licensing or other types of regulation (Rooks 2007). The long-established prevalence of nurse-midwifery, in the form of CNMs (Certified Nurse-Midwives), means that, being accredited and certified by the ANCM (American College of Nurse-Midwives), they are able to be reimbursed through Medicaid, Medicare or private health insurance.

Direct-entry midwifery and lay-midwifery arose out of the 1960s counter-culture's focus on homebirth and freedom from medicalisation and institutionalisation. In the United States in 1982 this group established MANA (Midwives Alliance of North America), which is open to all midwives, including those in Canada (MANA 2012). Unlike ANCM, MANA does not require a nursing qualification or background for recognition. As well as these two major groups, Certified Midwives (CMs) who have no nursing background, but equivalent education to CNMs, are recognised in some states (Rooks 2007).

Thus, the practice, qualifications and, hence, modes of entry into US midwifery vary hugely, giving rise to acrimonious relationships between ACNM and MANA (Kennedy 2009: 417). The rancour has reached such levels that conciliation was sought in 1998 by founding the 'Bridge Club' for those midwives seeking to heal the rift (Kennedy 2009: 418).

The close links between nurse-midwifery and nursing may be seen as disadvantageous, due to the limitations which such an orientation carries. The financial costs to the individual learner, whose aim is to become a midwife rather than a nurse, are similarly deterring. Judith Rooks argues that much of what the nurse learns may 'taint' her care by conveying an 'illness orientation' to midwifery practice (Rooks 2007: 15). Perhaps a conspiracy theorist, Rooks also warns of the indirect power over midwifery policy-making which nursing leaders may thus exert.

The importance of US nurse-midwives establishing a good relationship with a physician is emphasised by Rooks (2007). Although she omits to use the pejorative term 'physician-extender', the concept of the medical practitioner facilitating the practice of the nurse-midwife by providing 'back up' emerges clearly in Rooks' writing. Ivy Bourgeault and Mary Fynes, however, present a less sanguine portrayal of the relationship between the nurse-midwife and the physician (Bourgeault and Fynes 1997: 1060). These Canadian writers reflect on the tendency of physicians in both the United States and Canada to withdraw from obstetric practice, mainly on the grounds of litigation risks and costs but also to permit some personal life. This 'vacant jurisdiction' has provided midwives with a window of opportunity to step in to the empty niche and to establish their professional position (Bourgeault and Fynes 1997: 1060). The likelihood that the North American midwife is less costly, avoids expensive technology and intervenes less than the physician, also serve to make her attractive to clients and insurance agencies.

Summary

These two supremely wealthy countries show many similarities in their midwifery history, but currently operate very different systems of maternity. Canada appears to have been more successful than the United States in securing a woman-centred maternity service, through legalising self-regulating midwifery. The powerful nursing and medical input, together with internecine strife, are likely to have hindered the development of effective midwifery services in the United States. Canada's success is largely attributable nurse-midwives and lay midwives recognising the need to work together in order to achieve their common goal. Midwifery effectiveness is also partly attributable to the greater degree of state control over health service provision in Canada, as compared with the much-vaunted free market in health in the United States. Additionally, Canadian politicians recognised the need to display their woman-friendly credentials to their electorates (Bourgeault and Fynes 1997: 1061). The seemingly insurmountable differences which have driven wedges between the multiple factions in US midwifery, have served to squander the hard-won advances of the counter-culture and the women's movement (Bourgeault and Fynes 1997: 1061). So the Canadian midwifery system provides us with another example of the effectiveness of women collaborating with women politicians and with midwives for the benefit of childbearing women and their families.

Conclusion

This chapter has sought to focus on the 'good news' stories in the development of midwifery. To achieve this end, it has been necessary to assume a broad brush approach and to give less attention to the problems facing and encountered by those achieving some degree of success.

The political theme which emerges strongly out of these examples and which resonates throughout this chapter remains inescapable. This political message relates to the united front which has enhanced the achievements of the various groups of midwives to whom I have referred. This unity derives from midwives having honed their political skills for the common good. As a result, the midwives are all seen to be 'singing from the same hymn sheet'. Further, the midwives have identified and persuaded career politicians, usually women, of the rightness of their cause. Most significantly, women as service-users and voters have been recognised as a crucially important constituency to influence national, local and special interest politics.

Thus, although it was first used in New Zealand, the axiom 'Women need midwives need women' (Fleming 1996: 343) has been shown to be key to the success of the promising practices which midwives have advanced.

9 Conclusion

Introduction

Although party politics has come to assume a disproportionately burdensome part in our daily lives while not actually delivering what is needed, this book addresses aspects of politics more closely bound up with the lived experience of the childbearing woman and midwife. My focus has been the activities which the midwife and the woman encounter, and may be required to participate in, in the course of their everyday practice or experience of maternity care, respectively. I have written this book with the intention that it will assist the reader in negotiating her way through the elephant traps which litter maternity care, in her role either as a provider or service user. In this concluding chapter, I draw out and bring together the main themes emerging out of the discussion. At the same time, I also seek to emphasise and anticipate the ways in which this book will be used.

Communication and dialogue

The significance of communication surfaced in the Introduction, when I referred to the need for more effective communication systems to improve maternity care. I was also obliged to draw attention to the way that some occupational groups have honed their communication skills to their own advantage. The converse of this observation is that other occupational and other groups may be disadvantaged by their more limited familiarity with public and professional media. Following discussion, including material on the various interest groups involved in maternity, it is necessary to contemplate whether and how these groups communicate with each other. Some of the difficulties which are encountered emerged when I discussed the role and functioning of Maternity Services Liaison Committees (MSLCs; page 20).

Adopting a broad view of communication between professionals and service users at policy level, Charlotte Williamson identified some aspects of this potential minefield (Williamson 1998). Professionals dismiss the views of 'patients' because of certain preconceived assumptions, which Williamson recognised and which perpetuate themselves with successive generations of service providers. Unsurprisingly, medical practitioners attach immense value to medical knowledge, and Williamson reports that the converse applies; meaning that service users' knowledge passes unrecognised. Similarly, the breadth of experience among service user groups is unlikely to be credited. This lack of recognition and credit leads to consumers' views being dismissed as irrelevant. Further reasons for such dismissal relate to the need for service users who assume advocacy or activist roles to be articulate and speak a language comprehensible to service providers. Thus, the tendency for consumer representatives to be well-educated and possibly middle class engenders questions about their representativeness. Accusations are levelled that activists actually represent only themselves (Pievatolo 2005: 2). Because health care providers confuse representation with representativeness or typicality, they assume that this unrepresentativeness extends to activists' views being different from those they represent (Williamson 2010: 129). These assumptions mean that any users' questioning of service providers and their activities is all too easily dismissed as inconsequential.

Dismissing questioning is a relatively benign reaction to service users' probing. As Williamson observes, doctors' reactions include 'defensiveness, avoidance or aggressiveness' (Williamson 2010: 164). Such responses are associated with the confident arrogance, or 'bedside manner', deliberately cultivated by medical practitioners to allay patients' anxieties. It is this defensive response which threatens existing relationships with user groups and creates concern about effects on care.

Communication and dialogue with user groups has never reached the status of priority among health professionals. Williamson comments that, such indifference is linked to lack of esteem among care providers and may be due to medical practitioners' ignorance of the strength and validity of user groups' sources. Service providers know the evidence supporting their own case, but not that refuting it. Such limited understanding engenders dismissal of users' arguments. Medical practitioners' low esteem of user groups may also lead to other consequences; such as the tendency of what discussion there is to focus on uncontentious issues, rather than issues which really matter to service users. This tendency manifested itself in the topics addressed by the MSLC which Jacqueline Dunkley-Bent researched (Dunkley-Bent and Jones 2008). The discussion focused on small portion size, lack of decaffeinated coffee and the absence of leaflets about service organisation.

Thus, it is apparent that constructive communication and dialogue between service providers and user groups is little more than naïve aspiration. The political barriers erected, perhaps as a defensive shield, by health care providers are longstanding and firmly entrenched. While government publications may articulate well-intentioned clichés (SEHD 2001), there is clearly little understanding of defensive attitudes deeply engrained among service providers. Such seriously flawed form of communication appears to have deteriorated into a dialogue of the deaf. This phenomenon, Kjeld Møller Pedersen (2002) states, is established in the fields of health and healthcare due to the protagonists both holding and being unable to comprehend differing philosophies and views.

Drawing on personal observation, I have experienced such lack of communication operating in different ways. An example of such miscommunication would be the occasion when I was with a woman in early labour discussing her plans for the birth to be intervention-free. The consultant obstetrician and his entourage swept in to check progress and the woman bravely articulated her aspirations. She was blithely reassured: 'Yes, dear, an epidural will ensure that everything goes naturally for you'.

More generally, this dialogue of the deaf has become dishearteningly apparent in service providers' views of childbirth organisations and activists. The toxicity of their hostility surprised me when my otherwise splendid midwife colleagues in the labour ward reacted venomously to a new pamphlet by Shelia Kitzinger on the physical and emotional aspects of episiotomy (Kitzinger 1972). Practising in a setting in which elective episiotomy was supposedly routine for primigravid women, Kitzinger's insightful comments threatened the basis of our midwifery practice. The result was that her publication, credentials and NCT, as publisher, were pilloried mercilessly. Soon afterwards the RCT by Jenny Sleep and her colleagues clearly demonstrated the iatrogenicity of this routine practice (Sleep et al 1984).

More recent and equally disturbing examples of this dialogue of the deaf are when consumer groups, their members and birth activists have, effectively, been demonised by midwives. This reaction is due in part to midwives' perceptions of the consumer groups' and birth activists' influence over childbearing women, which happens when women choose a place or mode of birth differing from that espoused by the midwife. Choosing home birth is a significant example in the context of community midwives unconfident of their midwifery skills.

A personal example of miscommunication occurred when my interaction with the Royal College of Midwives (RCM) deteriorated due to my observations about statutory refresher courses provided by the RCM (Mander 1986a and b). Despite my endeavours to ensure a balanced presentation, I met personal criticism together with accusations of prejudice and partiality. It became apparent that the RCM was totally satisfied, to the point of complacency, with the educational opportunities it provided, despite a pervasive culture of 'bums on seats'. Refresher courses were abandoned soon afterwards, in favour of practitioner-centred post-registration education and practice (PREP; NMC 2011).

Such miscommunication would be historical were Robbie Davis-Floyd's 'post-modern midwife' to materialise. As well as being relativistic and organised, this fabulous being would bring articulacy, political skills and a consciousness of her 'cultural uniqueness' and 'global importance' (Davis-Floyd 2005: 33) to both her practice and her interactions with systematic challenges. Because this person would know about conflicting and discrepant systems of care, she would take advantage of aspects benefiting her client. Davis-Floyd anticipates that this is the person into whom midwives must morph to renegotiate identities, articulate new practice and, most importantly, survive (Davis-Floyd 2005: 34).

Political power

Inevitably closely associated with, even represented by, communicative strategies are the relationships between participants in maternity. While these relationships are likely to vary between individuals, the overall picture is one of unbalanced stability. This imbalance is most obvious in the hegemony of policy decision-makers and power brokers controlling the activities of fellow professionals and service users. These hegemonic relationships may be a feature of health care more widely and not just maternity; they may be associated with the gender or gendered attitudes of groups in whose hands power is vested. This established authority may be enhanced by the socio-economic background, including education, of the powerful elite.

On the other side of the equation are childbearing women seeking the birth experience which they hope may be achievable. Some childbearing women are sufficiently articulate or well-supported to voice their expectations, or may chance upon a health care provider able to understand and facilitate their hopes. Others, however, do not find themselves so well-placed. Thus a large proportion of service users are effectively disempowered by the services which they had anticipated would realise their aspirations. During childbearing most women are disinclined or unable to express their wishes, having more immediate concerns and little enthusiasm for disrupting the system. Afterwards the woman's disquiet may be cloaked by the plethora of other feelings and emotions. Women who don't 'speak the same language' or have least in common with care providers are those most vulnerable to having control wrested from them.

Throughout the health care system in general and the maternity services in particular, patriarchy diminishes the woman's position and her role in her own experience. The power exhibited by health care providers of both genders is underpinned by a masculinist orientation derived from medical attitudes. Systematic effects of patriarchy have been linked with interventions and behaviour regarded as, at best, unsupportive or, at worst, abusive (Kitzinger 2006).

The political environment featuring such abuse of power is not confined to clinical situations. As shown in Chapters 6 and 7, statutory regulatory bodies disempower not only the midwife, but also the childbearing woman, particularly if seeking the attendance of a sympathetic midwife. At the time of writing there is a degree of flux and uncertainty regarding the position in which the UK regulatory body finds itself. It is unlikely, though, that the underlying infrastructure will be resolved in the foreseeable future.

Stratified reproduction

The picture which I have presented of the political balance of power in maternity care early in the second millennium resonates powerfully with Shellee Colen's anthropological concept of 'stratified reproduction' (Colen 1994). This concept applies, not in the usual sense of developing countries' economic status, but pertaining to hierarchies based on gender, socioeconomic class, scientific knowledge and occupational orientation. I have demonstrated the reinforcement and intensification by powerful elites of the inequalities to which childbearing women and their midwife attendants are vulnerable. Thus, the differential accomplishment of childbearing activities and care are perpetuated by groups and occupations whose status endows them with hegemonic power. Such power is the legacy of outdated professional and cultural systems, which regarded women as lesser beings and their childbearing as inconsequential. So rather than recognising childbearing as crucial to both the woman's identity and establishment of the growing family, birth has been relegated to a series of medical interventions or a slot on the theatre list. Although woman centredness has gone the way of many governmental aphorisms, this all too obvious focus deserves retrieval and reinstatement.

Looking forward – the politics of autonomy

Through the medium of this book, particularly Chapter 8, I have shown that, although there are inevitably threats, midwives in certain settings have grasped opportunities to provide woman-friendly maternity services. These promising practices have demonstrated that political connectedness between them is crucial to advance the shared interests of the midwife and childbearing woman. While I have referred to autonomy many times in this book in a range of contexts, this 'connectedness' exemplifies a wider and more woman-friendly development of autonomy than is traditional. I have explored how the agency of both the midwife and childbearing woman are perceived as deficient; but there is a prospect that this situation may be rendered less hostile by collaborative strategies, reflecting a more *relational* form of autonomy, advanced by feminist ethicists (MacDonald 2006).

'Relational autonomy' seeks to dispense with the traditional ethical tunnel vision, which emphasises the individual's ability to determine her own environment in order to achieve 'self-government'. Such an essentially masculine focus on independence and self-reliance has been appropriately criticised (Baumann 2008: 446). This critique stems from there being many to whom such aspirations verge on fictional, including countless women, people with disabilities and black and minority ethnic groups. The result of these fictions is that the concept of autonomy risks being totally invalidated; so the feminist reinterpretation of autonomy in relational terms is welcome. Chris MacDonald has recounted its ready acceptance into the professional arena (MacDonald 2002), but midwifery has been less enthusiastic. Angela Thachuk, however, has shown the relevance of relational autonomy to interpersonal clinical aspects of childbearing (Thachuk 2007). It may be that midwifery remains too concerned with adjusting to the traditional interpretation of autonomy, and its real-life precursor consent, to embrace this newly-developed version.

Presenting an insightful analysis of autonomy, and its relational derivative, Lorraine Code draws on many issues already addressed in this book (Code 2000). She contemplates the regulatory systems operating in Western states which, in the name of autonomy, perpetuate longstanding and statutory oppression and disempowering behaviour; in this way capitalist patriarchy is maintained as the dominant ethos. Referring to traditional ideals of autonomy as 'individualistic' (Code 2000: 184), Code reflects that the associated hegemony is accessible only to members of well-defined and highly-advantaged social groups. Other, allegedly lesser, beings are subject to heteronomy, in the form of legislation and regulation created and imposed by others. Code's advocacy of relational autonomy is advanced through *ecological* thinking, and she seeks to persuade all levels of society of the limitations of 'white, affluent, Western, male' attitudes entrenched in aspirations to traditional autonomy (Code 2000: 198).

Writing in a North American context, Code probes health care providers' role in maintaining the medical *status quo* (Code 2000: 191); although she specifies nurses, her astute observations are relevant to some midwives. The health care hierarchy is depicted with the nurse, or midwife, occupying the middle ground between physician and childbearing woman. As a mediator, the nurse or midwife is positioned obsequiously, affirming the medical position atop the ranking. Probably inadvertently this position simultaneously and inevitably condemns the childbearing woman to the bottommost rung of the hierarchy.

The knowledge supporting maternity care is the product of traditionally autonomous knowers and researchers, with findings based on masculine experiences establishing scientific norms. That women's, and obviously childbearing women's, experiences differ fails to be confirmed by the highest scientific standards, making them suitable only to be disregarded as mere aberrations (Code 2000: 192). Thus, practices which have become established by custom and practice, despite having no research support and even less women's support, persist. Code supports her argument by listing a range of interested parties, including governments, multinational corporations, manufacturers and pharmaceutical companies, which fund research to refute the potentially toxic nature of products and activities.

An issue striking at the very root of the autonomy debate is the matter of the dependency culture, claimed by some to have evolved out of 'socialised medicine' or the welfare state (Code 2000: 195). Certain groups have effectively been stigmatised by politicians, ignorant of unemployment or deprivation, to endorse the dismantling of supportive structures. Traditional autonomy is firmly linked by such politicians to the rhetoric of self-reliance and 'hard working families'. That these politicians are not and can never be aware of the costs of impoverishment is all too clear.

The patriarchy which I have shown to be inherent in and to reinforce many systems of maternity care demonstrates the biological determinism ensuing from individualistic autonomy and keeping women 'in their place' (Code 2000: 200). Thus, these systems take advantage of women's innate caring abilities, which are misused to perpetuate their subjugation.

The solution to resolve these politically poisonous states is the establishment of communities which will enquire and deliberate in a collaborative *milieu*. Through this approach, experience will grow to achieve sufficient expertise to challenge hegemonic authorities so that the politics of knowledge in a maternity setting will become a force to be reckoned with. I suggest on this basis that Carol Hanisch's familiar and very relevant adage 'The Personal is Political' (Hanisch 1971) is updated. To make it relevant to women's issues in the twenty-first century, as I have shown through the medium of this book, this quotation needs to be refocused along lines envisaged by Mary Wollstonecraft (1792). Recognising the crucial role of childbearing women in negotiating the new political order, Wollstonecraft agued women's centrality by virtue of their innate reproductive power. I propose, therefore, that childbearing women and midwives collaborate to realise that 'The Perinatal is Political'.

References

Aaserud M, Lewin S, Innvaer S, Paulsen EJ, Dahlgren AT, Trommald M, Duley L, Zwarenstein M and Oxman AD (2005) 'Translating research into policy and practice in developing countries: a case study of magnesium sulphate for pre-eclampsia', *BMC Health Services Research* 5: 68

Abbott AD (1988) *The system of professions: an essay on the division of expert labor*, Chicago: University of Chicago Press

Abbott P and Meerabeau L (1998) 'Professions, professionalization and the caring professions' in P Abbott and L Meerabeau (eds) *The sociology of the caring professions*, London: Routledge

Abenhaim HA and Benjamin A (2011) 'Higher caesarean section rates in women with higher body mass index; are we managing labour differently?' *Journal of Obstetrics and Gynaecology Canada* 33:5 443–8

Abraham-Van and der Mark E (1993) 'Dutch midwifery, past and present: an overview', in E Abraham-Van der Mark (ed) *Successful home birth and midwifery: the Dutch model*, Westport, CT: Bergin and Garvey

Ahern EM (1978) *The power and pollution of Chinese women*, pp 269–90 in AP Wolf (ed) *Studies in Chinese society*, Stanford, California, Stanford University Press

Ahmed-Ghosh H (2005) 'Chattels of society domestic violence in India', *Violence Against Women* 10:1 94–118

AIMS (2006) 'Free-standing and proud', *AIMS Journal* 18:3

AIMS (2010a) Report: Southwark Council, *AIMS Journal* 22:3 16

AIMS (2010b) Critique of 'The London Project: A confidential enquiry into a series of term babies born in an unexpectedly poor condition' by the Centre for Maternal and Child Enquiries (CMACE Report), Accessed 08/12, http://www.aims.org.uk/Publications/CMACECritiqueAIMS.pdf

AIMS (2010c) 'King's overstretched': article run in the Daily Mail on 13 October 2010 *AIMS Journal* 22:34

AIMS (2011) 'What is AIMS?' Accessed 07/11, http://www.aims.org.uk/

AIMSI (2008) News Bulletin 'AIMS Ireland', Accessed 05/12, http://www.aimsireland.com/news/?topic=newsBulletin

AIMSI (2010) 'Birth groups say Nursing Bill will be the death of midwifery', Accessed 05/12, http://www.aimsireland.com/news/?topic=newsdropdown

Akhavan S and Lundgren I (2012) 'Midwives' experiences of doula support for immigrant women in Sweden – A qualitative study', *Midwifery* 28:1 80–5

Alfirevic Z, Devane D and Gyte GML (2006) 'Continuous cardiotocography (CTG) as a form of electronic fetal monitoring (EFM) for fetal assessment during labour', Cochrane

Database of SystematicReviews, Issue 3 Art No CD006066.DOI: 10.1002/14651858. CD006066

Allsop J, Jones K and Baggott R (2004) 'Health consumer groups in the UK: a new social movement?' *Sociology of Health & Illness* 26:6 737–56

Amnesty International (2010) *Deadly delivery: the maternal health care crisis in the USA,* Amnesty International Publications, Accessed http://www.amnestyusa.org/sites/default/files/pdfs/deadlydelivery.pdf, Accessed 01/13

Anderson T (2004) 'The misleading myth of choice: the continuing oppression of women in childbirth', in M Kirkham (ed) *Informed choice in maternity care,* Basingstoke: Palgrave Macmillan, pp 257–64

Anderson T (2006) 'Caesarean for non-medical reasons at term', *The Practising Midwife* 9:1 34–5

Anderson T (2007) 'Is this the end of independent midwifery?', *The Practising Midwife* 10:2 4–5

Antonovsky A (1979) *Health, stress, and coping,* San Francisco: Jossey-Bass

Antonovsky A (1987) 'The salutogenic perspective: toward a new view of health and illness', *Advances* 4:1 47–55

Antonovsky A (1996) 'The salutogenic model as a theory to guide health promotion' *Health Promotion International* 11:1 11–18

ARM (1986) *The vision,* Ormskirk, Lancashire: Association of Radical Midwives

Arnold PJ (2005) 'Disciplining domestic regulation: the World Trade Organisation and the market for professional services', *Accounting, Organizations and Society* 30 299–330

Aroian KJ (2001) 'Immigrant women and their health', *Annual Review of Nursing Research* 19:1 179–226

ARS/DoH (2010) Nurses and Midwives Bill 2010, *An Roinn Sláinte*/Department of Health, Accessed 05/12, http://www.dohc.ie/press/releases/2010/20100422.html

Arthur D and Payne D (2005) 'Maternal request for an elective caesarean section', *New Zealand College of Midwives Journal* 33 17–20

Ashton D (2003) Appendix 36: Memorandum by Dr David Ashton (OB 66), House of Commons Select Committee on Health Written Evidence

Aunos M and Feldman MA (2002) 'Attitudes towards sexuality, sterilization and parenting rights of persons with intellectual disabilities', *Journal of Applied Research in Intellectual Disabilities* 15:4 285–96

Baggott R, Allsop J and Jones K (2005) *Speaking for patients and carers: health consumer groups and the policy process,* Houndmills: Palgrave Macmillan

Baggott R and Forster R (2008) 'Health consumer and patients' organizations in Europe: towards a comparative analysis', *Health Expectations* 11:1 85–94

Baker D (1996) 'Use and effectiveness of interpreters in an emergency department', *Journal of American Medical Association* 275:10 783–8

Baker SR, Choi PYL, Henshaw CA and Tree J (2005) '"I felt as though I'd been in jail": women's experiences of maternity care during labour, delivery and the immediate postpartum', *Feminism Psychology* 15:3 315–42

Ball L, Curtis P and Kirkham M (2002) *Why do midwives leave?,* London: RCM Publications

Ballen LE and Fulcher AJ (2006) 'Nurses and doulas: complementary roles to provide optimal maternity care', *Journal of Obstetrical Gynecologic & Neonatal Nursing* 35:2 304–11

Bandura A (1977) 'Self-efficacy: towards a unifying theory', *Psychological Review* 84:2 191–215

Bangser M, Mehta M, Singer J, Daly C, Kamugumy C and Mwangomale A (2011) 'Childbirth experiences of women with obstetric fistula in Tanzania and Uganda and their implications for fistula program development', *International Urogynecology Journal* 22:1 91–8

Baraté P and Temmerman M (2009) 'Why do mothers die? The silent tragedy of maternal mortality', *Current Women's Health Reviews* 5:4 230–8

Barclay L (2008) 'Review: a feminist history of Australian midwifery from colonisation until the 1980s', *Women and Birth* 21:1 3–8

Barnard H and Turner C (2011) 'Poverty and ethnicity: a review of evidence', Joseph Rowntree Foundation York, Accessed 08/11 http://www.oneeastmidlands.org.uk/downloads/poverty-ethnicity-evidence-summary.pdf

Barnes HD (2012) 'Professional indemnity insurance for independent midwives', *AIMS Journal* 24:2 18–9

Barter R (2011) 'The rise of the gasman', *The History of Anaesthesia Society Proceedings* 44: 39–46

Basu AM and Koolwal GB (2005) 'Two concepts of female empowerment: some leads from DHS data on women's status and reproductive health' in S Kishor (ed) *A focus on gender collected papers on gender using DHS data*, Calverton: ORC Macro, pp 15–51 Accessed 12/11 http://pdf.usaid.gov/pdf_docs/PNADE016.pdf#page=22

Bates C (2004) 'Midwifery practice: ways of working' in M Stewart (ed) *Pregnancy, birth, and maternity care: feminist perspectives*, Edinburgh: Elsevier, pp 121–39

Batra N and Lilford RJ (1996) 'Not clients, not consumers and definitely not maternants', *European Journal of Obstetrics & Gynecology and Reproductive Biology* 64:3 197–9

Baulch B (2006) 'Aid distribution and the MDGs', *World Development* 34:6 933–50

Baumann H (2008) 'Reconsidering relational autonomy. Personal autonomy for socially embedded and temporally extended selves', *Analyse & Kritik* 30/2008 (c Lucius and Lucius, Stuttgart) pp 445–68, Accessed 07/12 http://www.analyse-und-kritik.net/2008–2/AK_Baumann_2008.pdf

Beck U (1992) *Risk society: towards a new modernity* (trans) M Ritter, London: Sage

Beech B (1985) 'The politics of maternity: childbirth freedom v obstetric control' in S Edwards (ed) *Gender, sex and the law*, London: Routledge, pp 50–78

Beech B (2009) 'Midwifery – running down the drain', *AIMS Journal* 21:3 3–5

Beech B (2010) 'Ignoring Albany Mums' *AIMS Journal* 22:3 21

Beech B (2011) 'Challenging the medicalisation of birth', *AIMS Journal* 23:2 4–10

Beech BL (2002a) 'Professional indemnity insurance – response to NMC consultation' 30th September, Accessed 03/12 http://www.aims.org.uk/Submissions/nmc.htm

Beech BL (2002b) 'State-sanctioned kidnapping: violation of a baby's human rights', *AIMS Journal* 14:2 1–3

Beech BL (2003) 'Challenging the illusion of choice', *AIMS Journal* 15:3 1, 3–4

Beech BL (2004) 'NICE guidelines for caesarean section', *AIMS Journal* 16:2 1–3

Beech BL and Thomas P (1999) 'The witch hunt: an international persecution of quality midwifery', *AIMS Journal* 11:2 1–4

Begley C, Higgins A, Lalor J, Sheerin F, Alexander J, Nicholl H, Lawler D, Keenan P, Tuohy T and Kavanagh R (2009) 'Women with disabilities: barriers and facilitators to accessing services during pregnancy', Childbirth and Early Motherhood National Disability Authority & TCD, Accessed 08/11 http://www.nda.ie/CntMgmtNew.nsf/DCC524B4546ADB3080256C700071B049/419BBFC356BC438A80257705003FA51D/$File/literaturereview.pdf

Belenky MF, Clinchy BM, Goldberger NR and Tarule JM (1997) *Women's ways of knowing: The development of self, voice, and mind*, New York: Basic Books

Benjamin W (2006) 'Paralipomena to "on the concept of history"' in H Eiland and M Jennings (eds) *Walter Benjamin, Selected Writings, Volume 4, 1938–1940*, Harvard: Harvard University Press

Benoit C, Wrede S, Bourgeault I, Sandall J, De Vries R and van Teijlingen ER (2005) 'Understanding the social organisation of maternity care systems: midwifery as a touchstone', *Sociology of Health & Illness* 27:6 722–37

Berndtson A (1970) 'The meaning of power', *Philosophy and Phenomenological Research* 31:1 73–84

Bettcher D and Lee K (2002) 'Globalisation and public health', *Journal of Epidemiology & Community Health* 56:1 8–17

Bewley S and Helleur A (2012) 'Rising maternal deaths in London, UK', *The Lancet* 379: March 31 1198

Bharj K (2007) 'Pollution: midwives defiling South Asian women' in M Kirkham (ed) *Exploring the dirty side of women's health*, London: Routledge, pp 60–71

Bick D and Sandall J (2010) 'Looking beyond the statistics for MDG 5', *Midwifery* 26:6 563–4

Billari FC, Goisis A, Liefbroer AC, Settersten RA, Aassve A, Hagestad G and Spéder Z (2011) 'Social age deadlines for the childbearing of women and men', *Human Reproduction* 26:3 616–22

Blaaka G and Eri TS (2008) 'Doing midwifery between different belief systems', *Midwifery* 24:4 344–52

Blomgren M and Sundén E (2008) 'Constructing a European healthcare market: the private healthcare company Capio and the strategic aspect of the drive for transparency', *Social Science and Medicine* 67 1512–20.

BMJ (1979) 'Briefing the Royal Commission on the NHS: the background', *BMJ Supplement* 28 July 288–9

Boero N (2007) 'All the news that's fat to print: the American "obesity epidemic" and the media', *Qualitative Sociology* 30:1 41–60

Boffey D (2012) 'Public services, big earners: a sector-by sector analysis' *Guardian* Saturday 25 February, Accessed 08/12 http://www.guardian.co.uk/society/2012/feb/25/public-services-private-sector?

Bogdan-Lovis EA and Sousa A (2006) 'The contextual influence of professional culture: certified nurse-midwives' knowledge of and reliance on evidence-based practice', *Social Science & Medicine* 62:11 2681–93

Bohra U, Donnelly J, O'Connell MP, Geary MP, MacQuillan K and Keane DP (2003) 'Active management of labour revisited: the first 1000 primiparous labours in 2000', *Journal of Obstetrics & Gynaecology* 23:2 118–20

Booth J, Hutchison C, Beech C and Robertson K (2006) 'New nursing roles: the experience of Scotland's consultant nurse/midwives', *Journal of Nursing Management* 14:2 83–9

Boseley S (2001) 'Caesarean births soar to one in five' *Guardian* Friday 26 October, Accessed 08/12 http://www.guardian.co.uk/society/2001/oct/26/NHS

Boseley S (2011) 'NHS maternity deaths patients still at risk, Care Quality Commission warns', *Guardian* Thursday 27 October, Accessed 12/12 http://www.guardian.co.uk/society/2011/oct/27/nhs-maternity-deaths-cqc-watchdog-report

Boukari SA (2011) 'Circumcision revisited: a universal practice', *International Journal of Humanities and Social Science* 1:14 51–67

Bourgeault IL and Fynes M (1997) 'Integrating lay and nurse-midwifery into the US and Canadian health care systems', *Social Science & Medicine* 44:7 1051–63

Bourgeault IL, Declercq E, Sandall J, Wrede S, Vanstone M, van Teijlingen E, DeVries R and Benoit C (2008) 'Too posh to push? Comparative perspectives on maternal request caesarean sections in Canada, the US, the UK and Finland', *Advances in Medical Sociology* 10:1 99–123

Bowen S (2001) *Language Barriers in Access to Health Care*, Ontario Canada: Health Canada.

Bowler I (1993) '"They're not the same as us": midwives' stereotypes of South Asian descent maternity patients', *Sociology of Health & Illness* 15:2 157–78

Brhlikova P, Jeffery P, Priti G and Khurana BS (2009) 'Intrapartum oxytocin (mis)use in South Asia', *Journal of Health Studies* II 33–50

Bricker L, Neilson JP and Dowswell T (2008) 'Routine ultrasound in late pregnancy (after 24 weeks' gestation)', Cochrane Database of Systematic Reviews, Issue 4, Art No CD001451. DOI: 10.1002/14651858.CD001451.pub3

Briggs Report (1972) Report of the Committee of Nursing (Chair Prof Asa Briggs), London: HMSO (Cmnd 5115)

Brims A (2011) Midwife, NHS Lothian, 12/11 Personal communication

Brocklehurst P, Hardy, P. et al (2011) 'Perinatal and maternal outcomes by planned place of birth for healthy women with low risk pregnancies: the Birthplace in England national prospective cohort study', *BMJ* 343:d7400

Brown HC, Paranjothy S, Dowswell T and Thomas J (2008) 'Package of care for active management in labour for reducing caesarean section rates in low-risk women', Cochrane Database of Systematic Reviews, Issue 4, Art No CD004907. DOI: 10.1002/14651858. CD004907.pub2

Brown J (1978) '"Social control" and the modernisation of social policy, 1890–1905' in P Thane (ed) *The Origins of British Social Policy*, London: Croom Helm

Brown S and Grimes D (1995) 'A meta-analysis of nurse practitioners and nurse midwives in primary care', *Nursing Research* 44:6 332–9.

Brown W (2001) *Politics out of history*, Princeton: Princeton University Press

Browne A (2005) 'Education and training of the maternity care assistant: developments from a BTEC diploma in maternity care', *RCM Midwives* 8:2 72–3

Bryar R and Sinclair M (2011) *Theory for midwifery practice* 2nd edn, London: Palgrave Macmillan

Buck D and Frosini F (2012) 'Clustering of unhealthy behaviours over time: Implications for policy and practice' London King's Fund, Accessed 08/12 http://www.kingsfund.org.uk/publications/unhealthy_behaviours.html

Burdett Trust (2006) *Who Cares Wins: Leadership and the Business of Caring*, London: The Burdett Trust for Nursing

Burke E (1909) 'Thoughts on the cause of the present discontents, 1770' in H Froude (ed) *The works of the Right Honourable Edmund Burke*, Vol 2 Oxford: Oxford University Press, p 83

Burtch B (1994) *Trials of Labour: The Re-emergence of Midwifery*, Montreal and Kingston: McGill-Queen's University Press

Byrne DL, Asmussen T and Freeman JM (2000) 'Descriptive terms for women attending antenatal clinics: mother knows best?', *British Journal of Obstetrics and Gynaecology* 107:10 1233–6

Cairoli E (2010) 'Medicalisation of childbirth in maternity health policies: Ethical evaluation of the use of medicalisation in the Dutch and British maternity policies', Unpublished Masters Thesis, University of Utrecht MA, Thesis Accessed 05/12 http://igitur-archive. library.uu.nl/student-theses/2010–0211-200251/MAthesis_EsterCairoli.pdf

Callaghan G and Wistow G (2006) 'Publics, patients, citizens, consumers? Power and decision making in primary health care', *Public Administration* 84:3 583–601

Callaghan H (2007) 'Birth dirt' in M Kirkham (ed) *Exploring the Dirty Side of Women's Health*, London: Routledge, 8–29

Campbell D (2010a) 'Midwives' leader warns against "baby factories"', *Guardian* Tuesday 4 May 2010, Accessed 08/12 http://www.guardian.co.uk/society/2010/may/04/maternity-services-nhs-midwives-factory?

Campbell D (2010b) 'Hospitals turned away 750 women in labour last year', *Guardian* Thursday 22 April 2010, Accessed 08/12, http://www.guardian.co.uk/society/2010/apr/22/hospitals-mothers-birth

Campbell D (2012a) 'NHS watchdog warns of midwife shortage', *Guardian* Thursday 28 June 2012, Accessed 08/12, http://www.guardian.co.uk/society/2012/jun/28/midwife-shortage-maternity-units-nhs

Campbell D (2012b) 'Close small maternity units and centralise care, demands leading doctor', *Guardian* Saturday 14 July 2012, Accessed 08/12, http://www.guardian.co.uk/society/2012/jul/14/maternity-units-care-doctor

Campbell D (2012c) 'NHS needs to close wards and hospitals to centralise care, says doctors' leader', *Guardian* Tuesday 24 July 2012, Accessed 08/12, http://www.guardian.co.uk/society/2012/jul/24/terence-stephenson-doctors-nhs

Campbell R and Macfarlane A (1987) *Where to be Born? The Debate and the Evidence*, Oxford: National Perinatal Epidemiology Unit

Care Quality Commission (2011) Investigation report, 'Barking, Havering and Redbridge University Hospitals NHS Trust Queen's Hospital, King George's Hospital', October 2011, Accessed 08/12, http://www.cqc.org.uk/sites/default/files/media/documents/20111026_bhrut_investigation_report_final_0.pdf

Care Quality Commission (2012) 'Challenges facing maternity services', Market Report (1) June 2012, Accessed 08/12, http://www.cqc.org.uk/sites/default/files/media/documents/20120626_cqc_market_report_issue_1_for_website_final_0.pdf

Carolan M (2003) 'The graying of the obstetric population: implications for the older mother', *Journal of Obstetric, Gynecologic & Neonatal Nursing* 32:1 19–27

Carr-Saunders AM and Wilson PA (1933) *The Professions*, Oxford: Clarendon Press

Carvel J (2003) 'NHS is race biased says Phillips', *Guardian* 30 April, p 10.

Casley-Ready K (undated) 'Audit Report, Version 1.2, for Kings College Hospital on outcomes from the Albany Maternity Group Practice during the period 31/03/06 to 31/10/08', unpublished

CBS (2012) Statline Centraal Bureau voor de Statistiek 2008/10, Accessed 05/12 http://statline.cbs.nl/StatWeb/publication/?DM=SLNL&pa=37302&d1=0–2&d2=a&vw=T

Chakladar A (2009) 'Encounter with a doula: is the system failing mothers?', *BMJ* 339:b5112 1316

Chalmers I (1993) 'Effective care in midwifery: research the professions and the public', *Midwives Chronicle* 106:1260 3–12

Chalmers I (2004) 'Globalisation and perinatal health care', *BJOG: An International Journal of Obstetrics & Gynaecology* 111:9 889–91

Chalmers I (2005) 'If evidence-informed policy works in practice, does it matter if it doesn't work in theory?', *Evidence & Policy* 1:2 227–42

Chalmers I, Enkin M and Keirse MJNC (1989) *Effective Care in Pregnancy and Childbirth*, Vols 1 & 2, Oxford: Oxford University Press

Chalmers I, Zlosnik JE, Johns KA and Campbell H (1976) 'Obstetric practice and outcome of pregnancy in Cardiff residents 1965–72, *BMJ* March 27:1 (6012) 735–8

Chapman L (2012) 'Evidence-based practice, talking therapies and the new Taylorism', *Psychotherapy and Politics International* 10:1 33–44

Cheung NF (2009) 'Chinese midwifery: the history and modernity', *Midwifery* 25:3 228–41

Cheung NF, Mander R and Cheng L (2005) 'The "doula-midwives" in Shanghai', *Evidence-Based Midwifery* 3:2 73–9

Cheung NF, Mander R, Cheng L, Chen VY and Yang XQ (2006) 'Caesarean decision-making: the negotiation between Chinese women and healthcare professionals', *Evidence Based Midwifery* 4:1 24–30

Cheung NF, Mander R, Wang X, Fu W, Zhou H and Zhang L (2011) 'Clinical outcomes of the first midwife-led normal birth unit in China: a retrospective cohort study', *Midwifery* 27:5 582–7 http://www.sciencedirect.com/science/article/pii/S026661381000080X

Cheung NF, Mander R, Wang X, Fu W and Zhu J (2009) 'The planning and preparation for a "homely birthplace" in Hangzhou, China', *Evidence Based Midwifery* 7:3 101–6

Chippington Derrick D (2004) 'The truth behind the NICE guidelines on caesarean section', *AIMS Journal* 16:3, Accessed 08/12 http://www.aims.org.uk/Journal/Vol16No3/CSGuideline.htm

CHRE (2012) 'Strategic Review of the Nursing and Midwifery Council: Final Report', Accessed 07/12 https://www.chre.org.uk/_img/pics/library/120702_CHRE_Final_Report_for_NMC_strategic_review_(pdf)_1.pdf

Christiaens W and van Teijlingen E (2009) 'Four meanings of medicalization: childbirth as a case study', *Salute e Societa* 8:2 123–41

Christiaens W, Verhaeghe M and Bracke P (2008) 'Childbirth expectations and experiences in Belgian and Dutch models of maternity care', *Journal of Reproductive and Infant Psychology* 26:4 309–22

Chummun H and Tiran D (2008) 'Increasing research evidence in practice: a possible role for the consultant nurse', *Journal of Nursing Management* 16:3 327–33

Clarke J (2004) 'Dissolving the public realm? The logics and limits of neo-liberalism', *Journal of Social Policy* January 2004 33:1 27–48

Clarke JB (1999) 'Evidence-based practice: a retrograde step? The importance of pluralism in evidence generation for the practice of health care', *Journal of Clinical Nursing* 8:1 89–94

Cleveland H (1972) *The Future Executive: A Guide for Tomorrow's Managers*, New York: Harper and Row

Cloake M (1991) 'Report on confidential enquiries into maternal deaths in the UK 1985–87: A summary of the main points', *Health Trends* 23:1 4–5

Clover B (2012) 'Mental health trust set to leave litigation scheme', *Health Services Journal* 2 April 2012, Accessed 08/12, http://www.hsj.co.uk/mental-health-trust-set-to-leave-litigation-scheme/5042919.article

CMACE (2011) 'Saving mothers' lives: reviewing maternal deaths to make motherhood safer: 2006–08, The eighth report on confidential enquiries into maternal deaths in the United Kingdom', *BJOG* 118:(Suppl. 1) 1–203

CMACE (undated) 'The London Project: a confidential enquiry into a series of term babies born in an unexpectedly poor condition', Centre for Maternal and Child Enquiries

CMB (1952) *Handbook Incorporating the Rules of the Central Midwives Board* 20th edn, London: Central Midwives Board

Cnattingius S, Bergström R, Lipworth L and Kramer MS (1998) 'Prepregnancy weight and the risk of adverse pregnancy outcomes', *New England Journal of Medicine* 338:3 147–52

CNOs (2010) *Midwifery 2020: Delivering Expectations*, Chief Nursing Officers of England, Northern Ireland, Scotland & Wales London: Department of Health

Cochrane AL (1972) *Effectiveness and Efficiency*, London: Nuffield Provincial Hospitals Trust

Code L (2000) 'The perversion of autonomy and the subjection of women: discourses of social advocacy at century's end' in C Mackenzie and N Stoljar (eds) *Relational Autonomy: Feminist Perspectives on Autonomy Agency and the Social Self*, Oxford: Oxford University Press, 181–209

Colen S (1994) '"Like a mother to them": stratified reproduction and West Indian childcare workers and employers in New York' in FD Ginsburg and R Rapp (eds) *Conceiving the New World Order: The Global Politics of Reproduction*, Berkeley: University of California Press, p 78

Committee on Nursing (1972) 'Report of the Committee of Nursing (Briggs Report)' London: HMSO (Cmnd 5115)

Connell R, Fawcett B and Meagher G (2009) 'Neoliberalism, new public management and the human service professions: introduction to the special issue', *Journal of Sociology* 45:4 331–8

Connolly S, Bevan G and Mays N (2010) 'Funding and performance of healthcare systems in the four countries of the UK before and after devolution', The Nuffield Trust London, Accessed 07/11, http://www.nuffieldtrust.org.uk/sites/files/nuffield/Funding_and_Performance_of_Healthcare_Services.pdf

Conrad O and Schneider JW (1980) 'Looking at levels of medicalization: a comment on Strong's critique of the thesis of medical imperialism', *Social Science & Medicine* 14A 75–9

Conrad P (1992) 'Medicalization and social control', *Annual Review of Sociology* 18 209–32

Cooke P (2004) 'Promoting partnerships in Paddington: a consultant midwife's role', *Midwives* 7:7 310–11

Cooper G and McClure J (2007) 'Anaesthesia' in G Lewis (ed) *Saving Mothers' Lives: The Confidential Enquiry into Maternal and Child Health (CEMACH). Reviewing Maternal Deaths to Make Motherhood Safer 2003–05. The Seventh Report of the United Kingdom Confidential Enquiries into Maternal Deaths in the United Kingdom*, London: CEMACH, pp 107–16

Coster S, Redfern S, Wilson-Barnett J, Evans A, Peccei R and Guest D (2006) 'Impact of the role of nurse, midwife and health visitor consultant', *Journal of Advanced Nursing* 55:3 352–63

CQC (2006) 'Investigation into 10 maternal deaths at, or following delivery at, Northwick Park Hospital, North West London Hospitals NHS Trust, between April 2002 and April 2005 Care Quality Commission', Accessed 08/11, http://www.cqc.org.uk/_db/_documents/Northwick_tagged.pdf

Croll E (2000) *Endangered Daughters: Discrimination and Development in Asia*, London: Routledge

Croll EJ (2001) 'Amartya Sen's 100 million missing women', *Oxford Development Studies* 29:3 225–44

Cronk M (1998) 'Keep your hands off the breech', *AIMS Journal* 10:3, Accessed 08/12, http://www.aims.org.uk/Journal/Vol10No3/handOffbreech.htm

Cronk M (2000) 'The midwife: a professional servant?' in M Kirkham (ed) *The Midwife–Mother Relationship*, Basingstoke: Macmillan Press

Crowhurst JA and Plaat F (2000) 'Labor analgesia for the 21st century'. *Seminars in Anesthesia, Perioperative Medicine and Pain* 19:3 164–70

Curtis P, Ball L and Kirkham M (2006) 'Ceasing to practise midwifery: working life and employment choices', *British Journal of Midwifery* 14:6 336–8.

Dale P and Fisher K (2009) 'Implementing the 1902 Midwives Act: assessing problems, developing services and creating a new role for a variety of female practitioners', *Women's History Review* 18:3 427–52

Davies C (1990) *The Collapse of the Conventional Career. The Future of Work and its Relevance for Post-registration Education in Nursing, Midwifery and Health Visiting*, London: English National Board for Nursing, Midwifery and Health Visiting

Davis D and Walker K (2010) 'Case-loading midwifery in New Zealand: making space for childbirth' *Midwifery* 26:6 603–8

Davies JW (2009) 'Giving birth to the maternity care assistant', *The Practising Midwife* 12:8 20–2

Davies S (2007a) 'Where next for the maternity services? A midwifery perspective', *Healthcare Risk Report* 13:2 13–14

Davies S (2007b) 'Standards must be embraced to improve safety and reduce litigation', *Healthcare Risk Report* 14:2 18–19

Davies S (2007c) 'Beware reconfiguration fever!', *The Practising Midwife* 10:5 4–5

Davies S (2009) 'Jury of your peers?' *AIMS Journal* 21:3 10–11

Davies S (2011a) 'Response: we need a new model for maternity care, not blame for individuals', *Guardian*, 11 November 2011, 45

Davies S (2011b) 'What is happening to Greater Manchester Maternity Services?', *Midwifery Matters* 128 2–3

Davies S (2012) Senior Lecturer, University of Salford Personal communication

Davies S and Edwards N (2010) 'Termination of the Albany Practice contract: unanswered questions', *British Journal of Midwifery* 18:4 260–1

Davies S, Edwards N, Kirkham M and Murphy-Lawless J (2012) Personal communication

Davies S and Rawlinson H (2012) 'Manchester maternity reconfiguration: claims of success are premature', *Health Service Journal*, 27 September 2012, http://www.hsj.co.uk/opinion/columnists/premature-celebrations/5048091.article

Davies S and Rawlinson H (2010) 'The case for retaining full maternity services in Salford', Keep Hope Maternity Open Campaign Group, Accessed 08/12, http://www.seek.salford.ac.uk/user/profile/publications/view.do?publicationNum=26355

Davis JAP (2010) 'Midwives and normalcy in childbirth: a phenomenologic concept development study', *Journal of Midwifery & Women's Health* 55:3 206–15

Davis-Floyd R (2001) 'The technocratic, humanistic, and holistic paradigms of childbirth international', *Journal of Gynecology & Obstetrics* 75 S1, S5–S23

Davis-Floyd R (2005) 'Daughter of time: the post-modern midwife', MIDIRS *Midwifery Digest* 15:1 32–9

Davis-Floyd R and Bonaro DP (2012) Joint Letter to Participants in the Human Rights in Childbirth Conference, Human Rights in Childbirth Conference, The Hague: International Conference of Jurists, Midwives and Obstetricians, pp 61–3

Davis-Floyd R, Pascal-Bonaro D, Davies R and Gomez Ponce de Leon R (2010) 'The International MotherBaby Childbirth Initiative: a human rights approach to optimal maternity care', *Midwifery Today* 94:12–4, 64–6

Davis-Floyd RE (1990) 'The role of obstetrical rituals in the resolution of cultural anomaly', *Social Science & Medicine* 31:1 175–89

Davis-Floyd RE, Barclay L, Daviss B-A and Tritten J (2009) (eds) *Birth Models that Work*, Berkeley: University of California Press

De Brouwere V and Van Lerberghe W (2001) 'Safe motherhood strategies: a review of the evidence studies in health services organisation and policy', 17, EC Directorate General DEV

de Kok B, Hussein J and Jeffery P (2010) 'Joining-up thinking: loss in childbearing from inter-disciplinary perspectives', *Social Science & Medicine* 71 1703–10

De Lee JB (1915) 'Progress towards ideal obstetrics', *Transactions of the American Association for the Study and Prevention of Infant Mortality* 6 114–38

De Muylder X (1993) 'Caesarian sections in developing countries: some considerations', *Health Policy and Planning* 8:2 101–12

de Swiet M, Williamson C and Lewis G (2011) 'Other indirect deaths', in CMACE 2011 *Saving Mothers' Lives: Reviewing Maternal Deaths to Make Motherhood Safer: 2006–08*. Centre for Maternal and Child Enquiries, *The Eighth Report on Confidential Enquiries into Maternal Deaths in the United Kingdom*, *BJOG* 118 (Suppl. 1), pp 119–31

De Vries R (2004) *A Pleasing Birth: Midwives and Maternity Care in the Netherlands*, Philadelphia: Temple University Press

De Vries R, Wiegers T, Smulders B and van Teijlingen E (2009) 'The Dutch obstetrical system: vanguard of the future in maternity care' in RE Davis-Floyd, L Barclay, B-A Daviss and J Tritten (eds) *Birth Models that Work*, Berkeley: University of California Press, 31–88

Deber RB, Kraetschmer N, Urowitz S and Sharpe N (2005) 'Patient, consumer, client, or customer: what do people want to be called?', *Health Expectations* 8:4 345–51

Declercq E and Viisainen K (2001) 'Appendix: The politics of numbers P267' in S Abram, R De Vries, H Marland, E Van Teijlingen and S Wrede (eds) *Birth by Design: Pregnancy, Maternity Care and Midwifery in North America and Europe*, London: Routledge

Declercq ER (1994) 'A cross-national analysis of midwifery politics: six lessons for midwives', *Midwifery* 10:4 232–7

Declercq ER, Sakala C, Corry MP, Applebaum S and Risher P (2002) 'Listening to Mothers: Maternity Center Association', New York, Accessed 12/09, http://www.childbirth connection.com/pdfs/LtMreport.pdf

Deery R, Hughes D and Kirkham M (2010) *Tensions and Barriers in Improving Maternity Care: The Story of a Birth Centre*, Oxford: Radcliffe Publishing

de Jonge A (2012) 'Paradox of the Dutch maternity care system' in H Hayes-Klein (ed) Conference papers, *Human Rights in Childbirth*, International Conference of Jurists, Midwives and Obstetricians, The Hague: Bynkershoek Publishing, pp 132–4

Denny K (1999) 'Evidence-based medicine and medical authority', *Journal of Medical Humanities* 20:4 247–63

DeVries R (1996) 'The midwife's place: an international comparison of the status of midwives' in SF Murray (ed) *Midwives and Safer Motherhood*, London: Mosby

DeVries R (2001) 'Midwifery in the Netherlands: vestige or vanguard?' *Medical Anthropology: Cross-Cultural Studies in Health and Illness* 20:4 Special Issue: Midwifery Part II pp 277–311

DeVries RG (1993) 'A cross-national view of the status of midwives' in E Riska and K Wegar (eds) *Gender, Work and Medicine: Women and the Medical Division of Labour*, London: Sage

DFID (2010) Millennium Development Goal Five, Department for International Development, Accessed 10/12, http://www.dfid.gov.uk/Global-Issues/Millennium-Development-Goals/5-Improve-maternal-health/S

DHSS (1980) 'Inequalities in Health': Report of a Research Working Group, London: Department of Health and Social Services, Accessed 07/11, http://www.sochealth.co.uk/Black/black.htm

Di Renzo GC (2003) 'Tocophobia: a new indication for cesarean delivery?', *Journal of Maternal-Fetal & Neonatal Medicine* 13:4 217

Dick-Read G (1933) *Natural Childbirth*, London: Heinemann.

Dimond B (1994) 'Reliable or liable?', *Modern Midwife* 4:4 6–7.

Dingwall R, Rafferty AM and Webster C (1988) *An Introduction to the Social History of Nursing*, London: Routledge

Dobash RE, Dobash RP, Cavanagh K and Lewis R (2000) *Changing Violent Men*, Thousand Oaks: Sage Publications Inc

DoH (1989) 'Working for patients', London: HMSO (Cm 555)

DoH (1993) 'Changing childbirth, Part 1, Report of the Expert Maternity Group', HMSO: Department of Health London Chair J Cumberlege

DoH (1998) 'European Working Time Directive', London, Accessed 10/11, http://webarc-hive.nationalarchives.gov.uk/+/www.dh.gov.uk/en/Managingyourorganisation/Work-force/Workforceplanninganddevelopment/Europeanworkingtimedirective/index.htm

DoH (1999) 'Nurse, midwife and health visitor consultants: establishing posts and making appointments' HSC 1999/217, London: Department of Health

DoH (2004) '*National Services Framework for Children, Young People and Maternity Services*', London: Department of Health

DoH (2006) 'National Guidelines for Maternity Services Liaison Committees (MSLCs)', London: Department of Health, Accessed 07/11, http://www.dh.gov.uk/prod_consum_dh/groups/dh_digitalassets/@dh/@en/documents/digitalasset/dh_4128340.pdf

DoH (2005) *Responding to Domestic Abuse: A Handbook for Health Professionals*, London: Department of Health, Accessed 12/11, http://www.dh.gov.uk/publications

DoH (2007a) 'NHS maternity statistics, England: 2002–03', Accessed 11/11, http://www.dh.gov.uk/en/Publicationsandstatistics/Statistics/StatisticalWorkAreas/Statisticalhealthcare/DH_4086521

DoH (2007b) 'Maternity matters: choice, access and continuity of care in a safe service', London: Department of Health

DoH (2010a) 'Equity and excellence: liberating the NHS Department of Health', Accessed 07/11, http://www.dh.gov.uk/en/Publicationsandstatistics/Publications/PublicationsPolicyAndGuidance/DH_117353

DoH (2010b) 'Healthy lives, healthy people: our strategy for public health in England', London: Department of Health

DoH and DCSF (2010) 'Teenage pregnancy strategy: beyond 2010', Department for Children, Schools and Families/Department of Health, Accessed 08/11, http://www.education.gov.uk/consultations/downloadableDocs/4287_Teenage%20pregnancy%20strategy_aw8.pdf

DONA (2011) 'History and Mission Doulas of North America International', Accessed 10/11, http://www.dona.org/aboutus/mission.php

Donnison J (1988) *Midwives and Medical Men: A History of the Struggle for the Ccontrol of Childbirth* 2nd edn, London: New Barnet Historical Publications

Douche JR (2008) 'Caesarean section in the absence of clinical indications: discourses constituting choice in childbirth', Unpublished PhD in Midwifery Thesis, Massey University of Palmerston North, Accessed 05/12, http://mro.massey.ac.nz/handle/10179/670

Doughty A (1987) 'Landmarks in the development of regional analgesia in obstetrics' in BM Morgan (ed) *Foundations of Obstetric Anaesthesia*, London: Farrand Press

Douglas J (1992) 'Black women's health matters: Putting black women on the research agenda' in H Roberts (ed) *Women's Health Matters*, London: Routledge, pp 33–46

Douglas M (1966) *Purity and Danger: An Analysis of the Concepts of Pollution and Taboo*, London: Routledge & Kegan Paul

Doula Consultancy (2011) 'Doula Training Courses, Accredited by Middlesex University In London', Accessed 10/11, http://findadoula.org.uk/doulatrainingbydoulaconsultancyac-creditedbymiddlesexuniversity/

Dowler C, Heritage A and Wallis S (2012) 'Labour of love: making a maternity services reconfiguration successful', *Health Services Journal* 6 March, Accessed 08/12, http://www.hsj.co.uk/resource-centre/best-practice/qipp-resources/labour-of-love-making-a-mater-nity-services-reconfiguration-successful/5041433.article

Downe S (2004) *Normal Childbirth: Evidence and Debate*, Edinburgh: Churchill Livingstone

Downe S (2010) 'Towards salutogenic birth in the 21st century' in D Walsh and S Downe (eds) *Essential Midwifery Practice: Intrapartum Care*, Chichester: Wiley Blackwell, pp 289–95

Doyal L (2001) 'Sex, gender, and health: the need for a new approach', *BMJ* 323:7320 1061–3

Drazek M (2009) 'North West Local Supervising Authority. Annual report to the Nursing and Midwifery Council on the statutory supervision of midwives & midwifery practice 2008–2009', NHS Northwest, Accessed 08/12, http://www.northwest.nhs.uk/document_uploads/lsa/LSA%20Annual%20Report%2008–09%20%20final.pdf

Drechsler W (2005) 'The rise and demise of the new public management', *Post-Qutistic Economics Review* 33:14, September 2005, Accessed 08/12, http://www.paecon.net/PAEReview/issue33/Drechsler33.htm

Drucker PF (1974) *Management: Tasks, Responsibilities, Practices*, London: Heinemann

du Plessis H and Johnstone C (2007) 'Obstetrics/pharmacology ethics and medico-legal aspects of obstetric anaesthesia', *Anaesthesia & Intensive Care Medicine* 8:8 337–9

Duerden J (2009) 'The supervisor of midwives' in R Mander and V Fleming (eds) *Becoming a Midwife*, London: Routledge

DUK (2011) 'About Doula UK', Doula UK, Accessed 10/11, http://doula.org.uk/content/about-doula-uk

Duley L, Matar HE, Almerie MQ and Hall DR (2008) 'Alternative magnesium sulphate regimens for women with pre-eclampsia and eclampsia (Protocol)', Cochrane Database of Systematic Reviews, Issue 4, Art No CD007388. DOI: 10.1002/14651858. CD007388.

Duncan S (2007) 'What's the problem with teenage parents? And what's the problem with policy?', *Critical Social Policy* 27:3 307–34

Dunkley-Bent J (2004) 'A consultant midwife's community clinic', *British Journal of Midwifery* 12:3 144–71

Dunkley-Bent J and Jones H (2008) 'Maternity Services Liaison Committee (MSLC) "walks the patch" to reflect the views of users', Midwives (online), Royal College of Midwives, Accessed 07/12, http://www.rcm.org.uk/magazines/papers/maternity-services-liaison-committee-mslcwalksthepatch

Dupree M (2011) 'James Young Simpson and the controversy over homoeopathy in Edinburgh' in A Nuttall and R Mander (eds) *James Young Simpson: Lad o Pairts*, Erskine: Scottish History Press

Dykes F (2009) '"No time to care": Midwifery work on postnatal wards in England' in B Hunter and R Deery (eds) *Emotions in Midwifery and Reproduction*, London: Palgrave

Dyson T and Moore M (1983) 'On kinship structure, female autonomy, and demographic behavior in India', *Population and Development Review* 9:1 35–60

Earle S and Church S (2004) 'Ethnicity and reproduction', *Practising Midwife* 7:6 34–7

Eberts M, Schwartz A, Edney R and Kaufman K (1987) *Report of the Task Force on the Implementation of Midwifery in Ontario*, Toronto: Queen's Park Printers

Editorial (1994) 'The AIMS Committee – what we do', *AIMS Journal* 6:1 3

Edwards N (1996) 'Is everything rosy in the MSLC garden? Part 1', *AIMS Quarterly Journal* 8:3 6–9

Edwards N (2004) 'Protection regulations and standards: enabling or disabling?', *RCM Midwives Journal* 7:3 116–19 and 7:4 160–3

Edwards N (2005a) *Birthing Autonomy: Women's Experiences of Planning Home Births*, London: Routledge

Edwards N (2005b) 'Promoting public participation: MSLC Workshops', *AIMS Journal* 17:2 16–17

Edwards N (2005c) 'Is public participation working for women?', *New Generation* 33

Edwards N (2006) 'Promoting public participation', *The Practising Midwife* 9:5 18–19

Edwards N (2008a) 'Women's emotion work in the context of current maternity services', in B Hunter and R Deery (eds) *Emotions in Midwifery and Reproduction*, London: Palgrave

Edwards N (2008b) 'Safety in birth: the contextual conundrums faced by women in a "risk society", driven by neoliberal policies', *MIDIRS Midwifery Digest* 18:4 463–70

Edwards N (2010a) 'Reclaiming birth rally', *AIMS Journal* 22:1

Edwards N (2010b) '"There's so much potential ... and for whatever reason it's not being realized" – Women's relationships with midwives as a negotiation of ideology and practice' in M Kirkham (ed) *The Midwife-Mother Relationship* 2nd edn, London: Palgrave-Macmillan

Edwards N (2012) Birth Activist, Pregnancy and Parent Centre, Edinburgh Personal communication

Edwards N, Murphy-Lawless J, Kirkham M and Davies S (2011) 'Attacks on midwives, attacks on women's choices', *AIMS Journal* 23:3 3–7

Eliason MJ (1996) 'Caring for the lesbian, gay, or bisexual patient: issues for critical care nurses', *Critical Care Nursing Quarterly* 19:1 65–72

Ellis N (2004) 'Birth experiences of south Asian Muslim women: marginalised choice within the maternity services', in M Kirkham (ed) *Informed Choice in Maternity Care*, Basingstoke: Palgrave, pp 237–55

Encarta (2011) Encarta on-line North American Dictionary, Accessed 07/11

ESRI (2012) 'Perinatal Statistics Report 2010', Economic and Social Research Institute, Accessed 07/12, http://www.esri.ie/news_events/latest_press_releases/perinatal_statistics_repo_4/index.xml

Etzioni A (1969) *The Semi-Professions and Their Organization: Teachers, Nurses, Social Workers*, New York: Free Press

EU (2011) 'The application of patients' rights in cross-border healthcare: Directive 2011/24/EU of the European Parliament and of the Council of 9 March 2011', *Official Journal of the European Union* L 88/45 4.4.2011

Ewing A (undated) 'About us', Accessed 03/12, http://www.calumny.demon.co.uk/scotbirth/Individuals/Allison.html

Ewing A (2012) Personal communication

Fahy K (2007) 'Discussion: an Australian history of the subordination of midwifery', *Women and Birth* 20:1 25–9

Fathalla MF (2006) 'Human rights aspects of safe motherhood', *Best Practice and Research Clinical Obstetrics and Gynaecology* 20:3 409–19

Fawole AO, Adekanle DA and Hunyinbo KI (2010) 'Utilization of the partograph in primary health care facilities in Southwestern Nigeria', *Nigerian Journal of Clinical Practice* 13:2 200–4

Fenwick J, Staff L, Gamble J, Creedy DK and Bayes S (2010) 'Why do women request caesarean section in a normal, healthy first pregnancy?', *Midwifery* 26:4 394–400

Fisher A (2008) 'Tackling obesity in Salford: a cross partnership strategy', Salford's Healthy Weight Strategy Salford Strategic Partnership, unpublished report

Fitzpatrick T (2001) *Welfare Theory: An Introduction*, London: Palgrave

Flandermeyer D, Stanton C and Armbruster D (2010) 'Uterotonic use at home births in low-income countries: A literature review', *International Journal of Gynecology & Obstetrics* 108 269–75

Fleming V (1998a) 'Women and midwives in partnership: A problematic relationship?', *Journal of Advanced Nursing* 27:1 8–14

Fleming V (1998b) 'Women-with-midwives-with-women: a model of interdependence', *Midwifery* 14 137–43

Fleming V (2000) 'The midwifery partnership in New Zealand: past history or a new way forward?' in M Kirkham (ed) *The Midwife-Mother Relationship*, Basingstoke: Macmillan Press, pp 193–206

Fleming VEM (1996) 'Midwifery in New Zealand: responding to changing times', *Health Care for Women International* 17:4 343–59

Flint C (1986) 'The know your midwife report', Flint, London

Foucault M (1973) *The Birth of the Clinic: An Archaeology of Medical Perception*, London: Tavistock.

Foucault M (1980) 'Power and strategies' in C Gordon (ed) *Michel Foucault: Power/Knowledge. Selected Interviews and Other Writings 1972–1977*, Brighton: Harvester Press

Foucault M (1982) 'The subject and power', *Critical Inquiry* 8:4 777–95

Foucault M (1990) 'Politics and reason' in L Kritzman (ed) *Michel Foucault: Politics, Philosophy, Culture: Interviews and Other Writings 1977–1984*, London: Routledge

Foucault M (1991) 'Politics and ethics: an interview' in P Rabinow (ed) *The Foucault Reader: An Introduction to Foucault's Thought*, London: Penguin

Foucault M (2001) *Fearless Speech*, Los Angeles (CA): Semiotext(e)

Foucault M (2002a) 'Governmentality' in J Faubion (ed) *Power: Essential Works of Foucault 1954–1984*, Vol 3, London: Penguin

Foucault M (2002b) 'The birth of social medicine' in J Faubion (ed) *Power: Essential Works of Foucault 1954–1984*, Vol 3, London: Penguin

Foucault M (2002c) 'The risks of security' in J Faubion (ed) *Power: Essential Works of Foucault 1954–1984*, Vol 3, London: Penguin

Foucault M (2004) '17 March 1976' in M Bertani and A Fontana (eds) *'Society Must be Defended': Lectures at the Collège de France, 1975–76*, London: Penguin

Fox RC (1977) 'The medicalization and demedicalization of American Society', *Daedalus* 106:1, 9–22

FPL (2011) 'The feasibility and insurability of independent midwifery in England', Accessed 04/12, http://www.nmc-uk.org/Documents/Midwifery-Reports/Feasibility-and-Insurability-of-Independent-Midwifery-in-England_September-2011.pdf

Fraser G (1995) 'Modern bodies, modern minds: midwifery and reproductive change in an African American community' in FD Ginsburg and R Rapp (eds) *Conceiving the New World Order: The Global Politics of Reproduction*, Berkeley: University of California Press, ch 3, pp 42–58

Fraser N (1989) *Unruly Practices: Power, Discourse and Gender in Contemporary Social Theory*, Cambridge: Polity Press

Frederickson HG (2007) 'Whatever happened to public administration? Governance, governance everywhere' in E Ferlie, L Lynn and C Pollitt (eds) *The Oxford Handbook of Public Management*, Oxford: Oxford University Press

Freeman L, Timperley H and Adair V (2004) 'Partnership in midwifery care in New Zealand', *Midwifery* 20 2–14

Freidson E (1970) *Profession of Medicine: A Study of the Sociology of Applied Knowledge*, New York: Dodd Mead

Friedman E (1954) 'The graphic analysis of labor', *American Journal of Obstetrics and Gynecology* 68:6 1568–75

Frigoletto FD (2007) 'Active management of labor – UpToDate', Waltham, Accessed 05/12, http://positivethinkers.web.officelive.com/Documents/Active%20management%20of%20labor.doc

Fullerton J, Navarro A and Young H (2007) 'Outcomes of planned home birth: An integrative review', *Journal of Midwifery & Women's Health* 52:4 323–33

Furstenburg FF, Brooks-Gunn JM and Morgan SP (1987) *Adolescent Mothers in Later Life*, Cambridge: Cambridge University Press

Gabrysch S and Campbell OMR (2009) 'Still too far to walk: literature review of the determinants of delivery service use', *BMC Pregnancy and Childbirth* 9:34

Gaines AD and Davis-Floyd R (2004) 'Biomedicine' in M Ember and C Ember (eds) *Encyclopaedia of Medical Anthropology*, Dordrecht: Kluwer Academic Publishers 95–109, http://www.cwru.edu/artsci/anth/documents/Biomed-GainesandDavis-F.PDF

Gamarnikow E (1978) 'Sexual division of labour: the case of nursing', in A Kuhn and AM Wolpe (eds) *Feminism and Materialism*, London: Routledge & Kegan Paul, pp 96–123

Garcia J and Garforth S (1989) 'Labour and delivery routines in English consultant maternity units', *Midwifery* 5:4 155–62

Garcia J, Kilpatrick R and Richards M (1990) *The Politics of Maternity Care: Services for Childbearing Women in Twentieth-century Britain*, Oxford: Clarendon

Garcia J, Kilpatrick R and Richards M (1990) 'Introduction' in J Garcia, R Kilpatrick and M Richards (eds) *The Politics of Maternity Care: Services for Childbearing Women in Twentieth-century Britain* Oxford: Clarendon Paperbacks

Gash T and Rutter J (2011) 'The quango conundrum' *The Political Quarterly* 82:1 95–101

Gaskin IM (1977) *Spiritual Midwifery*, Summertown (TN): The Farm

Gaudion A and Menka Y (2010) '"No decision about me without me": centering pregnancy', *The Practising Midwife* 13:1015–8.

Gaynor M, Laudicella M and Propper C (2012) 'Can governments do it better? Merger mania and hospital outcomes in the English NHS', January 2012 Working Paper No 12/281, Centre for Market and Public Organisation, Bristol Institute of Public Affairs, University of Bristol

George V and Wilding P (1994) *Welfare and Ideology*, Brighton: Harvester Wheatsheaf

Gibbons L, Belizán JM, Lauer JA, Betrán AP, Merialdi M and Althabe F (2010) 'The global numbers and costs of additionally needed and unnecessary caesarean sections performed per year: overuse as a barrier to universal coverage', World Health Report Background Paper No 30, Accessed 05/12, http://www.who.int/healthsystems/topics/financing/healthreport/30C-sectioncosts.pdf

Gilliland AL (2002) 'Beyond holding hands: The modern role of the professional doula', *Journal of Obstetrical Gynecological and Neonatal Nursing* 31:6 762–9

Global Health Watch (2011) *Global Health Watch 3: An Alternative World Health Report*, London: Zed Books

Godber G (1988) 'Forty years of the NHS: origins and early development', *BMJ* 297 37–43

Goode WJ (1971) 'Force and violence in the family', *Journal of Marriage and the Family* 33 624–636.

Gould D (2000) 'Normal labour: a concept analysis', *Journal of Advanced Nursing* 31:2 418–27

Gould D (2002) 'Subliminal medicalisation', *British Journal of Midwifery* 10:7 418

Gray JE (2010) 'Learning and the follow-through experience in three year Bachelor of Midwifery programs in Australia. "Placements with women, not institutions"', unpublished PhD Thesis, Sydney: University of Technology

Greater Manchester Children Young People and Families Network (2010) 'Making it better for children, young people, babies and families', A Network Approach to Achieving EWTD Compliance, End of Project Report, April 2010, http://www.makingitbetter.nhs.uk/./children-young-and-families-network

Green JM and Baston HA (2003) 'Feeling in control during labor: concepts, correlates, and consequences', *Birth* 30:4 235–47

Greer A and Hoggett P (1999) 'Public policies, private strategies and local spending bodies', *Public Administration* 77 235–256

Griffith R, Tengnah C and Patel C (2010) *Law and Professional Issues in Midwifery*, Exeter: Learning Matters

Groeschel N and Glover P (2001) 'The partograph used daily but rarely questioned', *Australian Journal of Midwifery* 14:3 22–7

Grosse RN and Auffrey C (1989) 'Literacy and health status in developing countries', *Annual Review of Public Health* 10:281–97

Guest DE, Peccei R and Rosenthal P et al (2004) *An Evaluation of the Impact of Nurse, Midwife and Health Visitor Consultants*, London: King's College

Guilliland K and Pairman S (1994) 'The midwifery partnership – a model for practice', *New Zealand College of Midwives Journal* 11:5–9.

Guilliland K and Pairman S (1995) *The Midwifery Partnership: A Model for Practice*, Wellington: Department of Nursing and Midwifery, Victoria University of Wellington, Monograph Series 95/1.

Gyte GML, Dodwell MJ and Macfarlane AJ (2011) 'Home birth metaanalysis: does it meet AJOG's reporting requirements?', *American Journal of Obstetrics and Gynecology* 204:4 e15

Hall J (2010) 'Editorial', *The Practising Midwife* 13:1 3

Hall J and Taylor M (2004) 'Birth and spirituality' in S Downe (ed) *Normal Childbirth: Evidence and Debate*, Edinburgh: Churchill Livingstone

Hamlin C (2009) 'Hamlin Fistula International', Accessed 01/12, http://www.hamlinfistula.org/what-is-a-fistula.html

Hanisch C (1971) 'The personal is political' in J Aget (ed) *The Radical Therapist*, New York: Ballantine Books

Hardt M and Negri A (2000) *Empire*, Cambridge (MA): Harvard University Press

Harper A (2011) 'Sepsis' in Centre for Maternal and Child Enquiries (CMACE). *Saving Mothers' Lives: reviewing maternal deaths to make motherhood safer: 2006–08*. The Eighth Report on Confidential Enquiries into Maternal Deaths in the United Kingdom. *British Journal of Obstetrics and Gynaecology* 118 (Suppl. 1): 1–203

Harris A, Gao Y, Barclay L and Belton S (2007) 'Consequences of birth policies and practices in post-reform China', *Reproductive Health Matters* 15:30 114–24

Harvey D (2005) *A Brief History of Neoliberalism*, Oxford: Oxford University Press

Hastings A, Bramley G, Bailey N and Watkins D (2012) *Serving Deprived Communities in a Recession*, York: Joseph Rowntree Foundation, Accessed 08/12, http://www.jrf.org.uk/sites/files/jrf/communities-recession-services-full.pdf

Hatem M, Sandall J, Devane D, Soltani H and Gates S (2008) 'Midwife-led versus other models of care for childbearing women', Cochrane Database of Systematic Reviews, Issue 4, No CD004667. DOI: 10.1002/14651858.CD004667.pub2.

Haverkamp AD, Thompson HE, McFee JG and Cetrulo C (1976) 'The evaluation of continuous fetal heart rate monitoring in high-risk pregnancy', *American Journal of Obstetrics and Gynecology* 125 310–17

Health Protection Agency (2012) 'Risk of infection from caesareans at nearly 10 per cent', 1 August 2012 press release, Health Protection Agency, Accessed 08/12, http://www.hpa.org.uk/webw/HPAweb&HPAwebStandard/HPAweb_C/1317135316315

Healthcare Commission (2006) 'Investigation into 10 maternal deaths at, or following delivery at, Northwick Park Hospital, North West London NHS Trust, between April 2002 and April 2005', London: Department of Health

Healthcare Commission (2007) 'Women's experiences of maternity care in the NHS in England: Key findings from a survey of NHS trusts carried out in 2007', Commission for Healthcare Audit and Inspection, Accessed 08/12, http://webarchive.nationalarchives.gov.uk/20090102094834/http://healthcarecommission.org.uk/_db/_documents/Maternity_services_survey_report.pdf

Healthcare Commission (2008) *Towards Better Births: A Review of Maternity Services in England*, London: Healthcare Commission

Healy E (2010) 'Nurses and Midwives Bill', *Irish Medical Times*, 12 May, Accessed 05/12, http://www.imt.ie/opinion/guests/2010/05/nurses-and-midwives-bill-2010.html

Heckel E (2012) 'Letter to the conference', in H Hayes-Klein (ed) *Conference Papers, Human Rights in Childbirth. International Conference of Jurists, Midwives and Obstetricians*, The Hague, Netherlands: Bynkershoek Publishing, pp 118–21

Heise LL, Pitanguy J and Germain A (1994) *Violence Against Women: The Hidden Health Burden*, Washington DC: The World Bank

Helman C (2007) *Culture, Health and Illness*, 5th edn, London: Hodder Arnold

Hemminki E and Merilainen J (1996) 'Long-term effects of cesarean sections: ectopic pregnancies and placental problems', *American Journal of Obstetrics & Gynecology* 174:5 1569–74

Hepple B (2010) 'The new single Equality Act in Britain', *The Equal Rights Review* 5 11–24

Hibbard BM and Scott DB (1990) 'The availability of epidural anaesthesia and analgesia in obstetrics', *British Journal of Obstetrics and Gynaecology* 97 402–5

Hill Collins P (2000) *Black Feminist Thought: Knowledge, Consciousness, and the Politics of Empowerment*, New York: Unwin Hyman

Hindin MJ (2005) 'Women's autonomy, status, and nutrition in Zimbabwe, Zambia, and Malawi' in S Kishor (ed) *A Focus on Gender: Collected Papers on Gender Using DHS Data*, pp 93–115, Calverton: ORC Macro, Accessed 12/11, http://pdf.usaid.gov/pdf_docs/PNADE016.pdf#page=22

Hirst P and Thompson G (1996) *Globalization in Question: The International Economy and the Possibilities of Governance*, London: Polity Press

HM Treasury (2010) 'Reforming arm's lengths bodies', Accessed 08/12, http://www.direct.gov.uk/prod_consum_dg/groups/dg_digitalassets/@dg/@en/documents/digitalasset/dg_186443.pdf

HMSO (1902) 'The Midwives Act' (*2 Edw. VII* c. 17), London: His Majesty's Stationery Office

HMSO (1979) 'Nurses, Midwives and Health Visitors Act c36', Accessed 05/12, http://www.legislation.gov.uk/ukpga/1979/36/pdfs/ukpga_19790036_en.pdf

Hobbs L (1997) *The Independent Midwife: A Guide to Independent Midwifery Practice*, 2nd edn, Cheshire: Books for Midwives

HOC (1992) 'House of Commons Select Committee on Maternity Services', 2nd Report, Vol 1, London: HMSO, Chair N Winterton

Hodnett ED, Downe S, Walsh D and Weston J (2010). 'Homelike versus conventional birth settings', Cochrane Database of Systematic Reviews, Issue 9, doi:10.1002/14651858.CD000012.pub3

Hodnett ED, Gates S, Hofmeyr GJ, Sakala C and Weston J (2011) 'Continuous support for women during childbirth', Cochrane Database of Systematic Reviews, Issue 2, Art No CD003766. DOI: 10.1002/14651858.CD003766.pub3

Hofberg K and Brockington I (2000) 'Tokophobia: An unreasoning dread of childbirth. A series of 26 cases', *British Journal of Psychiatry* 176 83–5

Hofberg K and Ward M (2007) 'Tokophobia: a profound dread and avoidance of childbirth (when pathological fear effects (sic) the consultation)', *Psychological Challenges in Obstetrics and Gynecology*, Part Two, 165–172

Hogg M, Penney G and Carmichael J (2007) 'Audit of care provided and outcomes achieved by Community Maternity Units in Scotland' 2005 SPCERH No 29, Aberdeen

Hoggett P (1996) 'New modes of control in public service', *Public Administration* 74 9–32

Holistic Community (2011) 'Maternity Support Therapist (doula) Programme', Accessed 10/11, http://www.holistic-community.co.uk/training-course/724/

Holmes JM (1955) 'Continuous intramuscular oxytocin', *The Lancet* 265: 23 April, 1191–3, Accessed 08/12, http://www.sciencedirect.com/science?_ob=MiamiImageURL&_cid=271773&_user=809099&_pii=S0305750X11002087&_check=y&_origin=&_coverDate=25-Sep-2011&view=c&wchp=dGLzVlS-zSkzk&md5=67547b2974741331ca18b2a24edf6c73/1-s2.0-S0305750X11002087-main.pdf

Hopkins C (2009) 'Independent midwives: working without professional indemnity insurance', *AvMA Medical & Legal Journal* 15:4 155–8

HPC (2009) 'Professional indemnity insurance', Health Professions Council London, Accessed 07/11, http://www.hpc-uk.org/assets/documents/1000274520090326-Council-enclosure9-professionalindemnityinsurance.pdf

Huang XH (2000) 'The present and future of Caesarean section' *The Journal of the Chinese Applied Obstetrics and Gynaecology* 16:5 259–61.

Hughes D (1995) 'Is midwifery safe in the embrace of the UKCC?', *Midwives* 108:1292 282.

Hulbert D (2011) 'Emergency medicine' in Centre for Maternal and Child Enquiries (CMACE) 'Saving Mothers' Lives: reviewing maternal deaths to make motherhood safer: 2006–8'. The Eighth Report on Confidential Enquiries into Maternal Deaths in the United Kingdom, *BJOG* 2011:118 (suppl 1): 1–203.

Hundley V, Cruickshank R, Lanf G and Glazener C (1994) 'Midwifery managed delivery unit: a randomised controlled comparison with consultant led care', *British Medical Journal* 309: 1401–4

Hunter B (1998) 'Independent midwifery: future inspiration or relic of the past?', *British Journal of Midwifery* 6:2 85–7

Hunter B (2004) 'Conflicting ideologies as a source of emotion work in midwifery', *Midwifery* 20:3 261–72

Hunter B, Berg M, Lundgren I, Ólafsdóttir Ó and Kirkham M (2008) 'Relationships: the hidden threads in the tapestry of maternity care', *Midwifery* 24 132–7

Hussain CJ and Marshall JE (2011) 'The effect of the developing role of the maternity support worker on the professional accountability of the midwife', *Midwifery* 27:3 336–41

IAC (2008) 'First Report of Conclusions and Recommendations: "Saving sanctuary"', London: Independent Asylum Commission, Accessed 08/11, http://www.independentasylumcommission.org.uk/pages/home.html

IAG (2010) 'Safe motherhood', Accessed 01/12, http://www.safemotherhood.org/priorities/initiatives.html

Ickovics JR, Kershaw TS, Westdahl C, Magriples U, Massey Z, Reynolds H and Rising S (2007) 'Group prenatal care and perinatal outcomes: a randomized controlled trial', *Obstetrics & Gynecology* 110:2 Pt 1 330–9.

Iganski P, Mason D, Humphreys A and Watkins M (2001) 'Equal opportunities and positive action in the British National Health Service: some lessons from the recruitment of minority ethnic groups to nursing and midwifery', *Ethnic and Racial Studies* 24:2 294–317

Illich I (1976) *Limits to Medicine: Medical Nemesis – the Expropriation of Health*, London: Boyars

Illich I (1995) 'Death undefeated: from medicine to medicalisation to systematisation', *British Medical Journal* 311 1652–3

IM-UK (2009a) 'Who we are', Accessed 03/12, http://www.independentmidwives.org.uk/?node=608

IM-UK (2009b) 'How much do independent midwives charge?', Accessed 03/12, http://www.independentmidwives.org.uk/?node=750

IM-UK (2009c) 'Professional indemnity insurance: the current situation', Accessed 05/12, http://www.independentmidwives.org.uk/?node=11615

Irvine LCG (2011) 'Ending female genital cutting: how have various approaches attempted to address the cultural significance of the practice and its impacts upon women's bodies?', University of Leeds: *POLIS Journal* 5, Accessed 12/11, http://www.polis.leeds.ac.uk/assets/files/students/student-journal/ug-summer-11/lucy-irvine.pdf

ISB (2011) 'Nurses and Midwives Act Number 41' Irish Statute Book, Accessed 05/12, http://www.irishstatutebook.ie/2011/en/act/pub/0041/index.html

Jack I (2009) 'The 12.10 to Leeds' in *The Country Formerly Known as Great Britain, Writings 1989–2009*, London: Jonathan Cape

Jackson C and Mander R (1995) 'History or herstory: the decline and fall of the midwife?', *British Journal of Midwifery* 3:5 279–83

Jackson N and Paterson-Brown S (2001) 'Physical sequelae of caesarean section', *Best Practice & Research Clinical Obstetrics & Gynaecology* 15:1 49–61

Janssen PA, Henderson AD and Vedam S (2009) 'The experience of planned home birth: views of the first 500 women', *Birth* 36:4 297–304

Jarman B (1989) 'Underprivileged areas: validation and distribution of scores', *BMJ* 289 1587–92

Jeffery P, Das A, Dasgupta J and Jeffery R (2007) 'Unmonitored intrapartum oxytocin use in home deliveries: evidence fom Uttar Pradesh', *India Reproductive Health Matters* 15:30 172–8

Jeffery P and Jeffery R (2008) '"Money itself discriminates": obstetric emergencies in the time of liberalisation', *Contributions to Indian Sociology* 42:1 59–91

Jeffery P and Jeffery R (2010) 'Only when the boat has started sinking: a maternal death in rural north India', *Social Science & Medicine* 71:10 1711–8

Jeffery P, Jeffery R and Lyon A (1989) *Labour Pains and Labour Power*, London: Zed Books

Jeffery P, Jeffery R and Lyon A (2002) 'Contaminating states: midwifery, childbearing, and the state in rural north India' in S Rozario and G Samuel (eds) *The Daughters of Hāritī: Childbirth and Female Healers in South and Southeast Asia*, London: Routledge, ch 4, pp 90–108

Jeffery R, Jeffery P and Lyon A (1984) 'Female infanticide and amniocentesis', *Social Science & Medicine* 19:11 1207–12

Jefford E, Fahy K and Sundin D (2010) 'A review of the literature: Midwifery decision-making and birth', *Women and Birth* 23 127–34

Jelliffe DB (1972) 'Commerciogenic malnutrition?', *Nutrition Reviews* 30 9199–205

Jentsch B, Durham R, Hundley V and Hussein J (2007) 'Creating consumer satisfaction in maternity care: the neglected needs of migrants, asylum seekers and refugees', *International Journal of Consumer Studies* 31:2 128–34

Jessop B (2002) 'Liberalism, neoliberalism, and urban governance: a state-theoretical perspective', *Antipode* 34:3 452–72

Johanson R, Newburn M and Macfarlane A (2002) 'Has the medicalisation of childbirth gone too far?', BMJ 324 892–5

Jones R, Swales HA and Lyons GR (2008) 'A national survey of safe practice with epidural analgesia in obstetric units', *Anaesthesia* 63:5 516–19

Jones SR and Jenkins R (2004) *The Law and the Midwife*, Oxford: Blackwell

Jordan RG and Murphy PA (2009) 'Risk assessment and risk distortion: finding the balance', *Journal of Midwifery & Womens Health* 54:3 191–200

Jowitt M (2008) 'Bystanding behaviour in midwifery: Machiavellian plot or unintended consequence of hospital birth?', *Midwifery Matters* 118 Autumn 11

Jowitt M (2009) 'Save the Albany', *Midwifery Matters* 123, Winter, Accessed 04/12, http://www.midwifery.org.uk/index.php?option=com_content&view=article&id=59:save-the-albany&catid=35:magazine-winter-2009&Itemid=116

Jowitt M (2010) 'Hypoxic ischaemic encephalopathy', *AIMS Journal* 22:3 13, Accessed 04/12, http://firstfamily.org.uk/wp-content/uploads/2011/03/AIMS223-Alb3-07.12.10_AIMS.pdf

Jowitt M and Kargar I (2009) 'Misgivings about the Nursing & Midwifery Council', *Midwifery Matters* 123:3 22–3, Accessed 04/12, http://www.midwifery.org.uk/index.php?option=com_content&view=article&id=58:misgivings-about-the-nursing-and-midwifery-council&catid=35:magazine-winter-2009&Itemid=116

Jowitt M and Montagu S (2009) 'HIE or NE? Differential diagnosis implications for maternity care', *Midwifery Matters* 123 20–2, Accessed 04/12, http://www.midwifery.org.uk/index.php?option=com_content&view=article&id=273:hie-or-ne&catid=99:issue-123-winter-2009& Itemid = 118

Kalra VS, Abel P and Esmail A (2009) 'Developing leadership interventions for Black and minority ethnic staff: A case study of the National Health Service (NHS) in the UK', *Journal of Health Organization and Management* 23:1 103–18

Kargar I (1987) 'Independent Midwives: threat or stimulus?', *Nursing Times* 83: 45, 69

Katbamna S (2000) *'Race' and Childbirth*, Buckingham: Open University Press

Kaufmann T (2004) 'Introducing feminism' in M Stewart (ed) *Pregnancy, Birth, and Maternity Care: Feminist Perspectives*, Edinburgh: Elsevier, 1–8

Keating A and Fleming VEM (2009) 'Midwives' experiences of facilitating normal birth in an obstetric-led unit: a feminist perspective', *Midwifery* 25:5 518–27

Kempe A, Noor-Aldin FA and Theorell AT (2010) 'Women's authority during childbirth and Safe Motherhood in Yemen', *Sexual & Reproductive Healthcare* 1:4 129–34

Kennedy HP (2009) '"Orchestrating normal": The conduct of midwifery in the United States', in RE Davis-Floyd, L Barclay, B-A Daviss and J Tritten (eds) *Birth Models That Work*, Berkeley: University of California Press, pp 415–39

Kennedy HP (2010) 'The problem of normal birth', *Journal of Midwifery & Women's Health* 55:3 199–201

Kennedy P (2010) 'Healthcare reform: Maternity service provision in Ireland', *Health Policy* 97:2–3 145–51

Kennedy P and Murphy-Lawless J (2003) 'The maternity care needs of refugee and asylum seeking women in Ireland', *Feminist Review* No 73, 'Exile and Asylum: Women Seeking Refuge in "Fortress Europe"', pp 39–53

Key E (1999) 'MSLCs – Where are they going now?', *AIMS Journal* 11:1 11

Kincaid JC (1975) *Poverty and Equality in Britain: A Study of Social Security and Taxation*, Harmondworth: Penguin

King H (1983) 'Bound to bleed: Artemis and Greek women' in A Cameron and A Kuhrt (eds) *Images of Women in Antiquity*, London: Croom Helm, pp 109–27

King's College Hospital NHS Foundation (2009) 'Albany Midwifery Practice', 14 December 2009, Accessed 08/12, http://www.kch.nhs.uk/news/media/press-releases/view/7987

King's Fund (2008) 'Safe births: everybody's business – an independent inquiry into the safety of maternity services in England', http://www.kingsfund.org.uk/publications/kings_ fund_publications/safe_births.html

Kirkham M (1999a) 'The culture of midwifery in the National Health Service in England', *Journal of Advanced Nursing* 30:3 732–9

Kirkham M (1999b) 'Exclusion in maternity care: midwives and mothers' in M Purdy and D Banks (eds) *Health and Exclusion: Policy and Practice in Health Provision*, London: Routledge, pp 78–104

Kirkham M (2000a) *Developments in the Supervision of Midwives*, Manchester: Books for Midwives

Kirkham M (2000b) *The Midwife–Mother Relationship*, Basingstoke: Macmillan Press

Kirkham M (2003) *Birth Centres: A Social Model for Maternity Care*, Manchester: Books for Midwives

Kirkham M (2004) *Informed Choice in Maternity Care*, Basingstoke: Palgrave Macmillan

Kirkham M (2010) *The Midwife–Mother Relationship* 2nd edn, London: Palgrave Macmillan

Kirkham M (2011) 'A duty of obedience or a duty of care?' *AIMS Journal* 23:3 13–14, Accessed 08/12, http://www.aims.org.uk/Journal/Vol23No3/dutyOfCare.htm

Kirkman S and Ferguson P (2007) 'Does being a principality with an assembly government help midwives in Wales to be free to practise?' in L Reid (ed) *Midwifery: Freedom to Practise – an International Exploration of Midwifery Practice*, Edinburgh: Churchill Livingstone, pp 100–18

Kishik D (2012) *The Power of Life: Agamben and the Coming Politics*, Stanford (CA): Stanford University Press

Kitzinger C (2005) 'Heteronormativity in action: reproducing the heterosexual nuclear family in after-hours medical calls', *Social Problems* 52:4 477–98

Kitzinger J (1990) 'Strategies of the early childbirth movement: a case study of the National Childbirth Trust', in J Garcia, R Kilpatrick and M Richards (eds) *The Politics of Maternity Care: Services for Childbearing Women in Twentieth-century Britain*, Oxford: Clarendon

Kitzinger S (1972) *Episiotomy: Physical and Emotional Aspects*, London: National Childbirth Trust

Kitzinger S (1987) *Some Women's Experiences of Epidurals: a Descriptive Study*, London: National Childbirth Trust

Kitzinger S (2005) *The Politics of Birth*, Edinburgh: Elsevier

Kitzinger S (2006) 'Birth as rape: there must be an end to "just in case" obstetrics', *British Journal of Midwifery* 14:9 544–5

Klein R (2007) 'Values talk in the (English) NHS', Ch 2 pp 19–28 in Greer SL, Rowland D (eds) *Devolving Policy, Diverging Values? The Values of the United Kingdom's National Health Services*. London: Nuffield Trust

KPMG (2008) 'Independent review of maternity and gynaecology services in the greater Dublin area', Dublin: Health Services Executive (HSE)

Kurinczuk JJ, Barralet JH, Redshaw M and Brocklehurst P (2005) 'Monitoring the incidence of neonatal encephalopathy – what next?', Report to the patient safety Research Programme, Oxford: NPEU

Lampinen R, Vehviläinen-Julkunen K and Kankkunen P (2009) 'A review of pregnancy in women over 35 years of age', *The Open Nursing Journal* 3 33–8

Lancet (1985) 'World Health Organisation: appropriate technology for Birth', *The Lancet* ii: 8452 436–7

Lane SD (2008) *Why are our Babies Dying? Pregnancy, Birth, and Death in America*, Boulder (CO): Paradigm Publishers

Larkin P, Begley C and Devane D (2009) 'Women's experiences of labour and birth: an evolutionary concept analysis', *Midwifery* 25:2 e49–e59

Lavender T (2003) 'NCT Evidence based briefing – use of the partogram in labour', *NCT New Digest*, 24 September, 14–16

Lavender T, Alfirevic Z and Walkinshaw S (1998) 'Partogram action line study: a randomised trial', *British Journal of Obstetrics & Gynaecology* 105 976–80

Leahy M, Löfgren H and De Leeuw E (2011) 'Introduction: consumer groups and the democratisation of health policy' in H Löfgren, M Leahy and E De Leeuw (eds) *Democratizing Health: Consumer Groups in the Policy Process*, Cheltenham: Edward Elgar, ch 1, 1–14

http://books.google.co.uk/books?hl=en&lr=&id=hl0UoO96ESoC&oi=fnd&pg=PR1&
dq=+%22Consumer+Groups+in+the+Policy+Process+%22&ots=gfelqbgtXK&sig=Tqo
eesZHfDxvyjMSALv49x1ap8k#v=onepage&q&f=false

Leap N (1996) 'Caseload practice: a recipe for burnout?', *British Journal of Midwifery* 4:6 329–30

Leap N and Hunter B (1993) *The Midwife's Tale: an Oral History from Handywoman to Professional Midwife*, London: Scarlet Press

Leap N, Sandall J, Buckland S and Huber U (2010) 'Journey to confidence: women's experiences of pain in labour and relational continuity of care', *Journal of Midwifery and Women's Health* 55:3 234–42

Lee ASM and Kirkman M (2008) 'Disciplinary discourses: Rates of cesarean section explained by medicine, midwifery, and feminism', *Health Care For Women International* 29:5 448–67

Lee E, Taylor J and Raitt F (2011) '"It's not me, it's them": how lesbian women make sense of negative experiences of maternity care: a hermeneutic study', *Journal of Advanced Nursing* 67:5 982–90

Leeman L (2005) 'Patient-choice cesarean delivery', *American Family Physician* 72:4 697, 700, 705

Leishman JL (2007) 'Introduction' in JL Leishman and J Moir (eds) *Pre-teen and Teenage Pregnancy: a Twenty-first Century Reality*, Keswick: M&k, ch 1, pp 7–24

Lentin R (2001) 'Responding to the racialisation of Irishness: disavowed multiculturalism and its discontents', *Sociological Research Online* 5:4, Accessed 08/11, http://www.socres online.org.uk/5/4/lentin.html

Levy D (2012) 'Centralising hospitals risks creating enclaves of excellence' *Guardian Letters* Wednesday 25 July 2012, Accessed 10/12, http://www.guardian.co.uk/society/2012/jul/ 25/centralising-hospitals-enclaves-of-excellence

Lewis G (2011a) 'The women who died 2006–2008', ch 1, pp 30–56 in Centre for Maternal and Child Enquiries (CMACE). 'Saving Mothers' Lives: reviewing maternal deaths to make motherhood safer: 2006–08'. The Eighth Report on Confidential Enquiries into Maternal Deaths in the United Kingdom, BJOG 2011; 118 (Suppl 1): 1–203

Lewis G (2011b) 'Deaths apparently unrelated to pregnancy from Coincidental and Late causes including domestic abuse', ch 12 in Centre for Maternal and Child Enquiries (CMACE). 'Saving Mothers' Lives: reviewing maternal deaths to make motherhood safer: 2006–08'. The Eighth Report on Confidential Enquiries into Maternal Deaths in the United Kingdom, BJOG 118 (Suppl 1): 1–203

Lewis G (2011c) Annex 12.1. 'Domestic abuse' in Centre for Maternal and Child Enquiries (CMACE). 'Saving Mothers' Lives: reviewing maternal deaths to make motherhood safer: 2006–08'. The Eighth Report on Confidential Enquiries into Maternal Deaths in the United Kingdom, BJOG 2011; 118 (Suppl 1): 1–203

Lewis G and Macfarlane A (2007) 'Which mothers died, and why', ch 1 in G Lewis (ed) The Confidential Enquiry into Maternal and Child Health (CEMACH). 'Saving Mothers' Lives: reviewing maternal deaths to make motherhood safer – 2003–2005'. The Seventh Report on Confidential Enquiries into Maternal Deaths in the United Kingdom.

Lewis K (2010) 'Editorial: The curate's egg', *British Dental Journal* 209, 151

Leys C and Player S (2011) *The Plot Against the NHS*, Pontypool: Merlin Press

Liebe M and Pollock A (2009) 'The experience of the private finance initiative in the UK's National Health Service', The Centre for International Public Health Policy, University of Edinburgh Update, Accessed 07/11, http://allysonpollock.co.uk/research/CIPHP_ 2009_Liebe_NHSPFI.pdf

Lloyd M (2001) 'The politics of disability and feminism: discord or synthesis?' *Sociology* 35:3 715–28

Locke A and Horton-Salway M (2010) '"Golden age" versus "bad old days": a discursive examination of advice giving in antenatal classes', *Journal of Health Psychology* 15:8 1214–24

Lowis GW and McCaffery PG (1999) 'Sociological factors affecting the medicalization of midwifery' in E van Teijlingen, G Lowis, P McCaffery and M Porter (eds) *Midwifery and the Medicalization of Childbirth: Comparative Perspectives*, New York: Nova Science, pp 5–41

Lukes S (2005) *Power: A Radical View* 2nd edn, Basingstoke: Palgrave Macmillan, Accessed 07/11, http://lib.myilibrary.com.ezproxy.webfeat.lib.ed.ac.uk/Open.aspx?id=85996&loc=&srch=undefined&src=0

Lundberg PC and Gerezgiher A (2008) 'Experiences from pregnancy and childbirth related to female genital mutilation among Eritrean immigrant women in Sweden', *Midwifery* 24 214–25

Lundgren I (2010) 'Swedish women's experiences of doula support during childbirth', *Midwifery* 26:2 173–80

Lundgren I, Karlsdottir SI and Bondas T (2009) 'Long-term memories and experiences of childbirth in a Nordic context: a secondary analysis', *International Journal of Qualitative Studies on Health and Well-being* 4 115–28

Lyons SM, O'Keeffe FM, Clarke AT and Staines A (2008) 'Cultural diversity in the Dublin maternity services: the experiences of maternity service providers when caring for ethnic minority women', *Ethnicity & Health* 13:3 261–76

Macdonald AM (1977) *Chambers Twentieth Century Dictionary*, Edinburgh: W & R Chambers

MacDonald C (2002) 'Relational Professional Autonomy', *Cambridge Quarterly of Healthcare Ethics* 11 282–9 http://myweb.dal.ca/mgoodyea/Documents/Ethics/Relational%20professional%20autonomy%20MacDonald%20Camb%20QHCE%202002%2011(3)%20%20282–9.pdf

MacDonald F (2006) 'Relational group autonomy: ensuring agency and accountability in the group rights paradigm', Annual Meeting of the Canadian Political Science Association http://www.cpsa-acsp.ca/papers-2006/MacDonald.pdf. Accessed 07/12

MacDonald ME and Bourgeault IL (2009) 'The Ontario midwifery model of care' in R Davis Floyd, L Barclay, J Tritten and BA Davis (eds), *Birth Models That Work*, London: University of California Press, ch 3, 89–118

Macfarlane A (2008) 'Reconfiguration of maternity units – what is the evidence?' *Radical Statistics* 96, Accessed 08/12, http://www.radstats.org.uk/no096/Macfarlane96.pdf

Macintyre S and Cunningham-Burley S (1993) 'Teenage pregnancy as a social problem' in A Lawson and DL Rhode (eds) *The Politics of Pregnancy: Adolescent Sexuality and Public Policy*, New Haven: Yale University Press, pp 59–73

Mackenbach JP (2011) 'Can we reduce health inequalities? An analysis of the English strategy (1997–2010)', *Journal of Epidemiology & Community Health*, Accessed 07/11, http://jech.bmj.com/content/early/2011/03/31/jech.2010.128280.full.pdf

MacKenzie Bryers H and van Teijlingen E (2010) 'Risk, theory, social and medical models: A critical analysis of the concept of risk in maternity care', *Midwifery* 26 488–96

Macvarish J (2010) 'Understanding the significance of the teenage mother in contemporary parenting culture', *Sociological Research Online* 15:4 3, Accessed 08/11, http://www.socresonline.org.uk/15/4/3.html

Magpie Trial Collaborative Group (2002) 'Do women with pre-eclampsia, and their babies, benefit from magnesium sulphate? The Magpie Trial: a randomised placebo-controlled trial', *Lancet* 359 1877–90

Mahmud S, Shah NM and Becker S (2012), 'Measurement of women's empowerment in rural Bangladesh', World Development 40:3 610–9 (doi:10.1016/j.worlddev.2011. 08.003) Accessed 12/11

Mahoney SF and Malcoe LH (2005) 'Cesarean delivery in Native American women: are low rates explained by practices common to the Indian Health Service?', *Birth* 32:3 170–8

Mair P (2006) 'Ruling the void? The hollowing of Western democracy', *New Left Review* 42 25–51

MANA (2012) Midwives Alliance of North America, Accessed 06/12, http://mana.org/

Mander R (1986a and b) 'Refresher courses: unfulfilled potential?' *Midwives Chronicle* 99: 1176 4–10 and 99: 1177 39–41

Mander R (1987) 'The employment decisions of newly qualified midwives', Unpublished PhD Thesis, University of Edinburgh

Mander R (1992) 'The control of pain in labour', *Journal of Clinical Nursing* July 1:4 219–23

Mander R (1995) 'The relevance of the Dutch system of maternity care to the United Kingdom', *Journal of Advanced Nursing* 22:6 1023–6

Mander R (1997) 'Choosing the choices in the USA: examples in the maternity area', *Journal of Advanced Nursing* 25:6 1192–7

Mander R (2001) *Supportive Care and Midwifery*, Oxford: Blackwell Science

Mander R (2004) *Men and Maternity*, London: Routledge

Mander R (2005) 'Perceptions of decision-making in relation to maternity care organisation and place of birth in New Zealand and Finland', unpublished Report to British Academy

Mander R (2007) *Caesarean: Just Another Way of Birth?* London: Routledge

Mander R (2008a) 'Baby friendly – mother friendly? Policy issues in breastfeeding promotion', MIDIRS 18:1 104–6 and 108

Mander R (2008b) Guest Editorial: 'Extricating midwifery from the elephant's bed', *International Journal of Nursing Studies* 45:5 649–53

Mander R (2010) Commentary: 'The politics of maternity care and maternal health in China', *Midwifery* 26:6 569–72

Mander R (2011a) 'The partnership model' in R Bryar and M Sinclair (eds) *Theory for Midwifery Practice* 2nd rev edn, Palgrave Macmillan, pp 304–14

Mander R (2011b) 'Commercialisation and entrepreneurialism in maternity services', *Midwifery* 27:4 393–8 http://dx.doi.org/10.1016/j.midw.2011.02.002

Mander R (2011c) MIDIRS Focus: 'Fat as a fatal issue: response to the "epidemic" of obesity among childbearing women', *Essentially MIDIRS* 2:4

Mander R (2011d) '"Saving mothers lives": the reality or the rhetoric?', *MIDIRS* 21:2 254–8

Mander R, Cheung NF, Wang X, Fu W and Zhu J (2010) 'Beginning an action research project to investigate the feasibility of a midwife-led normal birthing unit in China', *Journal of Clinical Nursing* 19:3–4 517–26

Mander R, Murphy-Lawless J and Edwards N (2009) 'Reflecting on good birthing: an innovative approach to culture change (Part 1)', *MIDIRS* 19:4 481–6

Mander R, Murphy-Lawless J and Edwards N (2010) 'Reflecting on good birthing: an innovative approach to culture change (Part 2)', *MIDIRS* 20:1 25–9

Mander R and Page M (2012) 'Midwifery and the LGBT midwife', *Midwifery* 28:1 9–13

Marland H (1993) 'The *"burgerlijke"* midwife: the *stadsvroedvrouw* of eighteenth-century Holland' in *The Art of Midwifery: Early Modern Midwives in Europe*, Wellcome Institute series in the history of medicine, London: Routledge, 192–213

Marland H (1995) 'Questions of competence: the midwife debate in the Netherlands in the early twentieth century', *Medical History* 39: 317–37

Marland H (1996) 'The guardians of normal birth: the debate on the standard and status of the midwife in the Netherlands around 1900' in E Abraham-Van der Mark (ed) *Successful Home Birth and Midwifery: the Dutch Model*, Amsterdam: Het Spinhuis, pp 21–44

Marshall H and Woollett A (2000) 'Fit to reproduce? The regulative role of pregnancy texts', *Feminism & Psychology* 10:3 351–66.

Matthews A and Kelly J (2008) 'Maternity services in Ireland', *AIMS Journal* 20:2, Accessed 05/12, http://www.aims.org.uk/Journal/Vol20No2/maternityServicesIreland.htm

May T (2010) *Contemporary Political Movements and the Thought of Jacques Rancière: Equality in Action*, Edinburgh: Edinburgh University Press

McClure J and Cooper G (2011) 'Anaesthesia', in G Lewis (ed) 'Saving mothers' lives', *BJOG: An International Journal of Obstetrics & Gynaecology* 118: s1, Accessed 11/11, http://onlinelibrary.wiley.com/doi/10.1111/j.1471-0528.2010.02847.x/pdf

McCourt C (2005) 'Research and theory for nursing and midwifery: rethinking the nature of evidence', *Worldviews on Evidence-Based Nursing* 2:2 75–83

McCourt C, Rance S, Rayment J and Sandall J (2011) 'Birthplace in England research Programme, Final Report', NIHR Service Delivery and Organisation Programme, Accessed 06/12, https://www.npeu.ox.ac.uk/birthplace

McCourt C and Stevens T (2008) 'Relationship and reciprocity in caseload midwifery', in B Hunter and R Deery (eds) *Emotions in Midwifery and Reproduction*, London: Palgrave

McHugh N (2009) 'The independent midwife' in R Mander and V Fleming (eds) *Becoming a Midwife*, London: Routledge, 154–66

McIntosh C (undated) 'Scottish Independent Midwives', Accessed 03/12, http://www.calumny.demon.co.uk/scotbirth/Individuals/carrie.html

McIntosh J and Tolson D (2009) 'Leadership as part of the nurse consultant role: banging the drum for patient care', *Journal of Clinical Nursing* 18:2 219–27

McIntyre MJ, Chapman Y and Francis K (2011) 'Hidden costs associated with the universal application of risk management in maternity care', *Australian Health Review* 35 211–15

McKendry R and Langford T (2001) 'Legalized, regulated, but unfunded: midwifery's laborious professionalization in Alberta, Canada, 1975–99', *Social Science & Medicine* 53:4 531–42

McLachan HL, Forster DA, Davey MA, Farrell T, Gold L, Biro MA, Albers L, Flood M, Oats J and Waldenström U (2012) 'Effects of continuity of care by a primary midwife (caseload midwifery) on caesarean section rates in women of low obstetric risk: the COSMOS randomised controlled trial', *BCOG*, DOI: 10.1111/j.1471-0528.2012.03446x

McNaughton D (2011) 'From the womb to the tomb: obesity and maternal responsibility', *Critical Public Health* 21:2 179–90

MCNZ (2005) 'Scope of Practice Midwifery Council of New Zealand', Accessed 05/12, http://www.midwiferycouncil.health.nz/midwifery-scope-of-practice/

MCNZ (2012) 'Competencies', Wellington Midwifery Council of New Zealand, Accessed 03/12, http://www.midwiferycouncil.health.nz/images/stories/pdf/competencies%20for%20entry%20to%20the%20register%20of%20midwives%202007.pdf

MCWP (2006) *Modernising Maternity Care: A Commissioning Toolkit for England*, 2nd edn, Maternity Care Working Party, The National Childbirth Trust, The Royal College of Midwives, The Royal College of Obstetricians and Gynaecologists

MCWP (2007) 'Making normal birth a reality', Consensus statement from the Maternity Care Working Party (The Royal College of Midwives, The Royal College of Obstetricians & Gynaecologists, The National Childbirth Trust), Accessed 02/12, http://www.rcog.org.uk.

Mead M (2004) 'Midwives' Practices in 11 UK maternity units' in S Downe (ed) *Normal Childbirth: Evidence and Debate*, Edinburgh: Churchill Livingstone, pp 71–84

Mead M and Newton N (1967) 'Cultural patterning of parental behaviour' in SA Richardson and AF Guttmacher (eds) *Childbearing: Its Social and Psychological Aspects*, Williams & Wilkins, pp 142–245

Mearns L (2009) 'Learning from the "stork nurse"', *The Practising Midwife* 12:8 25

Mcin-Smith P (1986) *Maternity in Dispute 1920–39*, Wellington (NZ.): VR Ward

Messent P (2002) 'Evaluating women's experiences for a MSLC', *British Journal of Midwifery* 10:10 626–30

Mezey GC (1997) 'Perpetrators of domestic violence' in S Bewley, J Friend and G Mezey (eds) *Violence Against Women*, London: RCOG Press, p 35

Milan M (2003) 'Childbirth as healing: three women's experience of independent midwife care', *Complementary Therapies in Nursing and Midwifery* 9:3 140–6

Miller B (1981) *The Endangered Sex: Neglect of Female Children in Northwest India*, Ithaca: Cornell University Press

Mills S, Ryan A, McDowell JP and Burke E (2011) *Disciplinary Procedures in the Statutory Professions*, Dublin: Bloomsbury Professional

Mitchell GJ (1997) 'Questioning evidence-based practice for nursing', *Nursing Science Quarterly* 10 154

Mogford E (2011) 'When status hurts: dimensions of women's status and domestic abuse in rural northern India', *Violence Against Women* 17:7 835–57

Moir DD (1973) *Pain Relief in Labour*, Edinburgh: Churchill Livingstone

Montagu S (2009) 'Torn between hatred and admiration', *Midwifery Matters* 121:22, Accessed 11/11, http://www.proactivesupportoflabor.com/index.php?option=com_fireboard&Itemid=2&func=view&catid=3&id=12

Moorhead J (2012) 'Midwives hope to deliver 1950s values of Call the Midwife in pilot scheme', *Guardian* 21 February 2012, Accessed 08/12, http://www.guardian.co.uk/society/2012/feb/21/midwives-revive-tv-series-values?INTCMP=SRCH

Moran AC, Wahed T and Afsana K (2010) 'Oxytocin to augment labour during home births: an exploratory study in the urban slums of Dhaka, Bangladesh', *BJOG: An International Journal of Obstetrics & Gynaecology* 117:13 1608–15

Morgan BM (1987) 'Mortality and anaesthesia' in BM Morgan (ed) *Foundations of Obstetric Anaesthesia*, London: Farrand Press

Morton A (2011) 'A Single European Market in Healthcare: The impact of European Union policy on national healthcare provision', *European Public Services Briefings* 3 European Services Strategy Unit, Accessed 08/12, http://www.european-services-strategy.org.uk/news/2011/a-single-european-market-in-healthcare/european-healthcare.pdf

Moscucci O (2003) 'History of medicine holistic obstetrics: the origins of "natural childbirth" in Britain', *Postgraduate Medical Journal* 79:168–173 doi:10.1136/pmj.79.929.168

Mossialos E, Allin S, Karras K and Davaki K (2005) 'An investigation of caesarean sections in three Greek hospitals: the impact of financial incentives and convenience', *European Journal of Public Health* 15:3 288–95

Munro J and Spiby H (2010) 'The nature and use of evidence in midwifery' in H Spiby (ed) *Evidence Based Midwifery: Applications in Context*, Chichester: Wiley-Blackwell, 1–16

Murphy MA (2010) 'Medicalization of birth: The social construction of caesarean section. A qualitative analysis', Unpublished PhD Dissertation, University of Michigan

Murphy-Black T (1992) 'Systems of midwifery care in use in Scotland', *Midwifery* 8 113–24

Murphy-Lawless J (1988) 'The silencing of women in childbirth or let's hear it from Bartholomew and the boys', *Women's Studies International Forum* 11:4 293–8

Murphy-Lawless J (2006) 'The language of government: does calling citizens "stakeholders" give them any more power?', *Bulletin of the Food Ethics Council* 3 15

Murphy-Lawless J (2011a) 'Stop Press: news on Ireland's midwifery unit closures', *AIMS Journal* 23:4 7

Murphy-Lawless J (2011b) 'Childbirth adrift in Ireland', *AIMS Journal* 23:3 22–4

Murphy-Lawless J (2011c) '"Ceiling caves in": the current state of maternity services in Ireland', *MIDIRS Midwifery Digest* 21:4 446–51

Murphy-Lawless J (2012) 'Empty promises: the dangers of risk discourses', in H Hayes-Klein (ed) *Conference Papers, Human Rights in Childbirth. International Conference of Jurists, Midwives and Obstetricians*, The Hague, Netherlands: Bynkershoek Publishing, pp 68–73

Mysak ED (1968) *Neuroevolutional Approach to Cerebral Palsy and Speech*, New York: Teachers College Press

Namey EE and Drapkin Lyerly A (2010) 'The meaning of "control" for childbearing women in the US', *Social Science & Medicine* doi:10.1016/j.socscimed.2010.05.024

NCT (1996) *Book of Pregnancy and Birth and Parenthood*, Oxford: Oxford University Press

NDS (2006) *National Disability Survey 2006: First Results*, Dublin: Stationery Office

Neal JL and Lowe NK (2012) 'Physiologic partograph to improve birth safety and outcomes among low-risk, nulliparous women with spontaneous labor onset', *Medical Hypotheses* 78 319–26

Neile E (1997) 'Control for Black and ethnic minority women: a meaningless pursuit' in M Kirkham and ER Perkins (eds) *Reflections on Midwifery*, London: Baillière Tindall, pp 114–34

Nelson-Piercy C, Mackillop L, Williams D and Williamson de Swiet M (2011) 'Maternal mortality in the UK and the need for obstetric physicians', *BMJ* 343:d4993 doi: 10.1136/bmj.d4993

Nevo I and Slonim-Nevo V (2011) 'The myth of evidence-based practice: towards evidence-informed practice', *British Journal of Social Work* 41 1176–97

Newman S and Lawler J (2009) 'Managing health care under New Public Management: a Sisyphean challenge for nursing', *Journal of Sociology* 45:40 419–32

NHS Wales (2006) 'All Wales clinical pathway for normal labour', Accessed 03/12, http://www.wales.nhs.uk/sites3/home.cfm?OrgID=327

Nicoll A (2006) 'Editorial: Definition', *AIMS Journal* 18:3 3

Nicoll A, Hoggins K and Winters P (2005) 'Waterbirth – changing attitudes', *AIMS Journal* 17:4 12–14

NMC (2007) 'The history of self-regulation', Accessed 07/12, http://www.nmc-uk.org/About-us/The-history-of-nursing-and-midwifery-regulation/

NMC (2008) *The Code: Standards of Conduct, Performance and Ethics for Nurses and Midwives*, London: Nursing & Midwifery Council

NMC (2010a) 'The history of nursing and midwifery regulation' Accessed 07/12' http://www.nmc-uk.org/About-us/The-history-of-nursing-and-midwifery-regulation/

NMC (2010b) 'Our strategic vision', Accessed 03/12, http://www.nmc-uk.org/About-us/Our-strategic-vision/

NMC (2010c) 'The code: standards of conduct, performance and ethics for nurses and midwives Nursing & Midwifery Council', Accessed 04/12, http://www.nmc-uk.org/Documents/Standards/The-code-A4-20100406.pdf

NMC (2010d) 'Conditions of practice', Accessed 04/12, http://www.nmc-uk.org/Documents/FTPOutcomes/COPList/20100916.%20Reed.pdf

NMC (2011) *The PREP Handbook*, Accessed 07/12, http://www.nmc-uk.org/Documents/Standards/NMC_Prep-handbook_2011.pdf

NMC (2012) 'Meeting of the Council 26 January 2012', London: Nursing and Midwifery Council, Accessed 04/12, http://www.nmc-uk.org/Documents/CouncilPapersAndDocuments/Council2012/NMC_Open-Council-Papers_26-January-2011.pdf

Nolan M (2007) 'Women supporting midwifery: influence of consumer organisations on best practice' in L Reid (ed) *Midwifery: Freedom to Practise*, London: Routledge, 282–304

Nuffield Trust (2011) 'NHS reforms: survey of public opinion, 9 March 2011. Media Summary: Results from the Ipsos Mori capibus survey', Accessed 08/12, http://www.nuffieldtrust.org.uk/sites/files/nuffield/document/Ipsos-MORI-Media-Briefing-100311.pdf

Nuttall A (2011) Personal communication

Nuttall C (2000) 'Caesarean section controversy. The caesarean culture of Brazil', *BMJ* 320:7241 1074

NZCOM (1990) 'Constitution', Unpublished, Christchurch: New Zealand College of Midwives

NZCOM (2012) 'Philosophy' Accessed 03/12, http://www.midwife.org.nz/index.cfm/1,179,529,0,html/Philosophy

NZLII (1983) 'Nurses Amendment Act 1983 (1983 No 147)' pp 1468–79 New Zealand Legal Information Institute, Accessed 05/12, http://www.nzlii.org/nz/legis/hist_act/naa19831983n147218/

NZLII (1990) 'Nurses Amendment Act 1990 (1990 No 107)' pp 1642–51, Accessed 05/12, http://www.nzlii.org/nz/legis/hist_act/naa19901990n107218/

NZLII (1971) 'Nurses Act' (1971 No 78), pp 1905–51, New Zealand Legal Information Institute, Accessed 05/12, http://www.nzlii.org/nz/legis/hist_act/na19711971n78138/

OAA (2011) Obstetric Anaesthetists' Association, Accessed 10/11, http://www.oaa-anaes.ac.uk/content.asp?ContentID=1

OALD (2011) *Oxford Advanced Learner's Dictionary*, Accessed 07/11, http://www.oxfordadvancedlearnersdictionary.com/dictionary/politics

Odent M (2003) *Birth and Breastfeeding: Rediscovering the Needs of Women During Pregnancy and Childbirth*, East Sussex: Clairview

O'Driscoll K, Jackson RJ and Gallagher JT (1969) 'Prevention of prolonged labour', *British Medical Journal* 2:477

O'Driscoll K and Meagher D (1980) *Active Management of Labour*, London: Saunders

O'Driscoll K, Meagher D and Boylan P (1993) *Active Management of Labour: The Dublin Experience*, 3rd edn, London: Mosby

O'Driscoll K, Stronge JM and Minogue M (1973) 'Active management of labour', *British Medical Journal* 3:135

OECD (2009) 'OECD StatExtracts', Accessed 10/11, http://stats.oecd.org/index.aspx?DataSetCode=HEALTH_STAT

Office of National Statistics (2010) 'Indices of deprivation 2010: Local Authority Summaries: Salford', Accessed 08/12, http://www.neighbourhood.statistics.gov.uk/

Ogunlesi TA, Dedeke OO, Okeniyi JAO and Oyedeji GA (2005) 'Infant and Toddler feeding practices in the Baby Friendly Initiative (BFI) era in Ilesa, Nigeria', *The Internet Journal of Nutrition and Wellness* 1:2

Ohaja M (2012) 'Contestations around safe motherhood and safe motherhood initiatives', *Essentially MIDIRS* 3:6 32–6

Ojanuga DN and Gilbert C (1992) 'Women's access to health care in developing countries', *Social Science & Medicine* 35:4 613–17

Olsen O and Jewell D (1998) 'Home versus hospital birth', Cochrane Database of Systematic Reviews, Issue 3, Art No CD000352. DOI: 10.1002/14651858.CD000352.

Orange C (1984) 'The treaty of Waitangi: a study of its making, interpretation and role in New Zealand history', Unpublished PhD Thesis, University of Auckland

O'Toole CJ (2002) 'Sex, disability and motherhood: access to sexuality for disabled mothers', *Disability Studies Quarterly* 22:4 81–101

Ozturk K (2004) 'Woman-centred care: how far have we come?', Paper presented at NZCOM Conference.

Ozturk KJL (2010) 'Becoming a homebirther ... smooth sailing or rocky road? An exploration of Pakeha women's experiences on the path to homebirth', Unpublished Master of Midwifery Thesis, Victoria: University of Wellington

Paech MJ (1999) 'A survey of parturients using epidural analgesia during labour. Considerations relevant to antenatal educators', *Australian & New Zealand Journal of Obstetrics and Gynaecology* 39:1 21–5

Page L (1996) 'The backlash against evidence-based care', *Birth* 23:4 191–2

Page M (2010) 'Embracing uncertainty: supporting normal birth', Unpublished PhD Thesis, Queen Margaret University

Page M (2012) Personal communication

Pairman S (1999) 'Partnership revisited: towards midwifery theory', *New Zealand College of Midwives Journal* 21 6–12.

Pairman S (2000) 'Woman-centred midwifery: partnerships or professional friendships?' in M Kirkham (ed) *The Midwife–Mother Relationship*, Basingstoke: Macmillan Press, pp 207–26

Pairman S (2006) 'Midwifery partnership: working "with" women' in LA Page and R McCandlish *The New Midwifery: Science and Sensitivity in Practice*, Edinburgh: Churchill Livingstone, pp 73–96

Palmer G (1993) *The Politics of Breastfeeding*, London: Pandora Press

Pardy M (1995) *Speaking of Speaking. Experiences of Women and Interpreting*, Collingwood UK: Clearing House for Migration Issues

Parekh B (2002) 'Foreword' in L Platt (2002) *Parallel Lives? Poverty Among Ethnic Minority Groups in Britain*, London: Child Poverty Action Group

Paterson S (2010) 'Feminizing obstetrics or medicalizing midwifery? The discursive constitution of midwifery in Ontario, Canada', *Critical Policy Studies* 4:2 127–45

Pearce DM (1993) 'Children having children' in A Lawson and DL Rhode (eds) *The Politics of Pregnancy: Adolescent Sexuality and Public Policy*, New Haven: Yale University Press, ch 2, pp 46–58

Pedersen KM (2002) 'The World Health Report 2000: dialogue of the deaf?', *Health Economics* 11:2 93–101

Pembroke NF and Pembroke JJ (2008) 'The spirituality of presence in midwifery care', *Midwifery* 24 321–7

Peng YS (2010) 'When formal laws and informal norms collide: lineage networks versus birth control policy in China', *American Journal of Sociology* 116:3 770–805,

Percival R (1970) 'The management of normal labour', *The Practitioner* 204:221 357–65.

Perkins BB (2003) *The Delivery Business: Health Reform, Childbirth, and the Economic Order*, New Brunswick NJ: Rutgers University Press

Peters BG (1982) 'Insiders and outsiders: the politics of pressure group influences on bureaucracy' in G McGrew and MJ Wilson (eds) *Decision Making: Approaches and Analysis*, Manchester: Manchester University Press, section 4.5 261–74

Peterson WE, Medves JM, Davies BL and Graham ID (2007) 'Collaborative maternity care in Canada: easier said than done', *Journal of Obstetrics & Gynaecology of Canada* 11 880–6

Philby C (2011) 'Who would be a midwife?', London: *Independent*, Saturday 26 November, Accessed 11/11, http://www.independent.co.uk/life-style/health-and-families/features/whod-be-a-midwife-6267307.html

Phillips M (2009) 'Woman centred care? An exploration of professional care in midwifery practice', Unpublished PhD thesis, University of Huddersfield, Accessed 03/12, http://eprints.hud.ac.uk/5764/1/PhD_THESIS_MARCH_2009.pdf

Philpott RH (1972) 'Graphic records in labour', *BMJ* 4:833 163–5

Phipps B (2010) 'The NCT view on the termination of the Albany Midwifery Practice contract', *The Practising Midwife* 13:8 34–5

Pieters A, van Oirschot C and Akkermans H (2010) 'No cure for all evils: Dutch obstetric care and limits to the applicability of the focused factory concept in health care', *International Journal of Operations & Production Management* 30:11 1112–39 http://dx.doi.org/10.1108/01443571011087350

Pievatolo MC (2005) 'Publicness and private intellectual property in Kant's political thought, 2008', in 10th International Kant Congress, São Paulo (Brasil), 4–9 September 2005, De Gruyter, pp.631–41, Accessed 08/12, http://eprints.rclis.org/handle/10760/13690?mode=full&submit_simple = Show+full+item+record

Pitt S (1997) 'Midwifery and medicine: gendered knowledge in the practice of delivery' in H Marland and AM Rafferty (eds) *Midwives, Society and Childbirth: Debates and Controversies in the Modern Period*, London: Routledge. 218–31

Plaat F and Wray S (2008) 'Role of the anaesthetist in obstetric critical care', *Best Practice & Research Clinical Obstetrics and Gynaecology* 22:5 917–35

Pollock A (2004) *NHS plc: The Privatising of our Health Care*, London: Verso

Pollock A (2012) 'It's a scandal that big hospital contracts are being awarded in private', Comment is Free, *Guardian* Friday 4 May 2012, Accessed 08/12, http://www.guardian.co.uk/commentisfree/2012/may/04/scandal-hospital-contracts-in-private

Pollock A and Price D (2000) 'Globalisation? Privatisation!', *Health Matters* 41: Summer 12–13

Pollock A, Price D, Roderick P, Treuherz T, McCoy D, McKee M and Reynolds L (2012) 'How the Health and Social Care Bill 2011 would end entitlement to comprehensive health care in England', *The Lancet* 379 387–89

Porter S, Crozier K, Sinclair M and Kernohan WG (2007) 'New midwifery? A qualitative analysis of midwives' decision-making strategies', *Journal of Advanced Nursing* 60:5 525–34

Pratten B (1990) *Power, Politics and Pregnancy*, London: Health Rights

Puthussery S, Twamley K, Harding S, Mirsky J, Baron M and Macfarlane A (2008) '"They're more like ordinary stroppy British women": attitudes and expectations of maternity care professionals to UK-born ethnic minority women', *Journal of Health Services Research and Policy* 13:4 195–201

Puthussery S, Twamley K, Macfarlane A, Harding S and Baron M (2010) '"You need that loving tender care": maternity care experiences and expectations of ethnic minority women born in the United Kingdom', *Journal of Health Services Research and Policy* 15:3 156–201

Qiu L, Lin J and Ma Y et al (2010) 'Improving the maternal mortality ratio in Zhejiang Province, China, 1988–2008', *Midwifery* 26 544–8

Raleigh VS Hussey D, Seccombe I and Hallt K (2010) 'Ethnic and social inequalities in women's experience of maternity care in England: results of a national survey', *Journal of the Royal Society of Medicine* 103:5 188–98

Ram K (2009) 'Rural midwives in South India: the politics of bodily knowledge' in *Science Across Cultures: the History of Non-Western Science* Vol 5, London, pp 107–22

Rancière J (1999) *Dis-agreement, Politics and Philosophy*, Minneapolis (MN): University of Minnesota Press

Rancière J (2007) *On the Shores of Politics*, London: Verso

Raynor MD and Morgan R (2000) 'Female genital mutilation unveiled and reconstructed' in D Fraser (ed) *Professional Studies for Midwifery Practice*, London: Elsevier, pp 45–62

Raynor MD, Marshall JE and Sullivan A (2005) *Decision Making in Midwifery Practice*, Edinburgh: Churchill Livingstone

RCM (1986) *Comments by the Royal College of Midwives on UKCC Project 2000: A New Preparation for Practice*, London: Royal College of Midwives

RCM (2000) 'Racism and the maternity services', Position Paper No 23, London: Royal College of Midwives, Accessed 07/11, www.rcm.org.uk/EasySiteWeb/GatewayLink. aspx?alId=12791

RCM (2009) *Annual Staffing Survey*, London: Royal College of Midwives

RCOG (2009) 'RCOG statement on the Saving Babies' Lives Report', Accessed 08/12, http://www.rcog.org.uk/what-we-do/campaigning-and-opinions/statement/rcog-statement-saving-babies-lives-report

Read JS and Newell ML (2005) 'Efficacy and safety of cesarean delivery for prevention of mother-to-child transmission of HIV-1', Cochrane Database of Systematic Reviews, Issue 4, Art No CD005479. DOI: 10.1002/14651858.CD005479.

Reed B (2008) 'An unplanned hospital birth', *The Practising Midwife* 11:11 24–5

Reed B (2007) 'Ten years, seven brothers and sisters', *The Practising Midwife* 10:7 31–3

Reed B (2010) 'Choices are not choices if you are not allowed to make them for yourself', *The Practising Midwife* 13:1 4–5

Reed B and Walton C (2009) 'The Albany Midwifery Practice' in R Davis-Floyd, L Barclay, J Tritten and BA Daviss (eds) *Birth Models That Work*, London: University of California Press, pp 141–58

Reid L (2011a) Personal communication, 18 July

Reid L (2011b) *Midwifery in Scotland: A History*, Erskine: Scottish History Press

Reiger K (1999) '"Sort of part of the women's movement. but different": Mothers' organisations and Australian feminism', *Women's Studies International Forum* 22:6 585–95

Reilly C (2011) '"They told me she was exaggerating – now she's gone" Rotunda neglected care of Bimbo Onanuga says partner', *Metro Éireann* 1–14 June, Accessed 08/11, http://www.metroeireann.com/article/they-told-me-she-was-exaggerating,2747

Reilly J (2011) 'Written answers – medical investigations', Dáil Éireann Debate Vol 733 No 3, Unrevised, Thursday 26 May, http://debates.oireachtas.ie/dail/2011/05/26/00094. asp Accessed 08/11

Relyea MJ (1992) 'The rebirth of midwifery in Canada: an historical perspective', *Midwifery* 8:4 159–69

Rennie AM, Gibb S, Hourston A, Bedford H and McNicol J (2009) 'The development of maternity care assistants in Scotland', *The Practising Midwife* 12:8 14, 16–19.

Reuwer P, Bruinse H and Franx A (2009) *Proactive Support of Labour*, Cambridge: Cambridge University Press

Reynolds B and White J (2010) 'Seeking asylum and motherhood: health and wellbeing needs', *Community Practitioner* 83:3 20–3

Rich A (1977) 'Of woman born: motherhood as experience and institution', London: Virago

Rich RF (1999/2000) 'Health policy, health insurance and the social contract', *Comparative Labor Law and Policy Journal* 21:2 397–422

Rising S and Lindell S (1982) 'The childbearing childrearing center: a nursing model', *Nursing Clinics of North America* 17 11–22

Robinson S (1990) 'Maintaining the independence of the midwifery profession: a continuing struggle' in J Garcia, R Kilpatrick and M Richards (eds) *The politics of maternity care: services for childbearing women in twentieth-century Britain*, Oxford: Clarendon, ch 4, pp 61–91

Roch S (1994) 'Independent midwives: why don't we give them more support?', 107 1278 247

Rodgers C (1999) 'The trial of Caroline Flint', *AIMS Journal* 11:2 8–9

Rogers J and Cunningham S (2007) 'A consultant midwives' clinic: a catalyst for change?', *MIDIRS Midwifery Digest* 17:2 201–6

Rogers J and Weavers A (2005) 'Consultant midwives: the next generation!', *Midwives* 8:4 172–3

Rooks JP (2007) 'Relationships between CNMs and CMs and other midwives, nurses, and physicians' in L Ament (ed) *Professional Issues in Midwifery*, Burlington (MA): Jones & Bartlett, pp 1–40, http://www.jblearning.com/samples/0763728365/Professional_ Issues_in_Midwifery_Ch1.pdf

Rose N (1998) 'Governing risky individuals: the role of psychiatry in new regimes of control', *Psychiatry, Psychology and Law* 5:2 177–95

Rose P (1993) 'Out in the open? How do nurses treat their patients and colleagues who are lesbians?', *Nursing Times* 89:30 50–2

Rosser J (2003) 'How do the Albany midwives do it? Evaluation of the Albany Midwifery Practice', *MIDIRS Midwifery Digest* 13:2 251–7

Rosser J (1994) 'World Health Organisation Partograph in management of labour', *MIDIRS Midwifery Digest* 4:4 436–7

Rothwell H (1996) 'Changing childbirth changing nothing', *Midwives* 109:1306 291–4

Rotter JB (1966) 'The Rotter internal-external locus of control', *Psychological Monographs* 80 609

Royal Commission on the NHS (1979) *BMJ Supplement*, 28 July, 284–7, 290–1

Rozario S (1992) *Purity and Communal Boundaries: Women and Social Change in a Bangladeshi Village*, London: Zed Books

Rundall P (1996) 'The commercial pressures against baby friendliness' in SF Murray (ed) *Baby Friendly Mother Friendly*, London: Mosby, pp 61–76

Rushwan H (2000) 'Female genital mutilation – FGM management during pregnancy, childbirth and the postpartum period', *International Journal of Gynecology & Obstetrics* 70 99–104

Sabarwal S (2007) 'Mother's education and female child survival: An empirical study from India', http://www.cid.harvard.edu/neudc07/docs/neudc07_s5_p06_sabarwal.pdf Accessed 01/12

Sackett DL, Rosenburg WMC, Gray JAM, Haynes RB and Richardson WS (1996) Editorial: 'Evidence based medicine: what it is and what it isn't', *British Medical Journal* 312:7023 71–2

Salford City Council (2008) Draft Obesity Strategy, services.salford.gov.uk/./SALFORD% 20OBESITY%20STRATEGY. Pdf.

Salford Star (2010) 'Salford baby unit reprieve: there's still hope!!!!', 1 December, Accessed 08/12, http://www.salfordstar.com/article.asp?id=78

Salvage J (1985) *The Politics of Nursing*, London: Butterworth-Heinemann

Sandall J (1995) 'Choice, continuity and control: changing midwifery, towards a sociological perspective', *Midwifery* 11 201–09

Sandall J (1996) 'Continuity of midwifery care in England: a new professional project?', *Gender, Work & Organization* 3:4 215–26

Sandall J, Davies J and Warwick C (2001) 'Evaluation of the Albany Midwifery Practice Final Report', King's College, London, Accessed 04/12, http://openaccess.city.ac.uk/ 599/2/albany_final_rpt.pdf

Sandall J, Morton C and Bick D (2010) 'Safety in childbirth and the three 'C's: Community, context and culture', *Midwifery* 26:5 481–2

Saunders TA, Stein DJ and Dilger JP (2006) 'Informed consent for labor epidurals: a survey of Society for Obstetric Anesthesia and Perinatology anesthesiologists from the United States', *International Journal of Obstetric Anesthesia* 15:2 98–103

Savage W (1986) *A Savage Enquiry: Who Controls Childbirth?* London: Virago

Savage W (1990) 'How obstetrics might change: Wendy Savage talks to Robert Kilpatrick' in J Garcia, R Kilpatrick and M Richards (eds) *The Politics of Maternity Care: Services for Childbearing Women in Twentieth-century Britain*, Oxford: Clarendon

Savage W (2007) *Birth and Power: A Savage Enquiry Revisited*, London: Middlesex University Press

Sawyer A-M, Green D, Moran A and Brett Judith (2009) 'Should the nurse change the light globe? Human service professionals managing risk on the frontline', *Journal of Sociology* 45:4 361–81

Scamell M and Alaszewski A (2012) 'Fateful moments and the categorisation of risk: midwifery practice and the ever-narrowing window of normality during childbirth', *Health, Risk and Society* 14:2 207–21

Scarry E (1985) *The Body in Pain: The Making and Unmaking of the World*, New York: Oxford University Press

Schindler RS and Jolivet R (2009) 'Circles of community: the CenteringPregnancy® Group Prenatal Care Model' in RE Davis-Floyd, L Barclay, B-A Daviss and J Tritten (eds) *Birth Models That Work*, Berkeley: University of California Press, pp 365–84

Schindler Rising S and Kennedy HP (2004) 'Redesigning prenatal care through CenteringPregnancy', *Journal of Midwifery & Women's Health* 49:5 398–404

Schmied VA, Duff M and Dahlen HG (2011) '"Not waving but drowning": a study of the experiences and concerns of midwives and other health professionals caring for obese childbearing women', *Midwifery* 27: 4 424–30

Schuler SR, Lenzi R and Yount KM (2011) 'Justification of intimate partner violence in rural Bangladesh: what survey questions fail to capture', *Studies in Family Planning* 42:1 21–8

Scottish Government (2009) 'Keeping Childbirth Natural and Dynamic Programme (KCND)', Accessed 03/12, http://www.scotland.gov.uk/Topics/Health/NHS-Scotland/nursing/naturalchildbirth

Scourfield P (2007) 'Client consumer or patient or partner social care and the modern citizen: client, consumer, service user, manager and entrepreneur', *British Journal of Social Work* 37:1 107–22.

Searle GR (1971) *The Quest for National Efficiency: A Study in British Politics and Political Thought, 1899–1914*, Oxford: Blackwell Press

Searle GR (2004) *A New England?: Peace and War, 1886–1918*, Oxford: Oxford University Press

SEHD (2001) 'Patient focus public involvement', Scottish Executive Health Department, Accessed 07/11, www.scotland.gov.uk/library3/health/pfpi-00.asp

Select Committee on Health (2003) 'Written Evidence Appendix 40 Evidence by the Southampton University Hospitals NHS Trust (MS 49) 5.3', Accessed 11/11, http://www.publications.parliament.uk/pa/cm200203/cmselect/cmhealth/464/464w41.htm

Sen A (2003) 'Missing women – revisited: Reduction in female mortality has been counter-balanced by sex selective abortions', *BMJ* 327: 507–8 6 December 1297–8

Sen A (1992) 'Missing women', *BMJ* 304 7 March

Sennett R (2008) *The Craftsman*, London: Allen Lane

SEU (1999) 'Teenage pregnancy', Social Exclusion Unit, Cabinet Office (CM 4342)

Shallow H (2003) 'The birth centre project' in M Kirkham (ed) *Birth Centres: A Social Model for Maternity Care*, Manchester: Books for Midwives

Sharma SK, Sawangdee Y and Sirirassamee B (2007) 'Access to health: women's status and utilization of maternal health services in Nepal', *Journal of Biosocial Science* 39:05 671–92

Shaw M, Smith GD and Dorling D (2005) 'Health inequalities and New Labour: how the promises compare with real progress', *BMJ* 330 1016–21

Shell-Duncan B, Wander K, Hernlund Y and Moreau A (2011) 'Dynamics of change in the practice of female genital cutting in Senegambia: testing predictions of social convention theory', *Social Science & Medicine* 73 1275–83

Shorter E (1983) *A History of Women's Bodies*, London: Allen Lane

Sibley LM, Sipe TA, Brown CM, Diallo MM, McNatt K and Habarta N (2007) 'Traditional birth attendant training for improving health behaviours and pregnancy outcomes', Cochrane Database of Systematic Reviews, Issue 3, Art No CD005460. DOI: 10.1002/14651858.CD005460.pub2.

Sidebotham M (2001) 'The consultant midwife role: will it make a difference?', *RCM Midwives Journal* 4:1 20–1

Siggins L (2011) 'Call for full reconfiguration of maternity services', *The Irish Times* Tuesday 6 December

Silverton L (1993) 'The elderly primigravida' in J Alexander, V Levy and S Roch *Midwifery Practice: A Research-based Approach*, London: Macmillan

Singer R (2012) 'Doctors are once again striking for more than themselves', *Guardian*, Monday 4 June, Accessed 08/12, http://www.guardian.co.uk/commentisfree/2012/jun/04/doctors-striking-nhs-industrial-action

Skinner J (1999) 'Midwifery partnership: individualism, contractualism or feminist praxis?', *New Zealand College of Midwives Journal* 21 14–17

Skinner J (2008) Editorial: 'Risk: Let's look at the bigger picture', *Women and Birth* 21 53–4

Skinner JP (2005) 'Risk and the midwife: A descriptive and interpretive examination of the referral for obstetric consultation practices and attitudes of New Zealand midwives', unpublished PhD thesis, Victoria: University of Wellington

Sleep J, Grant A, Garcia J, Elbourne D, Spencer J and Chalmers I (1984) 'West Berkshire perineal management trial', *BMJ* (Clin Res Ed). 289:6445 587–90.

Smith K (2005) 'Consuming passion: life as an MSLC rep', *The Practising Midwife* 8:8 40–1

Snowden A, Martin C, Jomeen J and Martin C (2011) 'Concurrent analysis of choice and control in childbirth', *BMC Pregnancy & Childbirth* 11:1

SOGC (2008) 'The Society of Obstetricians and Gynaecologists of Canada Joint Policy Statement on Normal Childbirth', *Journal of Obstetrics & Gynaecology of Canada* 221:1163–5

Sosa R, Kennell J, Klaus M, Robertson S and Urrutia J (1980) 'The effect of a supportive companion on perinatal problems, length of labor, and mother-infant interaction', *New England Journal of Medicine* 303:597–600

Spidsberg BD (2007) 'Vulnerable and strong – lesbian women encountering maternity care', *Journal of Advanced Nursing* 60:5 478–86

Spidsberg BD and Sørlie V (2011) 'An expression of love – midwives' experiences in the encounter with lesbian women and their partners', *Journal of Advanced Nursing* doi: 10.1111/j.1365-2648.2011.05780.x

Stacey M (2007) 'General anaesthesia and failure to ventilate' in D Dob G Cooper and A Holdcroft (eds) *Crises in Childbirth – Why Mothers Survive*, Milton Keynes: Radcliffe Publishing, pp 19–46

Stahl K and Hundley V (2003) 'Risk and risk assessment in pregnancy – do we scare because we care?', *Midwifery* 19 298–309

Stapleton H, Duerden J and Kirkham M (1998) *Evaluation of the Impact of the Supervision of Midwives on Professional Practice and the Quality of Midwifery Care*, London: English National Board for Nursing, Midwifery and Health Visiting

Stark E, Flitcraft A, Zuckerman D, Grey A, Robison J and Frazier W (1981) *Wife Abuse in the Medical Setting*, Domestic Violence Monograph Series 7 7–41

Steen M (2012) *Supporting Women to Give Birth at Home: A Practical Gguide for Midwives*, Abingdon: Routledge

Stephens L (2004) 'Pregnancy' in M Stewart (ed) *Pregnancy, Birth, and Maternity Care: Feminist Perspectives*, Edinburgh: Elsevier, pp 41–53

Stevens J, Dahlen H, Peters K and Jackson D (2011) 'Midwives' and doulas' perspectives of the role of the doula in Australia: A qualitative study', *Midwifery* 27:4 509–16

Stewart M (2004) 'Feminisms and the body' in M Stewart (ed) *Pregnancy, Birth, and Maternity Care: Feminist Perspectives*, Edinburgh: Elsevier, pp 25–38

Stockton A (2010a) *Gentle Birth Companions: Doulas Serving Humanity*, Dumfries: McCubbington Press

Stockton A (2010b) 'Mother's mouthpiece or clinician's curse: the doula debate continues', *MIDIRS Midwifery Digest* 20:1 57–8.

Stockton A (2012) 'NHS doulas' *AIMS Journal* 24:2 16–17

Strategic Review of Health Inequalities (2010) 'Fair society, healthy lives', *The Marmot Review*, Accessed 08/12, http://www.instituteofhealthequity.org/projects/fair-society-healthy-lives-the-marmot-review

Strong P and Robinson J (1990) *The NHS Under New Management*, Milton Keynes: Open University Press

Svensson J, Barclay L and Cooke M (2007) 'Antenatal education as perceived by health professionals', *Journal of Perinatal Education* 16:1 9–15

Symon A (2011) 'The Irish Nurses and Midwives Bill: legal changes and challenges', *British Journal of Midwifery* 19:3 193–4, http://www.nurse2nurse.ie/Upload/NA6912nurses%20and%20midwives%20bills.pdf

Symon A, Winter C, Donnan PT and Kirkham M (2010) 'Examining autonomy's boundaries: a follow-up review of perinatal mortality cases in UK independent midwifery', *Birth* 37:4 280–7

Symon A, Winter C, Inkster M and Donnan PT (2009) 'Outcomes for births booked under an independent midwife and births in NHS maternity units: matched comparison study', *BMJ* 338: Epub 2009 June 11.

Teakle B (2004) 'Don't blame women for the caesarean epidemic', *Birth Matters – Journal of the Maternity Coalition Inc.* 8:3 15.

Teate A, Leap N, Schindler Rising S and Homer CSE (2011) 'Women's experiences of group antenatal care in Australia – the CenteringPregnancy Pilot Study', *Midwifery* 27:2 138–46

Thachuk A (2007) 'Midwifery, informed choice, and reproductive autonomy: a relational approach', *Feminism & Psychology* 17:1 39–56, http://fap.sagepub.com/content/17/1/39.full.pdf+html

Thane P (1978) 'Introduction' in P Thane (ed) *The Origins of British Social Policy*, London: Croom Helm

Thomson A (1986) 'Patienthood and childbirth', *Midwifery* 2:4 163

Thomson G, Bilson A and Dykes F (2011) 'Implementing the WHO/UNICEF Baby Friendly Initiative in the community: a "hearts and minds approach"', *Midwifery* doi:10.1016/j.midw.2011.03.003

Thynne I (2006) 'Statutory bodies: how distinctive and in what ways?', *Public Organization Review* 6:3 171–84

Tian L, Li J, Zhang A and Guest P (2007) 'Women's status, institutional barriers and reproductive health care: A case study in Yunnan, China', *Health Policy* 84:2–3 284–97

Titmuss R (2001) 'The welfare state: images and realities' in P Alcock, H Glennerster, A Oakley and A Sinfield (eds) *Welfare and Wellbeing: Richard Titmuss's Contribution to Social Policy*, Bristol: The Policy Press

Traynor M (2002) 'The oil crisis, risk and evidence-based practice', *Nursing Inquiry* 9:3 162–9

Twamley K, Puthussery S, Macfarlane A, Harding S, Ahmed S and Mirsky J (2009) 'Recruiting UK-born ethnic minority women for qualitative health research – lessons learned from a study of maternity care', *Research, Policy and Planning* 27:1 25–38

UK Parliament (2010) 'Equality Act c 15', Accessed 08/11, http://www.legislation.gov.uk/ukpga/2010/15/contents

UN (2000) 'Millenium (sic) Declaration: Millennium Summit of the United Nations', New York: United Nations, Accessed 10/11, http://www.un.org/en/development/devagenda/millennium.shtml

UN (2011) 'World Population Prospects, the 2010 Revision' http://esa.un.org/unpd/wpp/Excel-Data/DB01_Period_Indicators/WPP2010_DB1_F03_CRUDE_BIRTH_RATE.XLS Accessed 01/13

UNICEF (2011) 'The baby friendly hospital initiative', Accessed 07/11, http://www.unicef.org/programme/breastfeeding/baby.htm

UNICEF (2012) 'The baby friendly initiative', Accessed 01/12, http://www.unicef.org.uk/babyfriendly/

Universities Scotland (2010) 'Race equality toolkit', Accessed 07/11, http://www.universities-scotland.ac.uk/raceequalitytoolkit/terminology.htm

Van de Bovenkamp HM and Trappenburg MJ (2010) 'Government influence on patient organizations', *Health Care Analysis* DOI 10.1007/s10728-010-0155-7 Accessed 07/11

van Teijlingen E (2005) 'A critical analysis of the medical model as used in the study of pregnancy and childbirth', *Sociological Research Online* 10:2, Accessed 11/11, <http://www.socresonline.org.uk/10/2/teijlingen.html>

van Teijlingen E and Hulst L (1994) 'Midwifery in the Netherlands: more than a semi-profession?' in T Johnson, G Larkin and M Saks (eds) *Health Professions and the State in Europe*, London: Routledge, p 109

van Teijlingen ER (1990) 'The profession of maternity home care assistant and its significance for the Dutch midwifery profession', *International Journal of Nursing Studies* 27:4 355–66

van Teijlingen ER (1994) 'Dutch model of maternity care may not suit Britain', *BMJ* 29: 308(6924) 342.

Varney Burst H (1983) 'The influence of consumers in the birthing movement', *Topics in Clinical Nursing* 5 42–54

VIL (1999) 'Verloskundig Vademecum Amstelveen Ziekenfondsraad', Accessed 05/12, http://europe.obgyn.net/nederland/?page=/nederland/richtlijnen/vademecum_eng_statement#Joint%20Statement

Villar J, Valladares E, Wojdyla D and Zavaleta N (2006) 'Caesarean delivery rates and pregnancy outcomes: the 2005 WHO global survey on maternal and perinatal health in Latin America', *The Lancet* 367: 1819–29

Visser R (2012) Birth: A Human Rights Issue? Human Rights in Childbirth Conference, The Hague: International Conference of Jurists, Midwives and Obstetricians, pp 143–5

Wackerhausen S (1999) 'What is natural? Deciding what to do and not to do in medicine and health care', *British Journal of Obstetrics & Gynaecology* 106:11 1109–12

Wade L (2011) 'Separating the heat from the light: lessons from 30 years of academic discourse about female genital cutting', *Ethnicities*, Accessed 12/11, DOI: 10.1177/1468796811419603 http://etn.sagepub.com/content/early/2011/09/19/1468796811419603

Wagner M (1994) *Pursuing the Birth Machine: The Search for Appropriate Birth Technology*, Camperdown (AU): ACE Graphics

Wagner M (1995) 'A global witch-hunt', *The Lancet* 346:8981 1020–2

Wagner M (2000) 'Choosing caesarean section', *The Lancet* 356:9242 1677–80

Wagner M (2001) 'Fish can't see water: the need to humanize birth', *International Journal of Gynecology & Obstetrics* 75 S25–S37

Wagner M (2002) 'Critique of the British RCOG National Sentinel Caesarean, Section Audit report of October 2001', *MIDIRS Midwifery Digest* 12:3 366–70

Wagner M (2006) *Born in the USA: How a Broken Maternity System Must be Fixed to Put Women and Children First*, Berkeley: University of California Press

Wagner M (2007) 'Birth and power' in W Savage (ed) *Birth and Power: A Savage Enquiry Revisited*, Middlesex: University Press London, Section 1 pp 35–44

Wahn EH, Nissen E and Ahlberg BM (2005) 'Becoming and being a teenage mother: how teenage girls in south western Sweden view their situation', *Health Care for Women International* 26:7 591–603,

Wainwright H and Little M (2009) *Public Service Reform ... But Not as We Know It!* Hove, Sussex: Picnic Publishing

Waldenström U (2007) 'Normal childbirth and evidence based practice', *Women and Birth* 20 175–80

Walker P (2002) 'Understanding accountability: theoretical models and their implications for social service organisations', *Social Policy & Administration* 36:1 62–75

Wall S (2008) 'A critique of evidence-based practice in nursing: challenging the assumptions', *Social Theory & Health* 6 37–53

Walsh D (2004) 'Feminism and intrapartum care: a quest for holistic birth' in M Stewart (ed) *Pregnancy, Birth, and Maternity Care: Feminist Perspectives*, Edinburgh: Elsevier, pp 57–67

Walsh D (2011) 'Nesting and Matrescence' in R Bryar and M Sinclair (eds) *Theory for Midwifery Practice*, Basingstoke: Palgrave Macmillan, pp 178–96

Walsh D and Devane D (2012) 'A metasynthesis of midwife-led care' Qualitative Health Research, Accessed 05/12, http://qhr.sagepub.com/content/early/2012/03/14/10497323 12440330

Walsh D and Downe S (2004) 'Outcomes of free-standing, midwifery-led birth centres: a structured review of the evidence', *Birth* 31:3 222–29

Walsh DJ (2010) Review article 'Childbirth embodiment: problematic aspects of current understandings', *Sociology of Health & Illness* 32:3 486–501.

Walt G (1998) 'Globalisation of international health', *The Lancet* 351:9100 434–7

Warren C (1994) 'Insurance – Why single out the independent midwife?', *Modern Midwife* 4:4 32–3

Warren KJ (1987) 'Feminism and ecology: making connections', *Environmental Ethics* 9:1 3–20

Warren KJ (1994) *Ecological Feminism*, Routledge: London

Wasserheit JN (1989) 'The significance and scope of reproductive tract infections among third world women', *International Journal of Gynecology & Obstetrics* 30 supp 145–68

Watchorn C (1978) 'Midwifery: a history of statutory suppression', Golden Gate U L Rev 9:2, Women's Law Forum, Accessed 07/11, http://digitalcommons.law.ggu.edu/ggulrev/vol9/iss2/11 631–42

Watkins S (2012) 'Presentism? A reply to T.J. Clark', *New Left Review* 74 77–102

Watson N and Mander R (1995) 'Advertising infant formula in the maternity area', *MIDIRS Midwifery Digest* 5:3 338–41

Wax JR, Lucas FL, Lamont M, Pinette MG, Cartin A and Blackstone J (2010) 'Maternal and newborn outcomes in planned home birth vs planned hospital births: a meta analysis', *American Journal of Obstetrics & Gynecology* 203:3:243.e1–8.

Wedin K, Molin J and Crang Svalenius EL (2010) 'Group antenatal care: new pedagogic method for antenatal care – a pilot study', *Midwifery* 26 389–93

Weig M (1993) 'Audit of Independent Midwifery 1980–1991', a Report Commissioned by the Department of Health, London, Royal College of Midwives

Whitfield D (2006) *New Labour's Attack on Public Services*, London: Spokesman Books

WHO (1981) *International Code of Marketing of Breast-milk Substitutes*, Geneva: World Health Organisation

WHO (1985) *Having a Baby in Europe*, Copenhagen: World Health Organisation

WHO (1994) 'World Health Organization partograph in management of labour', *The Lancet* 343:8910 1399–1404, World Health Organization Maternal Health and Safe Motherhood Programme

WHO (1996) *Care in Normal Birth: A Practical Guide*, Geneva: World Health Organisation

WHO (1997) *Care in Normal Birth*, Geneva: World Health Organisation WHO/FRH/MSM/96.24

WHO (2008) 'Closing the gap in a generation: health equity through action on the social determinants of health', Final Report of the Commission on Social Determinants of Health, Geneva: World Health Organization http://www.searo.who.int/LinkFiles/SDH_SDH_FinalReport.pdf Accessed 08/11

WHO (2012) 'World Health Statistics', Geneva: World Health Organisation, Accessed 05/12, http://www.who.int/gho/publications/world_health_statistics/EN_WHS2012_Full.pdf

Wickham S (1999) 'Evidence-informed midwifery. 1. What is evidence-informed midwifery?', *Midwifery Today* 51 42–3

Wiegers TA (2006) 'Adjusting to motherhood: maternity care assistance during the postpartum period: how to help new mothers cope', *Journal of Neonatal Nursing* 12:5 163–71

Wilkins R (2000) 'Poor relations: the paucity of the professional paradigm' in M Kirkham (ed) *The Midwife–Mother relationship*, London: Macmillan, pp 28–54

Wilkinson R and Pickett K (2010) *The Spirit Level: Why Equality is Better for Everyone*, London: Penguin

Williams J (1997) 'The controlling power of childbirth in Britain' in H Marland and AM Rafferty (eds) *Midwives, Society and Childbirth: Debates and Controversies in the Modern Period*, London: Routledge, pp 232–47

Williams R (1983) *Keywords: A Vocabulary of Culture and Society* 2nd edn, Oxford: Oxford University Press

Williamson C (1998) 'The rise of doctor-patient working groups', *BMJ* 317 1374–7

Williamson C (2007) 'Radical patient groups', *AIMS Journal* 19:2 5–8

Williamson C (2010) *Towards the Emancipation of Patients: Patients' Experiences and the Patient Movement*, Bristol: Policy Press

Wilton T (1999) 'Towards an understanding of the cultural roots of homophobia in order to provide a better midwifery service for lesbian clients', *Midwifery* 15:3 154–64

Wilton T and Kaufmann T (2001) 'Lesbian mothers' experiences of maternity care in the UK', *Midwifery* 17:3 203–11

Winter C (2002) 'How do independent midwives assess the progress of labour', Unpublished MSc Dissertation, University of Dundee, Accessed 05/12, http://discovery.dundee.ac.uk/bitstream/handle/10588/2613/Clare%20Winter%20MSc%20Dissertation.pdf?sequence=1

Winters P (2007) 'Holding up a mirror: the impact of user involvement', *AIMS Journal* 18:3, Accessed 08/12, http://www.aims.org.uk/Journal/Vol18No3/holdingUpAMirror.htm

Witz A (1990) 'Patriarchy and professions: the gendered politics of occupational closure', *Sociology* 24: 675–90

Witz A (1992) *Professions and Patriarchy*, London: Routledge

Wloch C, Wilson J, Lamagni T, Harrington P, Charlett A and Sheridan E (2012) 'Risk factors for surgical site infection following caesarean section in England: results from a multicentre cohort study', *BJOG* 2012; DOI: 10.1111/j.1471–0528.2012.03452.x.

Wolf-Phillips L (1987) 'Why "third world"? origin, definition and usage', *Third World Quarterly* 9:4 1311–27

Wolin S (2004) *Politics and Vision: Continuity and Innovation in Western Political Thought*, Princeton: Princeton University Press

Wolin S (2006) *Democracy Inc: Managed Democracy and the Specter of Inverted Totalitarianism*, Princeton: Princeton University Press

Wolin S (1994) 'Fugitive democracy', *Constellations* 1:1 11–25

Wollstonecraft M [1792] (1975) *Vindication of the Rights of Woman*, Harmondsworth: Penguin

WRA (2012) White Ribbon Alliance, http://www.whiteribbonalliance.org/index.cfm/the-issues/ Accessed 01/12

Yentis SM (2011) 'From CEMD to CEMACH to CMACE to ... ? Where now for the Confidential Enquiries into Maternal Deaths?', *Anaesthesia* 66:10 859–60

Yiannouzis K (2010) 'Reasons behind the decision to terminate the contract with Albany', *British Journal of Midwifery* 18:3 193–4

Young D (2006) '"Cesarean delivery on maternal request": was the NIH conference based on a faulty premise?', *Birth* 33:3 171–4

Young D (2009) 'What is normal childbirth and do we need more statements about it?', *Birth* 36:1 1–3

Zander L (2007) 'Preface' (pp xiii–xiv) in W Savage (ed) *Birth and Power: A Savage Enquiry Revisited*, London: Middlesex University Press

Index